D0466564

ART CENTER COLLEGE OF DESIGN

3 3220 00001 3743

THE DESIGN OF MEDICAL
AND DENTAL FACILITIES

*To Stuart
for cheerfully encouraging me
throughout this challenging
endeavor*

725.5
M251
1982

THE DESIGN OF MEDICAL AND DENTAL FACILITIES

JAIN MALKIN

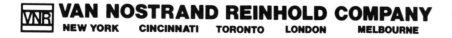 **VAN NOSTRAND REINHOLD COMPANY**
NEW YORK   CINCINNATI   TORONTO   LONDON   MELBOURNE

Copyright © 1982 by Van Nostrand Reinhold Company Inc.

Library of Congress Catalog Card Number: 81-10361
ISBN: 0-442-24493-2

All rights reserved. No part of this work covered by the copyright hereon may
be reproduced or used in any form or part or by any means—graphic, electronic, or
mechanical, including photocopying, recording, taping, or information storage
and retrieval systems—without permission of the publisher.

Manufactured in the United States of America

Published by Van Nostrand Reinhold Company Inc.
135 West 50th Street, New York, N.Y. 10020

Van Nostrand Reinhold
480 Latrobe Street
Melbourne, Victoria 3000, Australia

Van Nostrand Reinhold Company Limited
Molly Millars Lane
Wokingham, Berkshire, England

15 14 13 12 11 10 9 8 7 6 5 4 3 2

Library of Congress Cataloging in Publication Data

Malkin, Jain.
   The design of medical and dental facilities.

   Includes index.
   1. Health facilities—Design and construction.
2. Medical offices—Design and construction.
1. Title.
RA967.M36   725′.5   81-10361
ISBN 0-442-24493-2   AACR2

725.5
M251
1982

Preface

I decided to limit my design practice to the field of health care in 1970 because I realized that so little attention had been focused on it. I spent weeks at the library researching the literature relative to medical and dental space planning, color and its effect on patients, and the psychological aspects of illness—how do patients and visitors react to hospitals, why do people fear a visit to the doctor or dentist, what role does lighting play in patient rooms? Much to my surprise very little had been written on these topics. I found an occasional article here or there, sometimes in obscure publications and often dating from the 1940s. There were a few articles in *The American Journal of Occupational Therapy* on the effect of the environment on the patient, there were a few articles on the color preferences of various ethnic groups or cultural taboos with respect to color. A handful of articles on limited aspects of office space planning were scattered through medical or dental practice management magazines and Department of Health, Education, and Welfare publications. Furthermore, most medical and dental offices in 1970 harkened to the Dark Ages in their use of color and attractive furnishings. I concluded that I would have to do my own, albeit empirical, research in order to gather enough background on which to base my design work.

I spent the better part of a year visiting hospitals—interviewing the staff and patients and observing how patients were handled. I documented my visits with photographs of confusing signage, lobbies furnished with Salvation Army rejects, dismal lighting, corridors jammed with medical equipment, examination rooms that resembled concentration camp torture chambers. At the end of my research I had accumulated several thousand photos and reams of notes which I analyzed and from which I formulated my design philosophy. My dual major, psychology and environmental design, gave me the theoretical background by which I interpreted my data. As a result of my previous design experience with institutional projects, I was familiar with codes and the stringent requirements for sanitation and ease of maintenance. Although my studies had been primarily of hospitals, much of the information was relevant to the handling of patients in medical and dental offices as well.

In the eleven years since my entry into the health care field, I have designed hundreds of medical and dental offices and have served as design consultant to hospitals and medical equipment manufacturers. I have written many articles on humanizing the hospital environment and conducted seminars on medical and dental space planning. This book, then, is the culmination of my work in the field of health care. It is intended to be a general reference book for architects, interior designers, and health care professionals. Since I began my work in this field no reference book on medical space planning has been published and there is still only a scattering of articles, although the field has gained enormous recognition. Brilliant examples of intelligence and sensitivity in hospital design have been published in architecture and design magazines. And cheerful, tastefully designed medical and dental offices are gaining ground in all parts of the country. But we still have a lot to learn—this field is in its infancy.

To this end, I offer my book. A person with no prior experience in health care can pick up this book and become familiar not only with current philosophical issues, but also with medical procedures, equipment associated with each medical or dental specialty, room sizes, traffic flow, construction methods, codes, interior finishes, and more. I have attempted to synthesize my eleven years of research and experience so that others will not have to follow such a laborious course of study in order to enter this vital and exciting field.

The writer wishes to thank her colleagues, Marcia Hansen and Janice Smithey Howard, for their assistance in drafting the suite plan illustrations. Photographs of interiors in this book were primarily taken by either Michael Denny or the writer. The interior design work illustrated in these photos was done by the writer unless otherwise noted.

Jain Malkin

Introduction

We have come a long way since Hippocrates wrote his treatise on medical care, yet it is relatively recently that physicians have clustered their offices together in medical buildings. In ancient times, the physician offered his services in an open market place or traveled from town to town in search of patients.

At the end of the nineteenth century, many doctors tacked a shingle outside their homes and practiced medicine from there. This was particularly true in small towns. But in large cities physicians moved into commercial buildings, often above a bank or retail store. In the early part of this century, physicians in metropolitan areas occupied large multiuse general office buildings usually in the downtown core of a city. Before World War II many specialized buildings were erected exclusively for physicians, but after the war, doctors were among those attracted to the cheap land costs of the suburbs, and soon small owner-occupied medical office buildings sprouted—the forerunners of the large medical complexes now so familiar to us. The suburbs held other attractions: on-grade parking in a bucolic setting, the small scale, the residential character of the neighborhood, and the ability to bring medicine where the patient lived rather than make the patient endure the congestion of downtown traffic. In fact, the residential character of the suburban office parks was frequently reflected in their names—many were called "Doctors' Park" or "Medical Park."

Often physicians opened satellite offices in the suburbs while still maintaining the downtown location as their primary office. Specialists tended to remain in the urban setting in these early days of exodus to the suburbs, since they rely upon a large population and many referrals from primary physicians.

As land costs increased through the 1950's, it became more economically feasible to build larger buildings designed specifically for a medical tenant population. Hence the numerous small owner-occupied buildings gave way to large complexes composed of solo practitioners of various medical specialties. Of course the benefits of this were more than economic. In one building, primary care physicians and specialists, clinical labs, and radiology support services complemented each other. The proximity of these services amounted to great convenience for patients and physicians alike.

In the 1960's these buildings were increasingly located adjacent to hospitals so that physicians could shuttle back and forth between hospital and office without having to get into a car, thereby maximizing the time they could devote to patient care. Many hospitals even constructed medical office buildings on the hospital campus as an added incentive for their staff physicians to whom they leased space frequently at below-market-value rates, often with suite improvements all but underwritten by the hospital.

It is obvious today that conventional office buildings do not accommodate medical tenants. The physical structure does not permit efficient

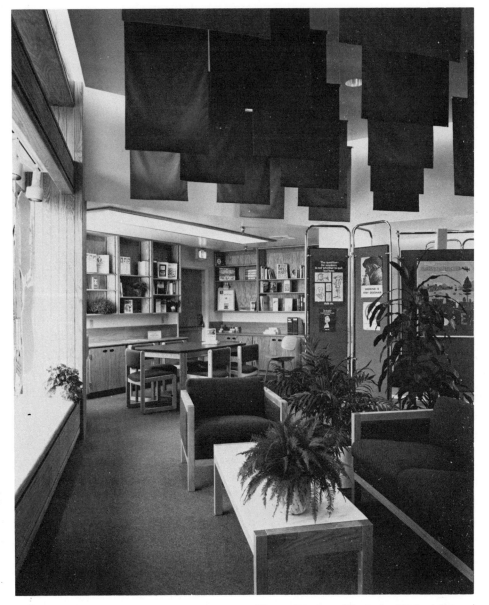

The well being. (Photo by Michael Denny)

utilization of space nor is it equipped with the required plumbing, electrical wiring, mechanical systems, or medical gases.

Great changes have occurred in the field of health care in the past ten years. The emphasis has shifted from treatment of disease to keeping people healthy. The trend is to prevent disease; to keep people out of the hospital through health education programs and holistic ideology, making persons responsible for their own health. Raising the general public's knowledge about the importance of proper nutrition, exercise, and the risks associated with alcoholism, drug abuse, and smoking is perhaps the most effective weapon in the battle against disease. Health education centers as adjuncts to hospitals and other health service agencies have sprung up recently in store fronts and shopping centers, making sound information accessible to the community.

Future social, economic, and political considerations will change the character of health delivery systems considerably. Good medical care is now considered the right of all citizens, rather than the privilege of a few. In addition, we have increased longevity, so more elderly persons will be around to need medical care. These two factors demand a comprehensive health planning system coordinated on a nationwide basis.

From the standpoint of economics, *prevention* of illness is more economical than disability and disease. Health maintenance organizations (HMOs) are based on this principle and have successfully demonstrated that a healthy profit can be realized while providing excellent health care benefits to subscribers. The healthy finance the treatment of the ill in a prepaid medical plan. The

Kaiser Foundation Plan is reputed to be the most successful HMO, and in many cities, there exists a waiting list of prospective subscribers.

Health maintenance organizations rely heavily on multiphasic screening facilities to detect and predict disease before it reaches advanced stages that would normally cause one to consult a physician. Mobile units carry programs for prevention of disease to residential and rural areas. Frequently parked at shopping centers, these mobile units can check blood pressure, do blood tests for diabetes, take chest X-rays for T.B. or lung cancer, or collect blood plasma donations.

There is presently a great emphasis on ambulatory and outpatient facilities. Many hospitals, instead of adding patient beds, are remodeling and adding day surgery centers, diagnostic and treatment units, and enlarged radiology and laboratory departments. The conditions under which insurance providers will pay for services will determine somewhat the extent of outpatient units constructed. If ambulatory patients can receive benefits without being hospitalized, health care costs will be lower and outpatient clinics and day surgery centers will multiply.

Rapid advances in medical technology are making outpatient diagnosis and treatment increasingly possible. As this equipment is very costly, it tends to be concentrated and centralized in hospitals, thereby forging an even stronger link between the hospital and the adjacent medical office building. Such equipment as Computerized Axial Tomography (CAT) body scanners has revolutionized medical diagnosis, providing greater accuracy than heretofore known and often eliminating a battery of procedures that were previously necessary.

Rehabilitation units located in or near general hospitals will aim their services at making patients more independent and able to provide better home care for themselves. These patients include diabetics, arthritics, the deaf, the mentally retarded, the blind, asthmatics, geriatric patients, the orthopedically handicapped, amputees, cancer patients, and those with cardiovascular or respiratory diseases.

There will be an increased need for highly specialized facilities such as cancer centers, alcoholism and narcotics treatment units, burn centers, kidney and eye banks. Yet, in contrast to these highly specialized structures, the general hospital must retain flexibility and be responsive to change. The speed with which new equipment, methods of practice, and other changes evolve demands flexibility.

The roles of health professionals will expand to include many more paramedical assistants. Much of the preliminary screening and routine medical procedures can be performed well by support staff, thus freeing the physicians for special examinations and diagnosis. Medical social workers will have expanded roles in an attempt to treat not just the patient, but also the family out of which came the alcoholic, the battered child, the drug abuser, or the unwanted elderly person. Again, the emphasis is on preventing future disease, rather than merely treating it when it occurs.

The trend of the 1970's for physicians to organize themselves in single or multispecialty groups will continue. The present inclination toward socialism in medicine and increasing government control has encouraged many solo practitioners to form group practices. Individual physicians can generally lower their overhead in a group practice where support staff, radiology and lab equipment, waiting room, and business office are shared by the group.

The 1980s carry forth a mandate of strict cost containment begun in the late 1970s when costs soared as hospitals frequently competed with each other for the latest equipment and often duplicated services available at a nearby facility, thereby leading to underutilization at both facilities. Lack of regional planning (to achieve better geographical distribution and coordination of health facilities), skyrocketing construction costs, and an unreasonable length of time for design and construction (somewhat ameliorated by "fast track" systems), are some of the problems that have led to the strict Certificate of Need requirements mandated by the Comprehensive Health Planning Organization.

Although the 1980s will bring enormous changes in the delivery of health care, it will continue to be one of the fastest growing categories of nonresidential building, supplying architects and interior designers with an unlimited number of challenging projects.

Contents

Color Plates

THE DESIGN OF MEDICAL AND DENTAL FACILITIES

Chapter 1
Psychology: Implications for Health Care Design

FORTRESSES AGAINST DISEASE

A critical look at our clinics, hospitals, and medical offices reveals that they are designed for ease of maintenance rather than human comfort. They seem to be resistant to human imprint—a definition of an institutional environment. The architecture, instead of embracing and welcoming inhabitants, seems to alienate and intimidate them. Hospitals, in particular, seem to be designed as a show of strength, fortresses against disease, which dwarf the individual and place him or her in a caste system in which the doctors and nurses are the ruling class and the patient or visitor is the serf. The language of the hospital is foreign to most people. They do not understand where to go or how to get there, and they need an interpreter to decode the medical jargon whispered all around them. It is not unlike a visit to a foreign country—nothing is familiar. The signage system in many hospitals is so inadequate and confusing that it only adds to the patient's or visitor's frustration and feeling of helplessness. It reduces the patient to a child who has to continually ask questions and beg for assistance.

A Labyrinth Of Corridors

All too many hospitals and nursing homes resemble a Kafkalike labyrinth of corridors—endless in their dimly lit pallor and multiple layers of chipped paint. Examination and treatment rooms are naked except for the snakes of electrical conduit lashed to the walls and the unfamiliar assortment of medical equipment with strange nozzles, dials, hoses. Antiseptic white walls. Is it any wonder patients are fearful and anxious? Who can fault them for letting a disease progress to an advanced stage before subjecting themselves to the terror inherent in a hospital confinement?

Exaggerated? Unfortunately, No.

And perhaps the saddest aspect of this tragedy is that patients have never paid more for health care services. Health care expenditures in the United States are approaching 10% of the gross national product or $1000 per capita. Yet large-scale changes in the delivery of health care have minimized the individual. It is increasingly more difficult for the individual to interface with the building structure or the medical system in general. Computer systems have reduced people to numbers and statistics.

Is There a Solution?

If we stop thinking of patients as inmates and view them as guests, hospitals could function more on the order of a hotel or restaurant. Why cannot the hospital lobby with its reception desk, reservations and cashier desks, gift shop, flower vendor, be as pleasant to visit as a hotel lobby, which accommodates precisely the same functions? If the individual can relate the medical environment to something else he or she has experienced with a positive association, much has been achieved toward reducing anxiety.

Human Factors Engineering

Hospitals are going to have to mend their ways for economic reasons, if not for humanitarian ones. In order to qualify for certain types of funding as well as Certificate of Need approval, hospitals in many states have to prove a census of 80% or better. Thus hospitals increasingly will be competing with each other for the community's patronage. They will have to rely on designers and architects to give them the competitive edge. And what is needed is more human factors studies indicating the patient's physiological and psychological responses to color, light, temperature, noise, the size and shape of a room. How do these same factors influence the staff's performance of routine tasks? Although very little is known about patients' and staff's reaction to their environment, dozens of hospitals have been designed in the past ten years that seem to be

sensitive to the patients' needs and are a visual treat owing, it seems, to the intuitive adeptness of the design team rather than to research. But dozens of hospitals out of a cast of thousands is just a beginning.

FEAR OF A VISIT TO THE DOCTOR OR DENTIST

Patients' anxiety is not confined to hospitals and nursing homes. A visit to the physician or dentist traumatizes many people. The basis for the fear, even more than lack of familiarity with procedures and a feeling of helplessness, stems from the invasion of one's personal space. Americans maintain larger territorial boundaries than most other groups. While an American may maintain an imaginary barrier 24 inches in front of him or her as a safe conversational distance for strangers, a person from the Middle East may reduce that safe boundary to 12 inches. Furthermore, we will tolerate a person at a closer distance to the side of us than in front of us. Another curious fact is that Americans physically remove themselves from a situation when they want solitude or privacy. Middle Easteners, by contrast, simply stop talking and ignore the presence of others nearby, allowing themselves to be isolated even when physically surrounded by others.

Nowhere is a person's privacy violated more than in a medical or dental examination, (see Fig. 1-1). One's territorial limits are invaded by strangers who poke, probe, and prod. And when the examination demands that the patient be naked, even the barrier of clothing ceases to protect. Is it any wonder that a visit to the dentist or physician can intimidate and can raise our basest fears? How, then, can practitioners break through

2

this barrier to respond to the patient with sensitivity and dignity?

Positive Aspects of Care

The patient must perceive the positive aspects of the care he or she is receiving through an understanding of the procedures and of how they will enhance his or her enjoyment of life. The relief of pain or the prevention of disease are joys in themselves. The diagnostic and therapeutic milieu must promote health rather than aggravate illness and feed anxiety. The environment must be clean, cheerful, and nonthreatening with contemporary furnishings, warm colors, and soothing textures. The staff just be neatly groomed, well trained, and interested in the patients' well-being.

Waiting Room Must Establish Rapport

The waiting room is the patient's introduction to the medical or dental office. It should establish immediate rapport and put the patient at ease. Out-of-date furniture, worn upholstery, tables with cigarette burns, and dirty spots on walls and woodwork tell the patient the doctor does not care about his or her comfort or that the doctor is too cheap to replace things when they wear out. It also suggests that the doctor may be a person who is outdated on medical matters as well. *Lack of confidence in the doctor breeds anxiety in the patient.*

Carpet Adds Warmth

Vinyl asbestos tile floors and vinyl upholstery fabric in the waiting room suggest that the doctor thinks his or her patients too sloppy to deserve carpeting and fabric upholstery.

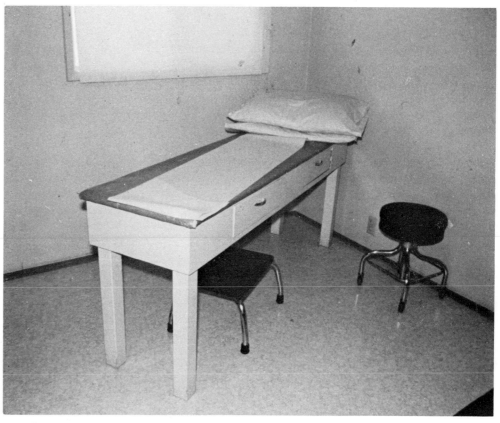

Fig. 1-1. Examination room. Diagnosis: dreary and frightening.

3

Live Plants Suggest Health

There is no substitute for live green plants. Plastic plants suggest that live plants probably could not survive the environment and the patient may fare no better.

Reception Window—To Welcome Patients or Close Them Out?

A closed, frosted sliding glass window with a buzzer for service tells the patients that they are not really welcome—they are intruding on the staff's privacy. The receptionist should always be in view of the patients and accessible to them.

Poor Illumination Hides Defects

A poorly illuminated waiting room not only makes it difficult to read but subliminally suggests to patients that the doctor is trying to hide something—perhaps the poor housekeeping, dust-encrusted baseboards, soiled carpet, finger-marked glass, or faded draperies. What else might be lurking in the dark?

Waiting Breeds Hostility

Waiting, unhappily, is one of the frustrations that accompanies a visit to the doctor. Patients who have an ailment that is frightening or that makes them uncomfortable will accept waiting in the realization that the doctor cannot always schedule appointments accurately. Well patients, however, such as those in a screening facility, have a different attitude and are not willing to accept discomfort or inconvenience without registering complaints. If that wait is in the waiting room (it is worse if it is in the exam room), a good assortment of current interesting magazines will make the time pass more quickly, as will attractive artwork on the walls. It is important that the delay be explained to the patient. An emergency at the hospital or the delivery of a baby are situations about which people will be forgiving. They understand medical emergencies. But when patients sit for an hour and are told nothing, they seethe with hostility wondering why the physician is so inconsiderate, why he or she has overbooked himself or herself, and why the physician is intent on making the patient late for work. When the patient finally does see the doctor, the latter should apologize for the delay. Not to do so is to treat the patient as a nonperson and as an inferior.

Perceived Status Difference

One of the main reasons patients feel intimidated is the perceived status difference between the physician or technician and themselves. The patient sits in a powerless position while being acted upon by others. The feelings of helplessness are accelerated when the physician is protected by a fortress-type desk and an imposing *executive* chair from which he appears to talk down to the patient, who is seated at a "safe" distance in a simple chair with no protective enclosure. Another example of patient intimidation occurs when a radiologist issues instructions to the naked patient on the X-ray table via loudspeaker from a remote control room—a humiliating experience. Every effort should be made to treat the patient as an equal, to explain each step of a medical or dental procedure, to make the patient a partner in his or her treatment, and to allow the patient as much dignity as possible during what can best be described as humiliating medical examinations: gastrointestinal X-ray studies, proctologic examinations, and so forth. An individual's most private bodily functions are scrutinized by strangers, causing great psychological stress.

Privacy Is Important

Examination rooms should have a dressing cubicle, a place where patients may disrobe, confident that the nurse or doctor will not barge in on them while naked. It also provides a place for patients to hang their undergarments out of view of strangers. The dressing cubicle should have a mirror, a chair, and hooks to hang the clothes. Similarly, radiology suites should have dressing rooms and a safe place to leave or lock up valuables. The floors should be carpeted so that patients do not have to walk barefoot on dirty cold floors to the radiography rooms.

Seating Arrangements

Americans, in particular, do not like to be touched by strangers. Middle Eastern and Latin cultures, by contrast, encourage closeness and touching. In the Arab world olfaction, as expressed by breathing in the face of a friend, is considered a necessary part of social grace. To deny a friend the smell of one's breath is a cause of shame. Middle Easterners and Latins will huddle together much more closely than will Americans in a crowd. Thus seating arrangements in a waiting room designed for Americans should not force strangers to sit together—this only intensifies the stress of visiting the physician or dentist. Individual chairs should be provided and arranged so that strangers do not have to face each other with a distance of less than eight feet between them. Chairs should be placed against walls or in configurations that offer a degree of security so that seated persons do not feel they are in jeopardy of being approached from behind.

Cultural Differences

If the medical office or clinic serves an ethnic population it is important to research how that group uses space. Mexican families, for example, tend to bring many relatives when one family member has to visit the doctor. Perhaps this is due to a distrust of "modern medicine" and a need for emotional security provided by the presence of the family. Perhaps they perceive that an individual might be swallowed up by the system, lost in a maze of floppy disks and high technology. The books by Robert Sommer and those of Edward T. Hall are excellent resources for the cultural use of space.

Body Language Indicates Stress

The patient's body language can indicate when the patient is uncomfortable with the physician, dentist, or technician. *Averted eyes*—looking away from the doctor is one sign. *Body positioned away* from the doctor is another. *Stereotyped behavior* (tapping toes, shaking a leg, or rocking) is another. At these signs, the doctor must reestablish contact with the patient and break the perceived-status-difference barrier. Taking the patient's hand and asking if he or she is okay is friendly and reassuring.

5

Seeing the Doctor as a Person

The consultation room (and sometimes the waiting room) should contain the doctor's personal memorabilia. Such items help the patient to see the doctor as a person with a family, hobbies, and interests outside of medicine. This reassures the patient that the doctor is a real person, not just a white coat with a stethoscope around the neck.

Style of Furnishings Should Not be Trendy

There is considerable leeway for the doctor to express his or her personality and style preferences in furniture. Indeed, for obstetricians, gynecologists, pediatricians, the sky is the limit. But most physicians, surgeons in particular, must carefully select furniture that will convey a solid, conservative image. A patient needs to feel that his or her surgeon is not impulsive—that he or she is a serious person not subject to frivolities and trendy decor.

Even if patients are not consciously aware of the message they are getting from the office design, they are subconsciously receiving it. The *body language of the office environment* tells patients things that might subconsciously undermine their confidence in the physician or dentist. Patients sometimes do abuse nice furnishings by putting their feet on the chairs and gum on the upholstery, but that is the price that must be paid to make patients feel comfortable. The replacement factor should be built into the office overhead. Most patients do not abuse the pleasant surroundings provided for them, so why make the many suffer for the transgressions of the few? The psychological benefits of an office designed to *serve* the patients far outweighs any liabilities.

Portions of this chapter have been adapted from an article I wrote for *Behavioral Medicine,* July 1980. (pub. by Magazines for Medicine, Inc., New York).

Chapter 2
General Parameters of Medical Space Planning

Efficient medical offices begin with an intelligently designed medical office building. All too often medical office buildings are planned by designers who are unfamiliar with the spatial requirements of medical suites; thus the structure of the building does not lend itself to an efficient layout of suites. The locations of the structural columns, the placement of stairs, elevators, mechanical shafts, public restrooms (if provided), and the window module either impede or facilitate the layout of the individual suites.

Other factors that influence the design of an MOB are the shape and size of the site, the specific requirements of a particular tenant or client, a beautiful view, or the architect's desire to impose a unique design on the project. All of these factors have to be weighed and balanced along with the applicable codes, zoning restrictions, and the client's budget. A building that is completely functional and efficient, but totally insensitive to aesthetics may not rent as quickly as the owners may wish. But an MOB designed primarily for aesthetic merit will prove to be a frustrating and costly exercise.

To begin with, an MOB should contain at least 10,000 to 11,000 square feet of rentable space per floor in order to accommodate suites of varying sizes and configurations as well as to locate efficiently the stairs and elevators. The services (elevator, stairs, mechanical equipment room, public restrooms) can be placed in the core with rental space wrapped around the perimeter (Fig. 2-1 and 2-2) or the services may be located at the ends of a double loaded public corridor (Fig. 2-3). The elevators may be placed in the center of the floor with the stairs on either end (Fig. 2-4). Figure 2-4 gives 88% rentable space and Fig. 2-1 gives 80% rentable, but it must be noted that Fig. 2-1 includes public restrooms, a mechanical equipment room, and a janitor's room. Were the services in Fig. 2-1 to be limited to stairs and elevators as in Fig. 2-4, the rentable space would be boosted to 12,879 square feet, or 88% rentable, and would permit a 45-foot-deep suite on two perpendicular sides of the building, and 32-foot 6-inch-deep suites on the other two perpendicular sides. Usually, it is most efficient to place the stairs and other intrusions into the rental space, at the ends of the building. It should be noted, however, that special attention must be paid to locating the stairwells when one tenant intends to lease an entire floor or half a floor. In

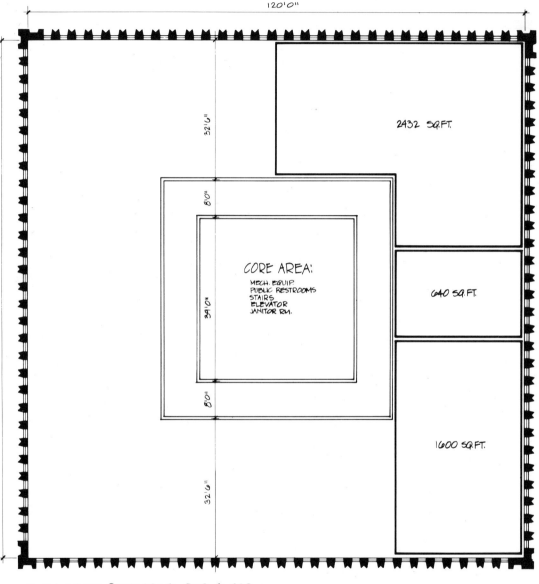

120'0"

32'6"

8'0"

39'0"

8'0"

32'6"

120'0"

2432 SQ.FT.

CORE AREA:
MECH. EQUIP.
PUBLIC RESTROOMS
STAIRS
ELEVATOR
JANITOR RM.

640 SQ.FT.

1600 SQ.FT.

11,484 SQ.FT. RENTABLE PER FLOOR

Fig. 2-1.

such case, the public exit stairwell may fall within an individual suite—a nonpublic space. There are several ways to handle this condition, but local fire codes must be consulted for exiting requirements.

The locations of structural columns should not affect the flexibility of the space if the building is engineered properly (unless the building is a high-rise with large columns). Most rooms are small; thus the density of partitions is high. Long spans are not necessary. The occurence of columns at intervals creating 20-foot-wide bays and at 32-foot centers through the depth of the building (Fig. 2–5) is typical. Were the spaces on both sides of the corridor a 32-foot depth, all columns could be contained in the public corridor walls with none occurring in the tenant space.

The depth of the building (or the depth of the spaces on either side of the public corridor) affects greatly the efficiency of suites of various square footage. A depth of 28 feet 6 inches is good for suites from 500 to 1800 square feet. This depth allows for a 4-foot clear center corridor and 12-foot-deep (11-foot 6-inch net) rooms on either side. Since a standard exam room is 8 x 12 feet (7–foot 6-inch x 11-foot 6-inch net) and a standard consultation room is 12 x 12 feet (11-foot 6-inch x 11-foot 6-inch net), this works well (Fig. 2–4). The ends of each corridor typically would have either a storage room or a toilet room. This functions well when the tenant expands into an adjoining suite because one has but to eliminate the storage room and the corridor continues to the new suite with no other remodeling necessary in the existing suite.

An office over 2000 square feet at a depth of 28 feet 6 inches requires too much corridor. A 32-foot depth is serviceable for suites of 1500 to 2400 square feet. This is the most common depth

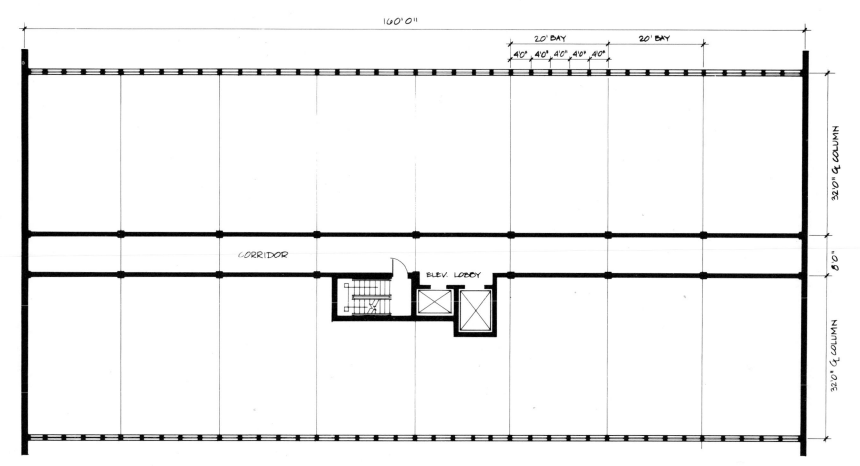

Fig. 2-2.

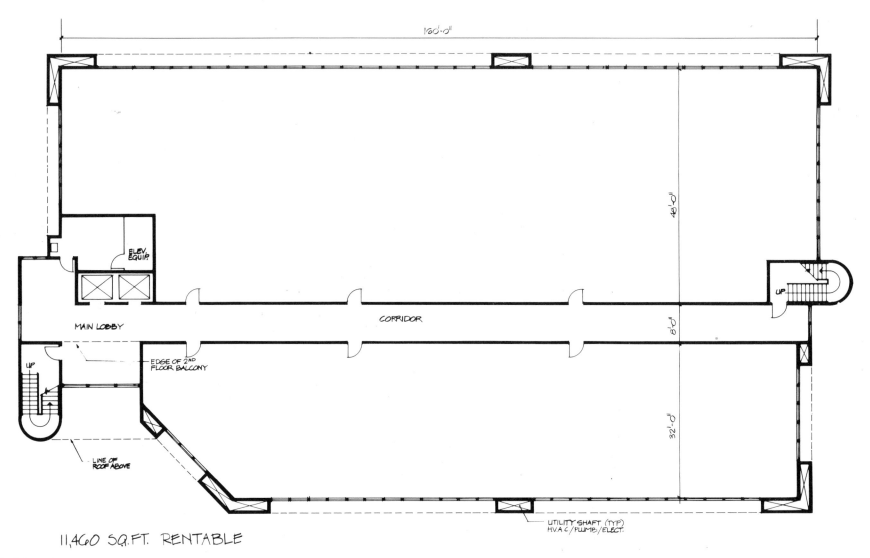

100'-0"

46'-0"

ELEV. EQUIP.

8'-0"

MAIN LOBBY

CORRIDOR

UP

EDGE OF 2ND FLOOR BALCONY

UP

32'-0"

LINE OF ROOF ABOVE

UTILITY SHAFT (TYP) H.V.A.C./PLUMB./ELECT.

11,460 SQ. FT. RENTABLE

Fig. 2-3.

10

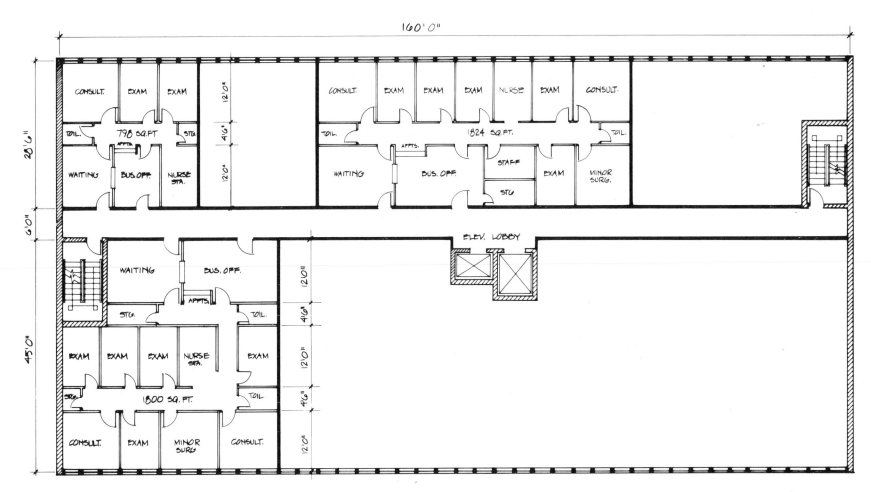

160'0"

20'6"

6'0"

45'0"

12'0"

4'6"

12'0"

12'0"

4'6"

12'0"

4'6"

12'0"

CONSULT. EXAM EXAM

TOIL. 798 SQ.FT. STG.

APPTS.

WAITING BUS. OFF. NURSE STA.

CONSULT. EXAM EXAM EXAM NURSE EXAM CONSULT.

TOIL. 1824 SQ.FT. TOIL.

APPTS.

STAFF

WAITING BUS. OFF. EXAM MINOR SURG.

STG.

ELEV. LOBBY

WAITING BUS. OFF.

STG. APPTS. TOIL.

EXAM EXAM EXAM NURSE STA. EXAM

STG. 1800 SQ. FT. TOIL.

CONSULT. EXAM MINOR SURG CONSULT.

11,256 SQ. FT. RENTABLE PER FLOOR

Fig. 2-4.

11

for suites in a medical office building. It permits a net 4-foot-wide interior corridor with a 12-foot-deep exam room or consultation room on one side and a 15-foot 6-inch-deep space for a waiting room, business office, or other room on the opposite side.

Suites over 2500 square feet and, depending on the individual requirements, sometimes under 2500 square feet (Fig. 2–4) are best served by a 45-foot-deep space. This allows for two 4-foot clear corridors with three rows of 12-foot-deep rooms (Fig. 2–4). The 45-foot depth will serve suites up to approximately 4000 square feet. Suites larger than that are unusual, but do occur. In such a case, the suite may be located across the end of the building, encompassing the public corridor and both the 32-foot 6-inch and the 45-foot-deep spaces, providing that the stairwell be located elsewhere. Or, a large suite may wrap around a corner as in Fig. 2–1. In Fig. 2–2, a large suite could be placed along one end of the building taking in three bays (a length of 60 feet) and the 8-foot public corridor plus the two 32-foot-deep spaces. This would create a suite of 4320 square feet without impinging upon public access to the stairwell and elevator lobby.

It is practical to design an MOB so that suites on one side of the public corridor have a depth of 28 feet 6 inches to 32 feet and the other a depth of 45 feet (Fig. 2–4). This permits a great deal of flexibility and allows the designer to place the tenant where the suite will lay out most efficiently. The 1824-square-foot suite in Fig. 2–4 located along the 28-foot 6-inch depth has 198 square feet of circulation, whereas the 1800-square-foot suite placed in a 45-foot-deep space has 236 square feet of circulation. It is possible to design a building so that one floor will accommodate suites of four different depths (Fig. 2–6).

The average medical suite for a solo practitioner would be 1000 square feet. Few suites are smaller than that. The bulk of suites the designer will encounter will fall into the range of 1200 to 2000 square feet. And there may be large orthopedic or internal medicine suites ranging from 3500 to 8000 square feet. Since the terms of financing often specify that the building must be largely preleased (documented by signed letters of intent) before construction begins, it is often possible to know who the large tenants with special needs will be, and the building can be shaped with those requirements in mind. An MOB constructed purely for speculation with little preleasing would be difficult to plan without a profile or feasibility study of the physicians in the area, their space needs *were they to lease space,* and their respective specialties.

Medical office buildings that are adjacent to and affiliated with hospitals have very special needs that will be touched on only briefly in this discussion. The major consideration lies in the interface with the hospital. Will the hospital actually be occupying space in the MOB? If so, and if inpatients have access to these facilities (an outpatient facility that also accommodates inpatients), the MOB will be classified as a hospital, with appropriate standards and codes applying, thereby greatly increasing the construction costs of the MOB. Will the building systems and layout be able to respond to future demands for change? Will the MOB by physically connected to the hospital? If so, great thought must be given to the configuration of each floor with regard to stairwells, elevators, and the point of entry to the hospital so that future expansion is not hampered and circulation between the hospital and the MOB is efficient. One disadvantage to physicians in a hospital affiliated MOB is that frequently the

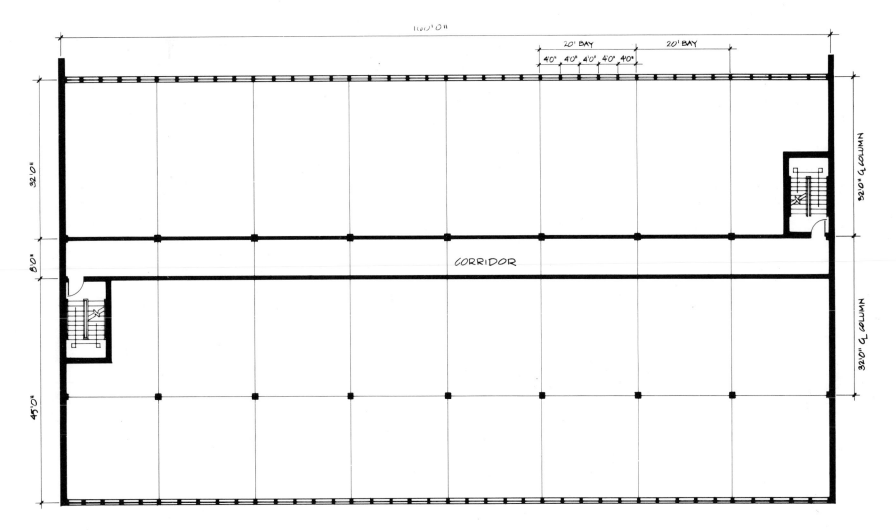

Fig. 2-5.

13

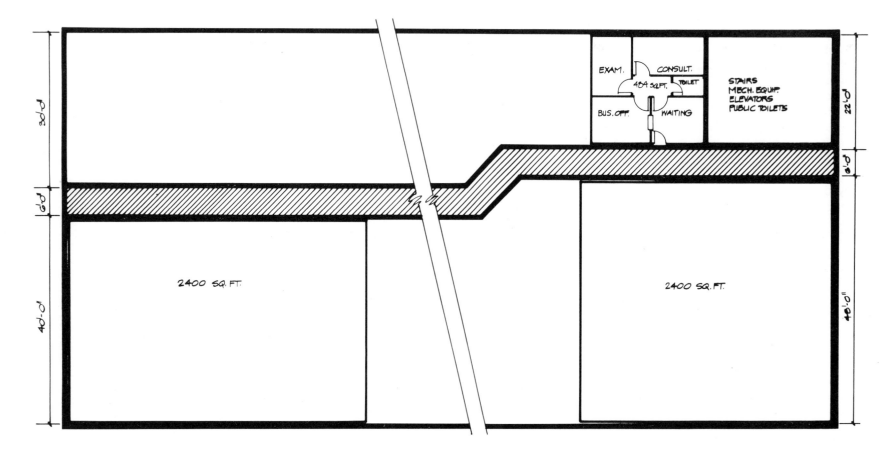

Fig. 2-6.

hospital imposes limitations upon the individual tenants whose services or practices are likely to compete with hospital departments. This is particularly true of diagnostic radiology, clinical lab, physical therapy, and pharmacy services.

At first glance, one might think that the way to approach the space planning of the individual suites would be via a grid. Grids do not work in this type building since physicians have strong opinions about the sizes of various rooms and they do not want to be told that the rooms are restricted to sizes that accommodate a grid. There is no module that really accommodates exam rooms, consultation rooms, special treatment rooms, toilets, and nurse stations. The functional sizes of each of these rooms is unique. However, the element that does affect space planning considerably is the window module. Unless one wishes to have partitions terminate in the middle of a panel of glass, the windows must conform to a certain module. Windows with mullions at 4 feet on center function well, permitting exam rooms to be 8 feet wide and consultation rooms along the window wall to be 12 feet wide. The 4-foot module can be reduced to a 2-foot module as in Fig. 2–1 as that permits even greater flexibility, but an increased construction cost. It is important that windows start at a minimum of 36 inches off the floor so that cabinets can be put under them and patient privacy in an exam room is not invaded. In fact, windows in exam rooms starting higher than 36 inches are to be desired. Even in a waiting room or lobby the windows should not start at the floor because it limits the area of seating. With a 4-foot window module, columns can be spaced at 20-foot to 24-foot intervals with transverse spans of 28 to 32 feet.

An 8-foot ceiling height is suitable for individual suites with the exception of a few individual rooms such as radiology, outpatient surgery, or physical therapy, which will require a 9-foot ceiling height. Modular ceiling systems do not work well because the rooms do not conform to a grid module, but a standard suspended 2 × 4 grid acoustic tile ceiling works well and permits access to the utilities above it. Lay-in four-lamp fluorescent fixtures function well.

When designing the individual suites, one will become aware of a basic problem: the conflicting goals of various groups with regard to tenant privileges and limitations. Of particular concern are the ownership of the building (whether the tenants may participate in ownership), the suite improvement allowances offered the tenants by the owners, and whether the tenants will be permitted to engage their own contractors. In essence, the owners want to give as little as possible but lease the building quickly and at high rents, and the tenants want to move into a custom suite designed according to their every whim, without having to foot any out-of-pocket expenses. The tug-of-war usually continues until the tenants actually take occupancy and then, little by little, the issues seem to resolve themselves. The designer is caught in the middle. If retained by the owner of the building to do the space planning for the tenants, the designer's obligation is to protect the rights of the owner; when employed by an individual tenant, the designer is forced to take on the owner on behalf of securing the greatest number of goods for the tenant. To be retained by both sides, is to court disaster.

The best way to approach the subject of suite improvement allowances is for the medical office building designer to be involved with the owners and developers of the project when the allowances and construction costs are being projected, so that a realistic appraisal can be made of how many lineal feet of partitions, how many electrical outlets or light fixtures, how many lineal feet of casework should be offered per 1000 square feet of rentable space. If a *realistic* budget is prepared and a *realistic* per-square-foot allowance is developed for these items, a tenant is less likely to receive a $40,000 bill for "extras" when he or she was originally told the suite improvement allowance would place him or her in the suite with minimal out-of-pocket expenses.

It is important for a building to provide a certain number of interior finishes. Since many physicians or dentists will choose to retain an interior designer, the building standard wall finish should be a semigloss enamel paint, with vinyl or other wallcoverings to be supplied and installed by the tenant. The standard floor finish may be vinyl asbestos tile with sheet vinyl in wet areas. The tenants often prefer to select their own carpet, in which case they would be credited for the VA tile or building standard carpet not used. The building may offer a standard commercial carpet for those tenants who desire it, but tenants appreciate being able to engage an interior designer and not be told they must accept the building's standard finishes. Window treatment is usually a standard and provided by the owners so that the building has a uniform appearance from outside. Party walls should be well insulated and constructed of staggered studs with half-inch soundboard nailed to the gypsum board (see Chapter 12). It should be a building standard that each interior partition must at least have fiberglass batting sound insulation.

Planning the space of a medical office building is a challenging endeavor. One must be not only a good designer, but also a skillful mediator. One must think about the relationships between the various suites and medical specialties. Radiology and clinical labs are usually best on the first floor, as are other high-volume suites, so that these patients do not have to use the elevator. The lowest-volume specialties fare well on the upper floors and in the least accessible locations. Conversely, the high-volume suites are best located, if not on the ground floor, then at least near the elevator to limit the foot traffic down the corridor. Specialties such as general practice or internal medicine, which utilize radiology and lab services a great deal, would be wisely located adjacent to the radiology and lab suites. Usually the radiology, lab, and pharmacy tenants would be the last to lease space in a building, since they depend on the other tenants for their livelihood. If the building is only 50% leased upon completion and they have to move in, they will suffer adversely. Also, they will want to know in advance of signing a lease, who the major tenants are so that they can project whether the composition of the building will net enough revenue for the type of equipment they have and the services they offer. One must remember that a fully equipped radiology suite may represent an investment of over a million dollars in equipment, not to mention the specialized rooms and the high construction cost for lead shielding, high ceilings, and reinforced walls and ceiling to support tube stands, and other accessories. And, such equipment is not easily relocated. It is understandable, then, that such tenants want very specific information on the other tenants in the building before committing themselves to a lease.

Chapter 3
The Practice of Medicine—Primary Care

The field of medicine is continually expanding as new knowledge and concepts are put into practice. But at the base level of the health care delivery sytem we begin with the "primary" fields of medicine: General Practice, Pediatrics, Family Practice, and Internal Medicine. Physicians in these areas are responsible for the total health care needs of their patients. They are termed "primary" medical specialties because they are normally the entry-level physician one would consult about a medical problem. If the problem requires a specialist, the general practitioner or internist will then refer the patient to a specialist— perhaps a urologist, a neurologist, orthopedist, or allergist. There are certain obvious exceptions to this primary care referral system. Persons frequently consult allergists, psychiatrists, plastic surgeons, dermatologists, obstetricians and gynecologists, and orthopedists on their own if they feel certain they have a problem that falls into that specialist's domain.

While a primary physician may refer a patient to a specialist to consult on a special problem, he or she will be in contact with the specialist and will retain overall responsibility for the patient's care. This provides for continuity of care—one physician who records a continuing health history for a patient and who oversees and coordinates his or her total health care over a period of years. This is particularly important for patients with long-term disabilities such as diabetes, heart disease, or hypertension.

Family practice is a new medical specialty. Doctors in this field have had at least three years' training and service in all major areas of medicine such as surgery, obstetrics and gynecology, pediatrics, internal medicine, and psychiatry. A general practitioner is a doctor who, having completed medical school and an internship, began his or her medical practice. A G.P. gains a broad general knowledge through experience that enables him or her to care for most of the problems his or her patients have. For the purpose of space planning, the needs of general practice and family practice physicians are identical.

GENERAL PRACTICE

The individual rooms that compose this suite, with modifications, form the specialized suites to be discussed in future chapters. Together, these rooms constitute the *basic* medical suite.

GENERAL PRACTICE

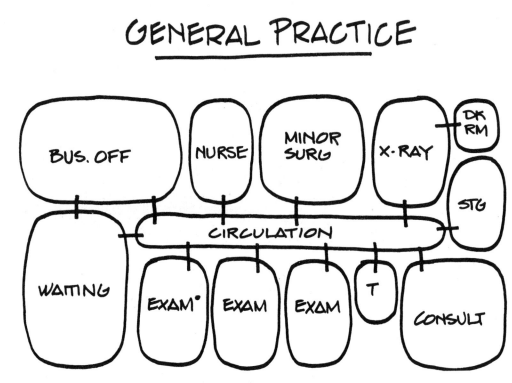

Fig. 3-1. Schematic diagram of a general practice suite.

Therefore the philosophy behind the design of these individual rooms (*waiting room, business office, exam room, consultation room, nurse station*) will be discussed in depth in this chapter.

The Functions of a Medical Suite:
1. Administrative
   A. Waiting and Reception
   B. Medical Records
   C. Business (Appointments, Bookkeeping, Insurance, Clerical)
2. Patient Care
   A. Examination
   B. Treatment/Minor Surgery
   C. Consultation
3. Support Services
   A. Nurse Station/Laboratory
   B. X-ray, Darkroom
   C. Storage
   D. Staff Lounge

The schematic diagram (Fig. 3–1) shows the relationship of rooms. The patient enters the waiting room, checks in with the receptionist via a communicating window between the business office and waiting room, and takes a seat in the waiting room. Since most medical offices require advance appointments (as opposed to walk-ins) the nurse will have pulled the patient's medical record prior to the patients entering the office. Later a nurse or assistant will call the patient to the examination area. Usually the nurse or assistant will then weigh the patient, sometimes take a urine sample, record blood pressure, and take a short history either before ushering the patient to an exam room or in the exam room. If the patient is acutely ill, the nurse will record the patient's temperature as well.

In the exam room, the nurse or aide will prepare the patient for the examination and will arrange the instruments the physician will need. The doctor will enter the room, wash his or her hands, chat with the patient about symptoms, make notes in the patient's chart, and proceed to examine the patient, often with a nurse or assistant in attendance. After examination the patient is asked to dress and meet the physician in the consultation room where a diagnosis and recommended treatment are discussed. The patient departs the office passing an appointment desk or window where future appointments may be booked and where payment for services may be made or arranged.

Obvious deviations to the above may occur when, for example, a patient breaks a limb. In this case, a patient may be sent to an X-ray room first and then proceed to a minor surgery room to have a cast applied, without ever entering an exam room. In high-volume practices, it slows down the physician to repeatedly have to return to a consultation room with each patient, so the doctor usually diagnoses and prescribes right in the exam room. With this brief outline, we shall turn to a detailed analysis of each area.

Waiting Room

The waiting room is the patient's introduction to a physician. One forms a first impression of the physician according to the image projected in the waiting room. This is where psychology plays a significant role. Dusty, antiquated furniture with torn and faded upholstery may simply be the result of a doctor's busy schedule and his or her reluctance to focus on it as an important aspect of patient care. But, whatever the actual reason,

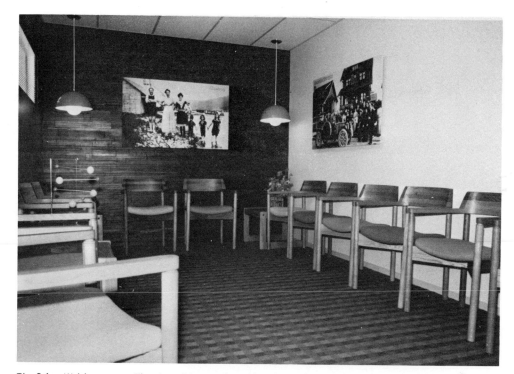

Fig. 3-1a. Waiting room: The photo blowups from historic archives reinforce the family theme.

19

such a neglected waiting room *conveys to a patient* that this is a doctor who is perhaps as outdated in his or her medical studies and technology as the waiting room evidences. The neglect of the waiting room generalizes to other areas, and patients tend to feel that this is a physician who might be neglectful in their care—a physician who manages to slide along with minimum standards. The need to design the waiting room as a comfortable, cheerful space with appealing colors, soft lighting, and attractive furnishings is paramount. These items are discussed in greater detail in Chapter 10.

In addition to the psychological aspects of the waiting room, above all, it must be functional. Unless the office is located in a warm climate, the waiting room should include a secure space for hanging coats and stashing boots and umbrellas. A patient must be able to enter the room and proceed directly to the receptionist's window without tripping over people or furniture. After checking in, the patient should be able to select a magazine from a conveniently located rack and find a seat. Should the patient be handicapped, the traffic aisles must be wide enough to accommodate a wheelchair and there must be an open space in the room where the person in a wheelchair can comfortably remain without clogging the traffic flow. The handicapped do not like to be made to feel they are a burden to the nonhandicapped population. They prefer to be independent. If we consider them in the planning stages of a project, their needs and their rights to access can be humanely and sympathetically handled. When called, the seated patient should be able to move quickly into the examination area without disturbing other patients.

The size of the waiting room can be determined after interviewing the physician and his or her staff (see Appendix for client interview form). The composition of the doctor's patient population and his or her work habits will dictate the parameters the designer must follow. Common sense dictates that a physician who sees people without advance appointments will need a much larger waiting room than one who follows an appointment schedule. Low-volume practices such as surgical specialties or psychiatry require smaller waiting rooms than do high-volume specialties such as general practice, orthopedics, pediatrics, internal medicine, and OB-GYN. In addition, practices that lend themselves to a large number of emergency cases need a larger waiting room. Accident cases will frequently be brought through the staff private entrance to avoid parading what might be a gory sight through the waiting room. The larger the patient volume, the larger the waiting room needs to be. A convenient formula for determining the number of seats follows.

$$2P \times D - E = S \qquad \frac{2P \times D}{2} = L$$

Where

P = Average number of patients per hour (per physician)
D = Number of doctors
E = Number of exam rooms
S = Seating
L = Late factor

The waiting room must accommodate at least one hour's patients. Thus if each doctor sees an average of four patients per hour and each G.P. has three examining rooms, and it is assumed that each patient is accompanied by one friend or relative, a solo practitioner would require five seats in the waiting room:

$$2(4) \times 1 - 3 = 5$$

Because this is a one-physician practice, it would be wise to assume that the doctor will run half an hour late, so the waiting room must accommodate one and one-half hour's patients. This expansion factor can be expressed as:

$$\frac{2P \times D}{2} = L \qquad \frac{2\,(4) \times 1}{2} = 4$$

Thus the waiting room should accommodate $S + L$ or nine persons, plus an area for children if space permits. The late factor can generally be reduced as the number of physicians is increased. It is important to understand that these formulas are only a guide. The specifics of each practice and the space limitations of the suite will often dictate the waiting room capacity. The formula and good common sense may tell you that ideally 45 seats should be provided, but the physical limitations of the space and the physicians' intent to squeeze in as many exam rooms as possible may limit the seating capacity to 25. In medical space planning, as in life, rarely does the ideal prevail. The designer has to skillfully juggle the client's requests, the client's budget, the building codes, the structural limitations of the given space, and the principles of medical space planning. Trade-offs and compromises are the reality out of which suites are built.

Once the number of waiting room seats has been estimated, the size of the room can be determined allowing 15 to 20 square feet per person. The author has found 18 square feet to be a workable guide for the average medical office. Nevertheless, the amount of space required for a comfortable waiting room will vary according to the room's configuration, and the location of the entry foyer and the reception window.

An area should be provided for children (Fig. 3-2). A table and chairs or a toy box is welcomed

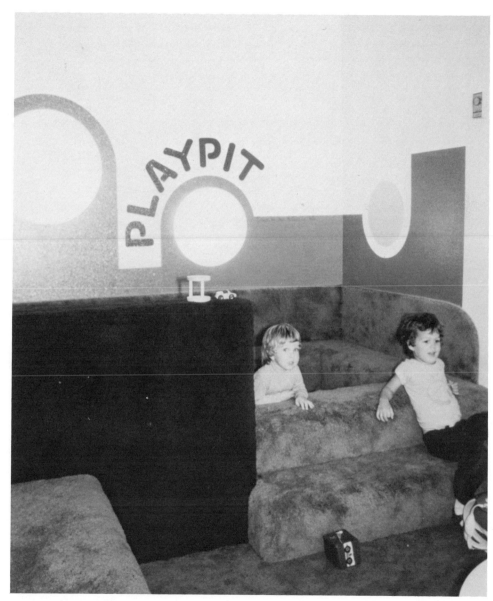

Fig. 3-2. Children's play area.

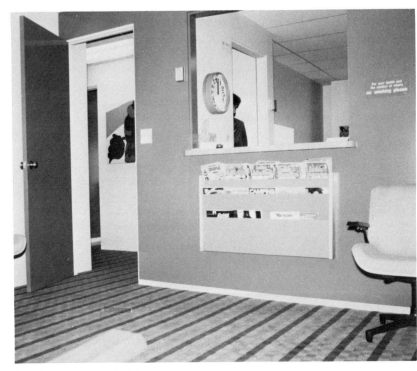

Fig. 3-3a. Reception window.

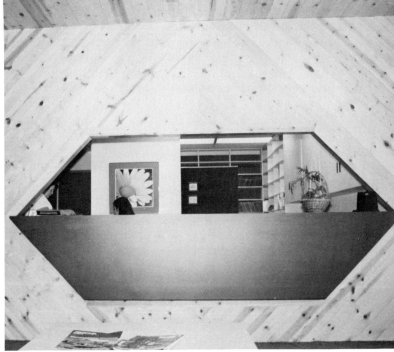

Fig. 3-3b. Reception window.

by parents. Special children's furniture can be fabricated (see Pediatrics) which will keep children busily occupied, quiet, and out of danger of being stepped on. Keep in mind that a children's corner must be located away from door swings or other hazards by which children might injure themselves. The children's area must be in sight of the receptionist, who is charged with keeping order.

Some physicians prefer maximum communication between front office staff and patients and favor a waiting room separated from the business office by only a low partition (see Fig. 3–3, Plate I). Although this may comfort the patient psychologically, it often results in a loss of privacy for the staff, who frequently have to discuss delicate matters with a patient. The patient might suffer embarrassment knowing that the adjacent waiting patients might be overhearing the conversation. Therefore the best policy seems to be a 4 to 6-foot-wide sliding glass window starting at 42 inches off the floor. Clear glass is preferable to obscure glass so that patients feel they have visual contact with the staff. (See Fig. 3a and 3b.)

22

There is a disagreement as to the practicality of providing a toilet room in the waiting area. It saves the staff the trouble of frequently directing patients into the bathroom of the examination area, but it has the disadvantage of patients emptying their bladders before the nurse can request a urine specimen. In pediatric offices, however, a toilet in the reception area is desirable to enable mothers to change a baby's diaper.

Medical Records

An important function of the business office is the storing of medical records. In order to protect the physician from legal complications as well as to provide continuity of care for patients, accurate records must be maintained and easy to retrieve. Primary physicians will keep more extensive and more detailed records than dermatologists or radiologists, who may see patients on a referral basis.

The preferred method of record storage is the lateral file cabinet (see Fig. 3-4). This may be a cabinet without doors or with retractable doors that store in the top of each shelf opening. The shelves may be stationary or they may pull out for easier access. They may also have wide drawers instead of shelves in which one can file front to back, rather than side to side laterally. These lateral files are considerably more economical of space when compared to the traditional pull-out drawer, deep file cabinets. When filing is done laterally, the file folder tab must be on the side so that it sticks out of the file cabinet. Color coded file jackets are the most efficient system for medical offices (Fig. 3-5). The standard file jacket accepts 8 1/2-x-11-inch papers, but radiology files require jumbo file jackets which are 14 1/2 x 17 1/2 inches. The patient's name may be encoded

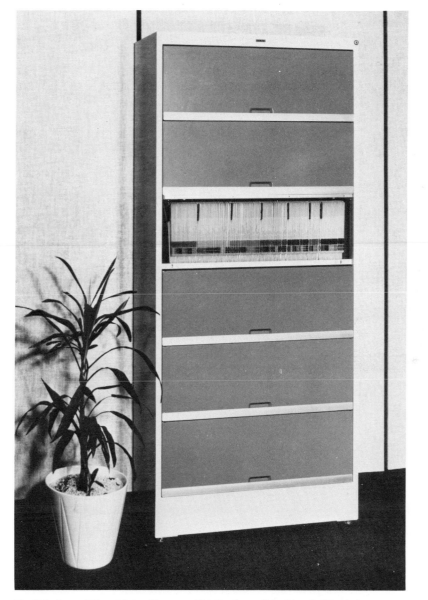

Fig. 3-4. Lateral file cabinet. (Courtesy Tab Products, Palo Alto, California.)

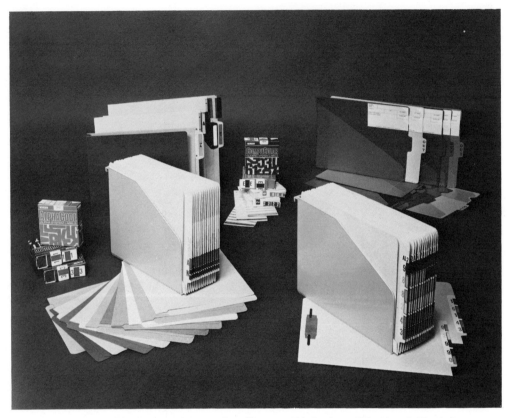

Fig. 3-5. Color coded file jackets and accessories. (Courtesy Tab Products, Palo Alto, California.)

alphabetically by color and/or number. Thus a misfiled folder immediately becomes obvious as the colors do not conform to the surrounding file jackets. Additionally one can encode by color special features such as the sex of the patient, certain unusual medical disorders, or the date the patient initially sought consultation. This facilitates pruning the files for inactive charts or selecting case studies of patients with various medical disorders for follow-up study. Various companies manufacture the specialized file jackets and color coding system. Ames Color-File (Somerville, Massachusetts) publishes a particularly good brochure explaining the details and refinements available with this system of medical record storage.

Group practices (several physicians and a high volume of patients) frequently utilize a large room for medical records with a mechanical retrieval system. This eliminates the need for aisles in front of all shelves since the files move to the operator and the access aisle is only in front of the operator (Fig. 3–6). This equipment can be purchased with manual controls or motorized (Fig. 3–7).

It is not necessary to buy factory fabricated file cabinets. They may be custom built on the job, particularly if the space allotted to medical chart storage does not accommodate standard file cabinet widths. These job-built file storage units would consist of open shelves with a clear height of 12 inches. However, steel file cabinets have the advantage of being able to be moved to another office, and they provide greater fire resistance and can be locked for security.

It is important for the designer to project the physician's future needs for storage space in the new office. The designer must ascertain from the client interview the number of new patients

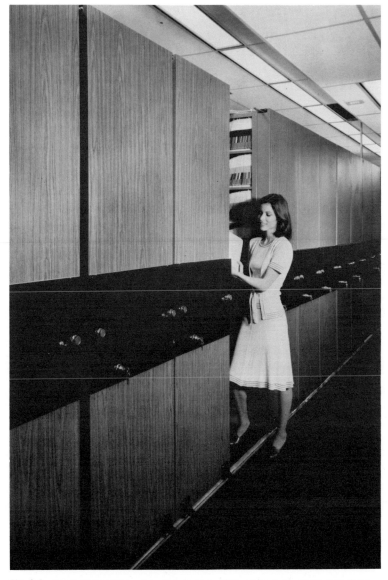

Fig. 3-6. Space-saving files, manual operation. (Courtesy Ames Color File Corp., Somerville, Massachusetts.)

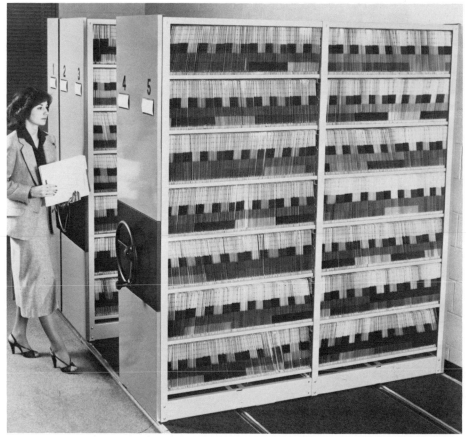

Fig. 3-7. Space-saving files, motorized. (Courtesy Ames Color File Corp., Somerville, Massachusetts.)

25

added to the practice each week or month. That number would be projected for 3 to 5 years (the length of most medical leases) and added to the existing number of medical charts. Charts should be pruned each year to eliminate patients who have not been seen in 3 years. These "aged" charts can be placed in storage at a local warehouse which offers a quick retrieval system for physicians.

Medical records should be located so that they are convenient to all of the staff. Charts are usually pulled in the morning for patients to be seen that day. The only other time the staff would need access to the charts would be primarily for phone calls or prescription refills. Medical records would normally be located in the business office but could be placed elsewhere in the suite. The bookkeeper needs convenient access to medical records for billing patients and filing insurance claims.

Business Office

Frequently referred to as the "front office" in medical jargon (versus the "back office" or examination area), this is the heart of the medical office. Appointments are scheduled here, patients are billed, medical records are stored here, patients are greeted from this room, and the routine insurance and bookkeeping duties are performed here. In a small practice, one or two people may perform all these tasks. In a large practice, three or more persons may occupy the business office. A convenient rule of thumb is one secretary for each two doctors in a low-volume practice and one secretary per physician in a high-volume practice. If a physician is seeing four to five patients per hour, the secretary may be spending more time with the patients than the doctor does since her work would involve arranging and rescheduling patient appointments on the telephone whenever the doctor is delayed or has to rearrange his or her daily schedule, filing medical charts, typing reports to referring physicians, billing patients, collecting money, filling out insurance forms, answering the phone, and ordering supplies.

A convenience in the business office is a gate door (just the lower portion) or a Dutch door (two halves that operate independently). In either case, the lower half of the door should have a shelf on it. This permits communication with patients as they are exiting the office and suffices for brief greetings or a routine discussion about a bill without the patient actually having to enter the bookkeeper's or the business office. Depending upon the width of the corridor (standard corridor width is 42 to 48 inches clear), the Dutch or gate door might be located in a recess or alcove so that a patient who stops to chat will not be blocking the traffic flow of the corridor. However, for longer conversations and more privacy, the patient would enter through that door and proceed to the bookkeeper's office. There ought to be a guest chair provided in the bookkeeper's office for this purpose. The shelf on the gate door serves several purposes. It can merely be a convenient place to rest one's elbows when chatting, or one can use it to write a check, or medical charts can be passed back and forth through it. Sometimes a box or container might be fastened to the shelf in which the medical charts for patients who have already been seen might be placed for refiling.

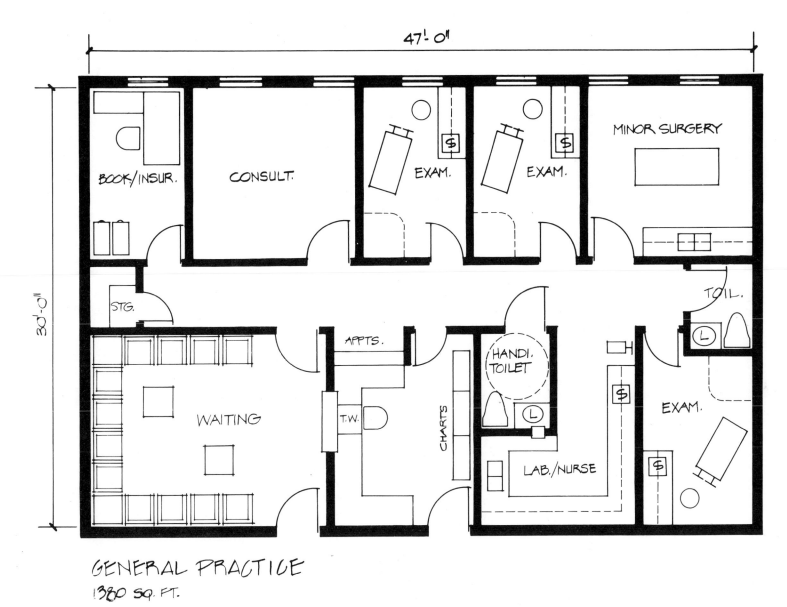

GENERAL PRACTICE
1380 SQ. FT.

Fig. 3-8. Suite plan for general practice, 1380 square feet.

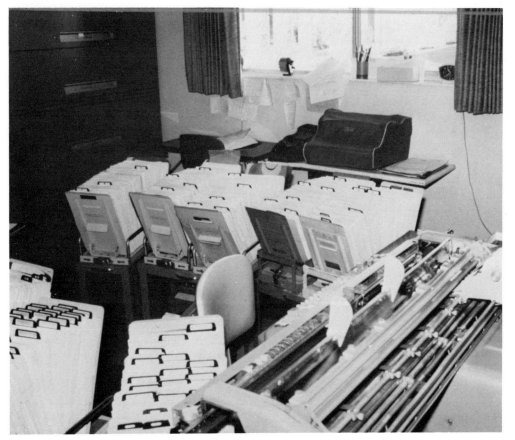

Fig. 3-9. Ledger files.

Reception

Since the receptionist maintains the appointment book, she must see the patient on arrival and just before leaving. She must also have a good view of the waiting room from her seat so that she can see who is waiting. The appointment book is usually quite large, particularly when open. Thus she needs approximately 6 lineal feet of counter-top work surface located in front of the reception window with a recess for a typewriter, a place for the phone and to write messages, a place for the appointment book, and if possible, an L-shaped return facing the corridor appointment window (Fig. 3-8) so that while remaining seated she can swivel around, greet an exiting patient, book an appointment, or accept payment for services. The front office personnel may also help in the back office, assisting the doctor in the examining room at times, weighing patients, or recording histories. But usually their duties will be confined to the business office.

Bookkeeping

The bookkeeper keeps a set of patient ledger cards upon which she posts the charges for treatment. Once a month she sends out statements. She needs to have a lowered countertop area (or floor space if on mobile carts) for the ledger card files, which are approximately 12 inches tall and are clamped into a metal holder that permits them to move in a fanlike manner, forward or back (Fig. 3-9). These ledger files can also be kept on a mobile cart which she moves up to her desk when she needs to refer to them. She needs a flat countertop work surface for the daily journal and for equipment having to do with posting charges, copying and mailing statements. She needs ample electrical outlets for these office machines, and she usually will have a typewriter and calculator as well.

A time-saving and widely used method of billing is the pegboard system. It is particularly well suited to the small office. The pegboard is a hard covered binder with "pegs" along one side upon which one aligns a statement, ledger card, and daily journal sheet. Since the forms have carbon backing, one entry for each transaction will reproduce on all forms. There are combinations of pegboard and photocopy billing. Medium-volume practices which send over 500 statements per month may post and bill by a computerized bookkeeping machine that uses ledger cards (Fig. 3-10). NCR and Burroughs Co. make small computers and other data processing units for the larger medical office (Figs. 3-11 and 3-11a). The space requirements vary considerably, so it is necessary to ascertain what type of equipment the client intends to use before laying out the bookkeeping office (see also Fig. 3-11b).

Large-volume practices that do not have data processing units may use a combination of old-style posting machine and photocopy. If the machine posts one entry per minute and it takes another minute to photocopy the ledger sheet for use as a statement (eliminating the need to address the statements each month), then one bookkeeper can prepare approximately 200 statements per day or 4000 per month. An envelope stuffer and postage meter can further increase output.

The designer must compute the projected number of monthly statements and analyze the type of bookkeeping system (and equipment) in

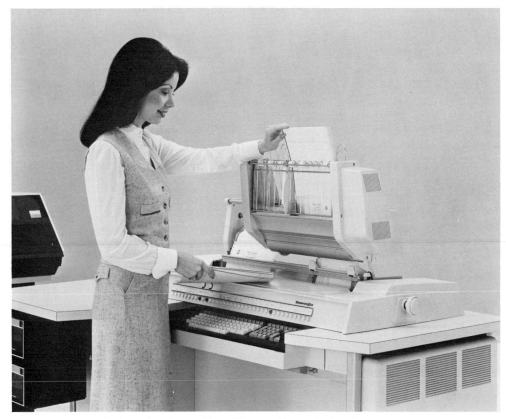

Fig. 3-10. Computerized bookkeeping machine. (Courtesy Burroughs Corp.)

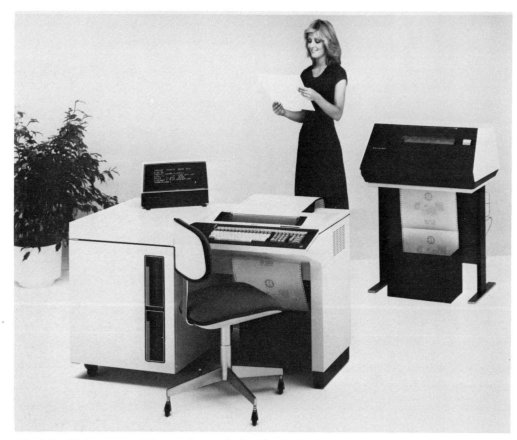

Fig. 3-11. Mini-computer. (Courtesy Burroughs Corp.)

order to know how many work stations to provide. Some practices use an outside bookkeeping service. The daily charges for service and payments received are recorded in a log and forwarded to the service, which transfers the information to a journal and mails the statements. These bookkeeping services use a computer to process the work for their clients. A monthly computer statement of all transactions would then be sent to the physician. These large computer printouts do not fit on standard 12-inch-deep shelves. The designer must provide space for these and determine whether they are to fit in large binders on a shelf or to hang.

Within the next ten years it will be increasingly common for medical offices to own their own computer. Presently only large practices own their own computer or time-share. By the end of the 1980s, it is likely that even small medical offices will have abandoned the more traditional bookkeeping methods in favor of computer systems. Since computer systems vary considerably in size and complexity of components, the designer must study the specific system used by the client before determining the space to be allotted and the relationship of personnel and machines. Basically, there are these items: a computer, a printer, and one or more CRT terminals with displays, storage for floppy disks (unless a hard disk is used). The terminal looks like a typewriter with a T.V. screen attached. It is from this unit that material is entered into the computer and is accessed from it. The computer should be in an air-conditioned room, and carpet, if used, should be permanently antistatic, such as Antron III nylon.

In large offices, the bookkeepers are in a separate room adjacent to but not part of the business office/reception area. The insurance

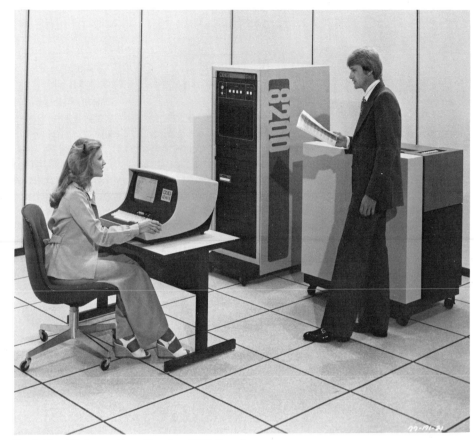

Fig. 3-11a. Mini-computer. (Courtesy NCR Corp.)

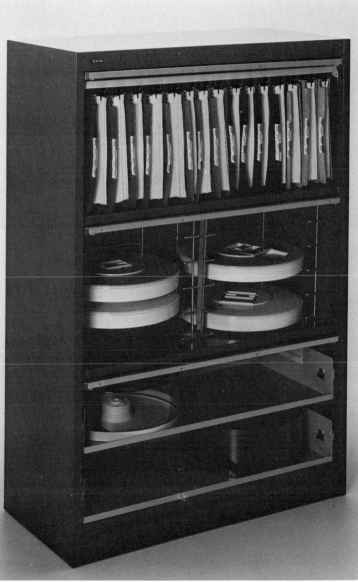

Fig. 3-11b. Computer accessories storage cabinet.
(Courtesy Tab Products, Palo Alto, California.)

secretary may also have a separate office to provide working conditions with fewer interruptions. The designer must remember that the business office of a busy practice is an extremely hectic place: Phones ring continually, people are rushing around. It is not a good place for people who work with figures. If space permits, it is always better to protect the bookkeeper and insurance secretary by giving them separate offices.

The physician may wish to have a safe for storage of cash and the ledger files. Most medical offices take in little cash, so that is not much of a problem. But ledger cards should be locked up each night and put in a fire-resistive safe. Since the cards are stacked so tightly together when in the closed position they, themselves, offer a good deal of resistance to fire, but a safe should be considered. In addition, most offices would have fire extinguishers mounted on the wall where they are easily accessible. The carbon dioxide or dry powder type is preferred.

Insurance

Most medical treatment is paid by third-party endorsers—the insurance companies. This amounts to a great deal of paperwork, and a medical office of any size usually has a full-time employee doing nothing but insurance forms. She requires a desk with a typing return, a calculator, access to the medical records, access to the copy machine, and proximity to the patients' ledger cards. File cabinets are needed as well as open shelf storage for a multitude of business forms and stationery. A guest chair should be provided for a patient. As government control increases, more and more procedures will be

covered by third-party endorsers, and the personnel required to process the forms will increase.

Medical Transcription

Medium-volume to large-volume practices often have a part-time or full-time medical transcriptionist who works from dictation tapes and transcribes the physician's notes. The transcription typing equipment is very noisy and is best accommodated in a separate room with good insulation in the walls. Only a countertop work surface is required. It should be at 26-inch height for comfortable typing. Some physicians send their tapes out of the office for transcription, or a physician may have a dictation line to a word processing unit on his or her telephone. The notes would be recorded and the typed manuscript would be delivered to the physician's office. Some medical offices have a dictation niche or kiosk (Fig. 3–12, Plate 2) outside each bank of exam rooms so that a physician may dictate notes after examining each patient, rather than at the end of the day.

Office Manager

Large offices frequently have an office manager or a business manager (Fig. 3–13). This person hires the personnel, may order supplies and drugs, and may assist the physicians in special secretarial or business matters in the capacity of an executive assistant. The office manager should have a private office. It need not be large—10 x 10 feet is adequate—and it should be located so that it faces the business office. In fact, the walls facing the business office should have glass starting at 48 inches off the floor so that the manager can oversee the staff at all times (Fig. 3–27).

Private Entrance

A medical office, regardless of size, must have two entrances—one for patients and a private one for the doctor so that he or she can enter the office without meeting patients in the waiting room. In large suites, usually over 3000 square feet, the local building code may require two exits separated by a distance equal to no less than one-half the length of the maximum overall diagonal dimension of the area served, measured in a straight line between exits. It is important to check local building codes when planning medical offices. These codes vary from city to city and state to state. (See Chapter 13.)

The Examination Room

Good traffic flow is imperative for the efficiency of a medical office. Several factors influence the location of the exam rooms:

1. It is the nurse's responsibility to control traffic to and from the exam rooms, so the nurse station and the exam rooms should be clustered together. This enables the nurses to prepare the patients in each room quickly while traveling back and forth to the nurse station to clean instruments or obtain materials needed for the examination.
2. The exam rooms must be close to the consultation room to save the physician unnecessary steps, but it is preferable that patients not pass the consultation room when making their way to the exam room.
3. The exam room corridor(s) should be arranged so that patients must pass the business office when exiting the suite. This provides control so that future appointments may be booked, medications explained, and payment for services discussed.

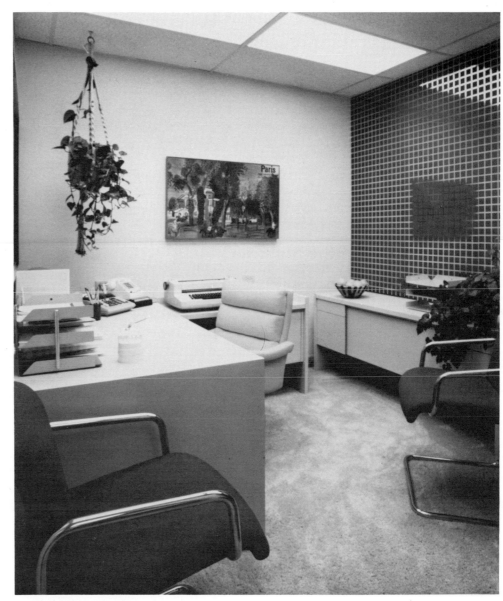

Fig. 3-13. Office manager.

33

The exam room is the background for diagnosis. As such, it should be designed very functionally with an understanding of the equipment that needs to be provided for and the psychological needs of the patient (refer to Chapter 1). If the amenities of the room can aid the patient in relaxing (wallcovering, flooring, color, and artwork), it will make the examination easier for the physician. It is desirable that patients have their life functions (blood pressure, pulse, etc.) at normal levels prior to an examination. Anxiety, due to fear generated by a clinical and unfamiliar environment, elevates the patient's life functions and may give a false reading.

The first functional consideration is size: 8 × 12 feet is the ideal size for exam rooms (gives a clear dimension of 7 feet 6 inches × 11 feet 6 inches inside the room) as it comfortably allows for a full-size exam table, a built-in sink cabinet with storage above, a dressing area, a small writing desk (usually wall mounted), a stool on casters for the doctor, a guest chair for the patient, a treatment stand (if required), and perhaps a small piece of portable medical equipment. If the room is used for purposes other than routine examinations such as stress testing, in which case the room would contain an EKG unit and a treadmill, it should be larger than 8 × 12 feet; 9 × 12 feet or 10 × 12 feet might be more appropriate. If a dressing area is not required, the length of the room can be shortened to 10 feet. If space permits, it is desirable to provide a dressing area for patients. This need be no more than a 3 × 3-foot surface-mounted drapery cubicle track at the ceiling (with a radius corner), a built-in bench or a freestanding chair, a few clothes hooks, hangers, a mirror, and perhaps a shelf for disposable gowns. It provides patients with more privacy in undressing. The alternative is that patients must disrobe in the open exam room with the fear that the nurse or doctor may walk in on them while they are naked or while they are squeezing into a girdle or panty hose. Older persons tend to be more sensitive about this than younger persons, as are those with orthopedic girdles or braces and other less-than-beautiful undergarments. There is also the possibility of creating a private dressing alcove with a 30-inch-wide door or panel hinged to the wall. It is perpendicular to the wall when in use and folds flat against the wall when not in use. The freestanding chair can be used either inside the dressing area when the hinged panel is extended, or outside when the panel is folded flat against the wall. With certain medical specialties, for example, ear-nose-throat (ENT) or orthopedics, the patients rarely undress, or if they do so, they primarily undress just to the waist, so private dressing cubicles would not be a priority in these practices.

The second functional consideration is the position of the examining table. The foot or stirrup end of the table should be angled away from the door (Fig. 3–14) as well as the wall so that the doctor has access to all sides of the patient and the patient is out of the view of passersby in the corridor when the door is opened. The door to an exam room should be hinged so that it opens *away* from the wall (does not stack against the wall). While this might seem awkward in most rooms, it is desirable in a medical exam room because it shields the patient from corridor traffic should the door be opened accidentally, and gives the patient more privacy when dressing since one has to literally walk around the open door to enter the room.

Right-handed physicians (and many left-handed ones) examine patients from the patient's right side. Thus a "right-handed" exam room will

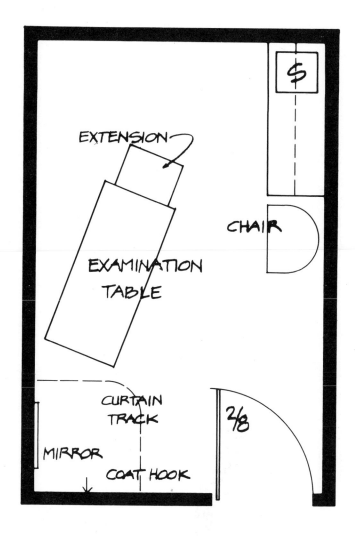

EXTENSION

CHAIR

EXAMINATION
TABLE

CURTAIN
TRACK

MIRROR

COAT HOOK

2/8

TYPICAL EXAM ROOM

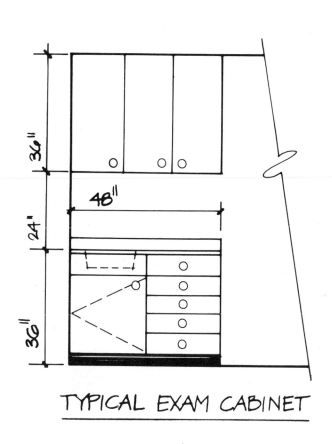

36"

48"

24"

36"

TYPICAL EXAM CABINET

Fig. 3-14. Standard examination room layout.

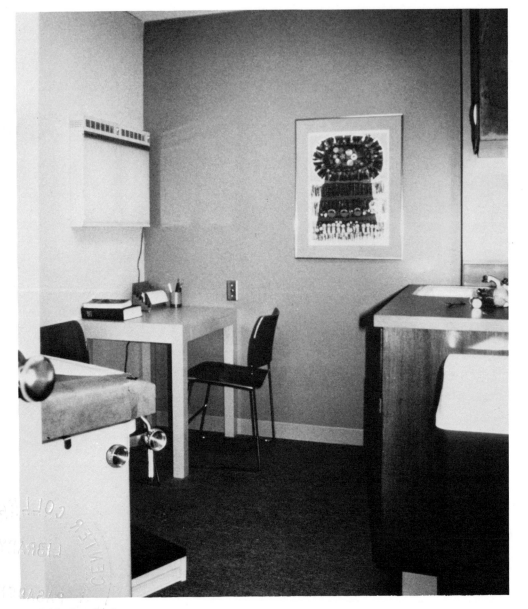

Fig. 3-15. Examination room.

have the entry door on the right side of the room with the exam table on the left as one would face the room upon entering. The sink cabinet may be located either on the wall with the door or on the long wall to the right as one enters the room. The latter position is preferable in a room in which pelvic or proctologic examinations are done so that the doctor can examine the patient with the right hand and reach for instruments with the left hand, enabling him or her to pick up and discard instruments conveniently. A sink cabinet on the long wall also has the advantage that the physician upon entering the room can, without walking around the door, quickly walk to the sink cabinet, wash hands, turn around, and be in position to examine the patient.

It is poor economy to locate sink cabinets in exam rooms back to back (mirror image) in order to reduce plumbing costs. This creates one "right-handed" room and one "left-handed" room—a most inefficient layout. For greatest efficiency, all exam rooms should be identical so that a physician can quickly move from room to room, with eyes closed, be able to orient himself or herself. The sink cabinet need only have a small sink (a 12 x 12-inch stainless steel bar sink works well) as instruments will be washed at the nurse station or lab. In addition, the sink should have a single-lever faucet control. The sink cabinet should be a minimum of 48 inches long and should be 24 inches deep and 36 inches high. If space permits, it might have a built-in compartment for trash with a hinged "trash slot" cut into the face of the cabinet door.

An upper cabinet should be provided (48 inches long, 12 inches deep, 36 inches high) over the base cabinet for storage of disposable gowns, sheets, and other paper products (Fig. 3-14). Shallow drawers in the base cabinet store instruments, syringes, surgical gloves, dressings, tongue depressors, and the like. Paper towel and liquid soap dispensers should be mounted on the wall near the sink. These items are often provided by the large paper or supply companies that service the units.

Obstetricians and gynecologists often like to warm their specula prior to examinations. For this purpose an electrical outlet may be provided in the drawer in which the specula are kept. The more expensive pelvic examination tables have a built-in warmer for specula.

A small wall-hung writing shelf should be provided in an exam room so that the physician can complete most examinations in the exam room without returning to the consultation room. If the sink cabinet is located on the long wall, the countertop can be extended and lowered from 36 inches to 30 inches to serve as a writing desk. A rolling stool that stores under the "desk" when not in use should be provided for the physician. The patient may sit on the exam table or on a guest chair while the physician is taking a patient history or writing a diagnosis. Frequently slots for prescription pads are built into the desk top (Fig. 4–77).

If the sink cabinet is located on the door wall, the writing desk should be placed on the long wall. If space permits, a freestanding Parson's style table can serve well as a writing desk (Fig. 3–15). The cabinetry and desk should be faced with plastic laminate, rather than painted. The additional cost when fabricating the cabinets is minimal and well worth it when one considers the abuse of the painted surfaces of such a cabinet and the inconvenience and cost of repainting it.

Some physicians may request a connecting door between examining rooms and their consultation room. This is usually not a good idea.

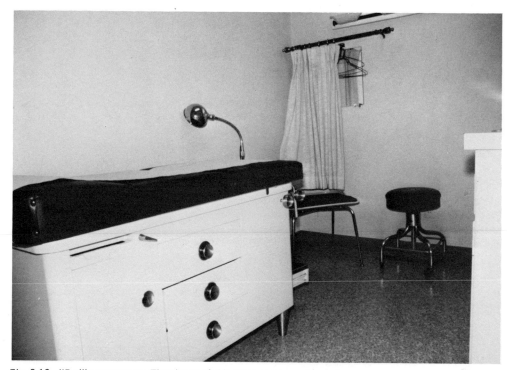

Fig. 3-16. "Bad" exam room: The charm of this room needs no description.

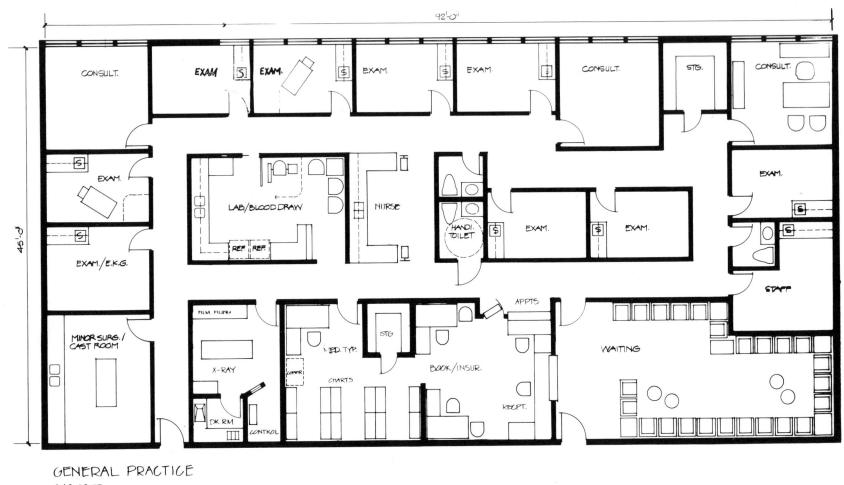

GENERAL PRACTICE
4140 SQ FT.

Fig. 3-17. Suite plan for general practice, 4140 square feet.

Considerable space is lost in the exam room by installing an extra door, there is a loss of privacy in the consultation room via sound transmission through the door into the exam room, and there is then the tendency of the physician to bring each patient into the consultation room, which greatly reduces the number of patients the physician can see in a day.

There is controversy over the benefit of windows in exam rooms. There is no need for natural light in an exam room for most specialties (it is recommended for dermatology exam rooms), so the inclusion of windows would be either a matter of the physician's preference or a "given" of the building's architecture. If present, the glass should start at a height sufficient to afford the patient a measure of privacy. Gray glass is superior to bronze since the latter casts an unhealthy tint on patient's skin. Narrow-slat metal window blinds are particularly well suited to windows in exam rooms for the slats can be tilted to provide privacy without cutting off the light or view entirely. Too many windows in a medical building can make it difficult to lay out the rooms efficiently unless one wishes to have partitions that terminate in the middle of a window, instead of at a wall or a mullion. This is particularly common when the architect who designed the building was not familiar with medical space planning and a window module was designed that is not compatible with the size of rooms in a medical office—basically a 4-foot module.

Three grounded duplex electrical outlets should be provided within an exam room—one above the cabinet countertop, one at the foot of the table, and one near the head of the table. Except for the outlet over the countertop, which would be at a height of 44 inches, the other outlets may be at a standard 12-inch height. Rooms used for ophthalmic or ENT examinations have special electrical requirements to be discussed in Chapter 4. Certain exam rooms, such as pediatric or orthopedic exam rooms, often require only two electrical outlets, one over the countertop and the other near the foot of the exam table. Outlets in a pediatric exam room must be carefully guarded and located where a child cannot reach them. It may be necessary to shield a specialized exam room (one used for electrocardiograph machinery or diathermy, for example) against electrical interference from surrounding medical offices or equipment.

The standard exam table is 2 x 4 feet with stirrups at the foot (Fig. 3–18) if it is to be used for pelvic, procto, or urologic examinations. If not used for these examinations, the table will probably have just a pull-out foot board that extends the length of the table to about 5 feet.

The examining room as described above will be suitable for most physicians, but some medical specialties require modifications and these are discussed in future chapters. Most notably, orthopedic surgeons use a 6-foot-long exam table which is often placed against a wall. Pediatricians, also, place their exam tables against the wall. The combination consultation room and examination room popularized by the Mayo Clinic is an alternative that has a place in some practices—very low volume practices. Whatever the design of the exam room, the formula for a productive and efficient office is in the relationship of exam rooms to consultation rooms to nurse station and ancillary facilities.

Treatment/Minor Surgery

Each family practice or general practice suite will have a minor surgery room. It is sometimes labeled *Treatment Room*. It is a large exam room (usually 12 × 12 feet) which serves a variety of purposes. It may be used as a cast room, in which case a plaster trap should be provided in the sink, and cabinets should contain a bin for plaster and for the remains of casts that have been removed (see Chapter 4 under *Orthopedic Surgery*). It may be used as an EKG room, an operating room for minor surgical procedures utilizing local anesthetics, and as an emergency exam room for accident cases. In an accident case, the physician may need one or more aides in the room plus certain medical equipment not usually stored in the other exam rooms. Add to that the relatives who accompany the patient and frequently wish to remain in the treatment room, and the need for an oversized multipurpose exam room becomes clear.

A minor surgery room should have a 10-foot to 12-foot length of upper and lower cabinets—one full wall of built-ins. Usually this room will have a ceiling-mounted surgical light over the treatment table in addition to the normal fluorescent lighting. Adequate illumination is mandatory for this room. If the suite is so situated within the layout of the medical building as to make possible a direct entrance into the minor surgery room, it is desirable. Accident cases or those with contagious diseases do not have to walk through the waiting room if they can enter the minor surgery room directly. This would be an unmarked door in the public corridor of the medical building provided with a buzzer, or the door might simply state *Emergency Entrance—Ring bell for service.*

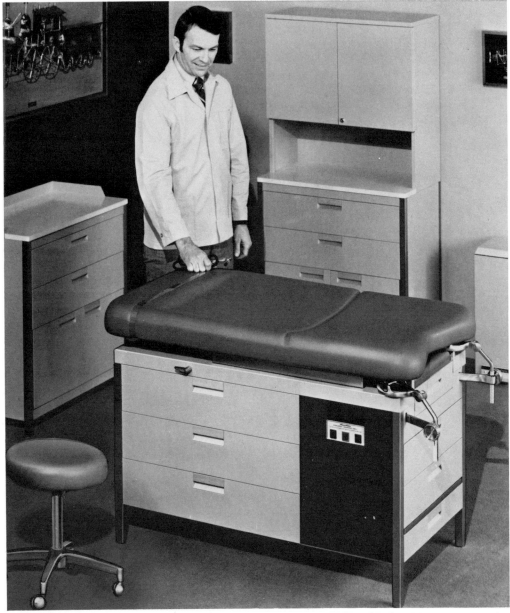

Fig. 3-18. Examination table. (Courtesy Hamilton Industries.)

The receptionist taking the phone message would explain to the patient that he or she should go to the door marked *Emergency Entrance* and ring the bell.

The Consultation Room

This room functions as a private office for the most part, but some physicians do consult with patients here. Routine consultation can be handled in a well-designed exam room, saving the physician the trouble of continually returning to his or her private office between patients. Certain physicians (for example, internists, neurologists) spend a good deal of time interviewing the patient on his or her initial visit. In such a case the physician may feel that the consultation room provides a more conducive atmosphere for establishing the relationship. Surgeons also tend to use their private offices for consultation with patients. But this remains a matter of individual preference for each physician.

The consultation room is also used by the physician for reading, returning phone calls, dictating notes, or just relaxing. The minimum size for this room is 10 × 12 feet, but 12 × 12 feet is better. The room must accommodate a desk, credenza, bookshelves for the doctor's library, two guest chairs, a coat closet (optional), and perhaps a private bathroom. The room should be furnished like a living room with cut pile carpet, warm colors, textured wallcoverings or wood paneling, and fabric upholstery. If the doctor has a hobby that lends itself to expression in room decor, this is the one room in the suite that can be highly personalized. Family photos, armed forces honors, diplomas, and personal memorabilia humanize the doctor's image and provide a clue to him or her as a person apart from his or her medical practice.

A consultation room should have natural light if possible. In addition, table lamps or indirect lighting may add to the room's homelike ambience. It is desirable to locate the consultation room at the rear of the suite so that the physician has more privacy and so that patients do not pass it on their way to the examining room. Still, some aggressive patients find their way to the consultation room uninvited and unannounced.

Frequently it is possible to locate a door to the outside in the private office. The physician may thus enter or leave the office without being seen by patients. If such a door is not possible, then a private rear entrance to the suite, as previously discussed, is mandatory.

In certain suites, such as pediatrics, the consultation room is used so minimally that several physicians may share a consultation room. Their combined medical library would be stored here and each doctor would have a small desk and telephone (Fig. 3–36). At the other extreme, occasionally a physician will request a consultation room with a sofa large enough to sleep on, a table with reading lamp, a refrigerator and bar, and a bathroom with shower, in addition to the usual components of a private office. Such an office may serve a cardiac surgeon who, due to many emergency surgeries, may have to spend the night at his office (if it is near the hospital) or just catch up on sleep during the day between surgeries.

Nurse Station/Laboratory

The nurses' station is an area where the doctor's nurse or aides perform a variety of tasks such as weighing patients, sterilizing instruments, dispensing drug samples, giving injections, taking a patient's temperature, performing routine lab tests, communicating with patients by telephone, or handling office paperwork. The nurse station may be only a 6-foot length of countertop (with cabinets below and above) recessed in a niche in the corridor (Fig. 3–26), or it may be an 8 × 12-foot room adjacent to the exam rooms (Fig. 3–17). The size of the nurses' station/laboratory depends on the number of aides who will use it, the type of medical practice, and the functions to be performed by the aides.

The number of aides can be estimated on the basis of each doctor requiring one or two aides depending on whether the practice is a high-volume specialty. The aide may assist the physician in the exam room or may actually perform certain examinations herself. Obstetricians and gynecologists have been using assistants in this expanded role for routine pelvic and gynecologic examinations. Called *nurse practitioners,* these women are registered nurses who take an additional study program that prepares them to examine patients. Since OB-GYN is a very high volume specialty, the use of nurse practitioners saves the physician's time on routine examinations and permits him or her to concentrate on patients with special or unusual medical problems.

Therefore the nurses' station in an OB-GYN suite must be large enough to accommodate the nurse practitioners and other aides who need a knee space for sitting down and writing notes, one or two scales (all OB-GYN patients are weighed each visit) with a writing shelf nearby. Sometimes the scales are recessed into the floor if practical in terms of cost and construction parameters. This recess in the concrete slab can be carpeted with the adjacent floor carpet. An area of approximately 24 inches should be allowed for each scale—this is not the size of the recess but the floor space necessary to accommodate a standard medical scale with balance rod.

There is an advantage to locating the nurse station near the front of the suite in a small office (under 2000 square feet). The nurse has easy access to patients as she leads them from the waiting room to the exam room, and she can cover for the business office staff when they are momentarily away from their desks. In larger suites each doctor may have his or her own aide working from a nurse station convenient to his or her pod of exam rooms (Fig. 3–27).

In some medical offices the nurse station is combined with the laboratory. In otolaryngology (ENT), for example, this is true since there are few lab tests performed in the office. The nurse station/lab would be used for preparing throat cultures and for cleanup of instruments in the sink or for sterilizing instruments. With the widespread use of disposable syringes, gowns, sheets, and even many examination instruments, there are relatively few items that have to be washed or sterilized. In an OB-GYN practice, the laboratory would generally be a separate room because a good deal of lab work is processed in the suite. Each patient supplies a urine sample for urinalysis, which is performed in the lab, and each patient having a pelvic exam and Pap smear will have a tissue culture that will have to be prepared for sending to a cytology lab. There are a number of other routine tests that would be performed within the lab, plus many gynecologists do D & Cs and other types of minor surgical procedures in a well-equipped minor surgery room in their office. These procedures can be messy and require an adequate area for cleanup and good-sized nurse station and lab support facilities.

A lab should have a double-compartment sink, a knee-space area for a microscope, a full-size refrigerator if necessary (otherwise an under-counter one), and a facility for blood draw. The blood draw area may be nothing more than a chair in the lab or it may be a special prefabricated tablet arm blood draw chair. It is advisable to shield the patient whose blood is being drawn from the sight of other patients who often become faint upon observing the procedure. It is desirable to have at least one toilet room adjacent to the lab so that a specimen pass-through door in the wall can give the lab technician access to urine specimens without his or her leaving the lab (Fig. 3–8). The reader is referred to Chapter 5 for more detailed specifications of a small laboratory and to the Appendix for a diagram of a specimen pass-through.

The nurse station of an orthopedic surgery suite would need to be minimal since there are no lab tests performed and no blood is drawn. The supplies needed for examinations or for making or removing casts would be stored in the respective rooms, and very little would have to be carried into a room for a procedure. By contrast, a family practice or G.P. suite would tend to have a good-sized nurse station. Since such a wide variety of medical procedures are dealt with and there is such a wide range of patients, it would be impractical to store in each exam room all the supplies one might need for the range of examinations that might be performed, so the nurse will prepare the exam room with any special supplies, injections, dressings, and instruments that she anticipates will be required. A good many of these items will be stored in the nurse station, and each nurse station might have its own autoclave for sterilization of instruments. In addition, the nurse might give allergy or other injections at the nurse station, blood might be drawn for tests to be done in the suite's own lab or sent out to a lab for processing, patients are weighed at each visit, and many other routine duties are carried out here.

A nurse station should always have a sink and often has an under-counter refrigerator and a knee-space work area with telephone. Most nurse stations have a scale space with a nearby shelf for writing the weight in the patient's chart. The reader is referred to Chapter 4 for nurse station requirements for each medical specialty. As regards the laboratory, it is the physician's decision whether to do lab tests within the office or send the work out. Some physicians do not even like to draw blood in their office but prefer to send the patient to a lab if one is conveniently located in the medical building. Sometimes the physicians who are tenants or owners of the medical building own the lab jointly and agree to send all of their lab work there for their mutual benefit. This also generates the type of lab income that enables them to buy more sophisticated equipment for their jointly owned lab than any of the individual physicians could afford to purchase for their own use. The automated clinical analyzers (Fig. 3–19) perform over 20 different lab tests from one blood sample in a matter of minutes.

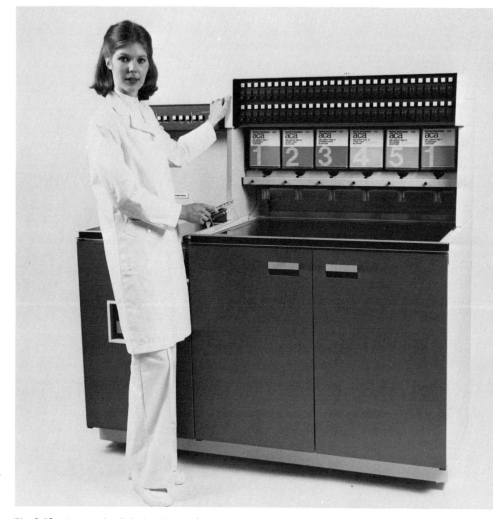

Fig. 3-19. Automatic clinical analyzer. (Courtesy The DuPont Co., Clinical Systems Div.)

X-ray Room

This discussion will focus on the one-room X-ray unit that can be found in a G.P. or internal medicine suite. Rather simple radiographic procedures are performed here—films of extremities, chests, gallbladders, appendixes, etc. More complicated procedures will be performed in a radiologist's office. A large internal medicine practice might have a suite of radiographic rooms within its facility with a full-time radiologist on staff. But usually a patient who requires G.I. (gastrointestinal) studies, thyroid scans, Computerized Tomography (CAT scans), radiation oncology therapy, or other specialized or complicated radiographic procedures will be referred to a local hospital on an outpatient basis or to a nearby radiology clinic.

A 10 x 12-foot room is adequate (not taking into account the dressing area and darkroom) for most X-ray machines used in a G.P.'s or internist's office. Usually a 9-foot ceiling height is required. The room should have a place for a patient to dress (ideally a 3 x 4-foot alcove with a drapery for privacy), a control area for the technician, and a place to process the film. Although the equipment breaks down into components, it is advisable to provide a minimum 3-foot-wide door in this room for ease in moving the equipment. The radiography room does not need a sink or prep area unless G.I. studies are performed or contrast media are used. In such cases a bathroom must be located close to the radiographic room (Fig. 5–8).

Two or more walls of an X-ray room will have to be·shielded with lead to protect passersby from radiation scatter. It is necessary to obtain a radiation physicist's report, based upon the type of equipment and the location of the room within the suite and within the medical office building, in order to know which walls must be shielded, the thickness of the lead, and the height of the lead panels. Frequently the door to the room must also be lead lined. Such a door is very heavy and must have a good-quality door closer controlling it. The control partition, if located within the room, must also be lead lined. It is possible to buy prefabricated, freestanding, lead-lined control partitions with glass viewing panels from X-ray supply houses.

If the control area is located outside the X-ray room, there must be a lead-lined glass window provided to enable the operator to observe the patient at all times. The control area need not be large (3 feet square), but should be based upon the manufacturer's recommendations for that brand of equipment. There are considerable variations in size of equipment, power requirements, lead shielding requirements, and other specifications from one manufacturer to another. Therefore it is advisable to obtain a brochure of specs with photos of each piece of equipment and a layout template before proceeding. A valuable reference in laying out radiology rooms is the catalog of radiology supplies and accessories marketed by each manufacturer. General Electric Co. has a particularly good one in which thousands of items are pictured with dimensions and pertinent data. The designer can immediately become familiar with the many accessory items such as cassette pass boxes, film illuminators, film dryers, automatic processors, etc., which must be accommodated in a radiology room or suite.

A lead-lined cassette pass box should be located in the wall between the darkroom and the procedure room. The pass box is used for passing exposed and unexposed film back and forth from the darkroom to the procedure room.

The manufacturer's literature will guide the designer as to the required electrical connections and critical distances between equipment. Sometimes wood blocking is needed in the ceiling to support the tube stand. Usually the X-ray unit, if new, will be supplied by a local distributor and the installer can assist the designer in locating the equipment in the room. Or, if the physician is relocating existing equipment in a new office, it will usually be moved and reinstalled by a skilled technician who can offer assistance as to the equipment's requirements. In any case, the designer should not hesitate to enlist the aid of the equipment vendor to verify the room layout and mechanical specifications.

Darkroom

A small darkroom must be provided. If an automatic film processor is not used, a "wet" and a "dry" side should be set up in the darkroom. A 4 x 6-foot room is the minimum size. The room should have two 4 to 5-foot counters either parallel to each other or at right angles. The wet side contains the sink and developing tank, while the dry side is used for loading cassettes. A lightproof metal film storage bin should be located under the dry side of the counter. Ideally the cassette pass box would be positioned in the wall close to the film storage bin. Films may be hung in a rack over the counter to air dry or they may be placed in a electric film dryer. The film dryer may be a countertop unit or one that fits under the counter. Sometimes a rack for storage of cassettes is provided. A floor drain must be located near the tanks. One outlet should be provided over the counter on both the wet and dry sides. An outlet is needed for the film dryer as well. The tanks require hot and cold water and a temperature control mixing valve.

Local codes normally require a vacuum breaker on piping to darkroom tanks to prevent the chemical waste from backing up into the water supply. Also, acid-resistant pipe is recommended since the chemical waste is very corrosive.

The room must have an exhaust fan and some codes require that the door have a lightproof louver ventilation panel. The darkroom door should open inward so that if someone tries to enter while developing is in process, the technician inside the room can put a foot against the door to prevent it from opening. Some darkrooms have a red warning light that is activated when developing is in process. In a small office, the staff usually know when someone is in the darkroom, and there is not a sufficient volume of X-rays to warrant a more complicated warning signal system. The door to the darkroom need be only 24 inches wide and it must have a light seal.

The darkroom must have two sources of light. A 100-watt incandescent fixture either recessed or surface mounted to the ceiling will suffice for normal work. But a safelight must be provided for working with exposed film. The safelight can be plugged into an outlet at 60 to 72 inches off the floor and it can work by a pull chain or be wired into a wall switch. If the latter, the switch should be located away from the incandescent light switch so that the technician does not confuse them and hit the wrong one while the film is exposed. Any recessed light fixtures and the exhaust fan must have a light-sealed housing.

The counters and cabinets in a darkroom may be at a 36-inch or 42-inch height according to personal preference. A 6-inch to 10-inch-deep shelf mounted 12 to 14 inches above the countertop is convenient for bottles of chemicals. There is no need for "closed" storage in the darkroom. All shelves should be open shelves.

A small viewing area should be provided outside the procedure room near the darkroom. This may consist of nothing more than a double-panel view box illuminator either surface mounted to the wall or recessed. The technician can check the films for resolution and clarity before handing them to the physician for diagnosis. If the film is not good, the patient is still at hand with little time lost in having to take the film again. In a larger X-ray suite of rooms, the viewing area will be larger, with several banks of film illuminators and a place for two or more persons to sit down.

Some physicians will have an automatic film processor if they have a sufficient volume of films. They may still have manual developing tanks as a backup measure in case the automatic processor is out of order. The automatic processor may be a small tabletop unit such as dentists or facial plastic surgeons use, or it may be a large piece of equipment that sits outside the darkroom with a "tongue" that fits through the wall into the darkroom (Fig. 5–7). Such units are discussed in detail in Chapter 5 under *Radiology*.

Storage

Medical offices should have a storage room at least 5 feet square. Two or more walls should have adjustable shelves for storage of office supplies, sterile supplies, pharmaceutical items, housekeeping supplies, and cartons of toilet paper, hand towels, and facial tissue. If the office does not use a janitorial service, this is usually where the vacuum cleaner and mop and pail are stored.

Staff lounge

Any suite with more than three employees should have a staff lounge if space permits. The room need not be larger than 8 × 12 feet with a built-in sink cabinet 4 to 6 feet in length, an under-counter refrigerator, perhaps a hot plate, and a small table and chairs. A larger staff lounge should include a cot or sofa where an employee may lie down. This is a private room where the staff can take coffee breaks, eat their lunch, or smoke. A staff lounge is not a must in a small of-fice, but it is an amenity that pleases the employees and makes their job a little more plea-sant.

Table 3–1. Analysis of Program.
General Practice

No. of Physicians:	1	2	3
Consultation	12 × 12 = 144	2 @ 12 × 12 = 288	3 @ 12 × 12 = 432
Exam Rooms	3 @ 8 × 12 = 288	6 @ 8 × 12 = 576	9 @ 8 × 12 = 864
Waiting Room	12 × 14 = 168	14 × 18 = 252	20 × 24 = 480
Business Office	12 × 14 = 168	14 × 16 = 224	18 × 30 = 540[a]
Nurse Station	8 × 10 = 80	10 × 12 = 120	12 × 12 = 144
Toilets	2 @ 5 × 6 = 60	2 @ 5 × 6 = 60	3 @ 5 × 6 = 90
Storage	4 × 6 = 24	6 × 8 = 48	8 × 10 = 80
Cast Room	Use Minor Surgery	Use Minor Surgery	12 × 12 = 144
EKG	Use Minor Surgery	Use Minor Surgery	8 × 12 = 96
Staff Lounge	—	8 × 12 = 96	10 × 12 = 120
Minor Surgery	12 × 12 = 144	12 × 12 = 144	12 × 12 = 144
X-ray Area[b]	—	12 × 20 = 240	12 × 20 = 240
Laboratory	—	8 × 10 = 80	16 × 16 = 256[c]
Subtotal	1076 ft^2	2128 ft^2	3630 ft^2
15% Circulation	161	319	545
Total	1237 ft^2	2447 ft^2	4175 ft^2

[a] Includes insurance clerk, bookkeeper, and office manager.
[b] Includes darkroom, control, film filing, and dressing area.
[c] Includes lab, waiting, and blood draw.

INTERNAL MEDICINE

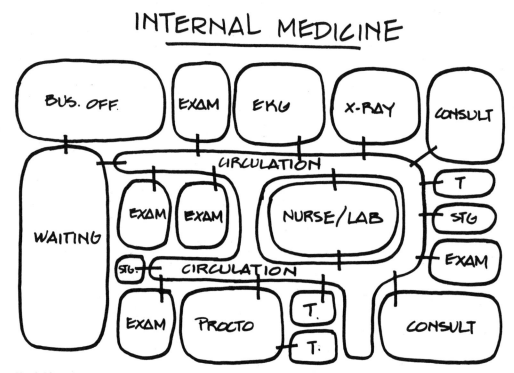

Fig. 3-20. Schematic diagram of an internal medicine suite.

INTERNAL MEDICINE

The practice of internal medicine is broad. It encompasses many subspecialties such as pulmonary disease, nephrology, oncology, hematology, endocrinology, and cardiovascular disease—the major emphases. Before planning an internal medicine suite it is important to analyze the physicians' respective specialties and practice schedules. With such a broad range of areas of expertise, it is common for internists to practice in groups rather than as solo practitioners. A designer must also understand the structure of a physician's workday. Physicians tend to visit their hospitalized patients in the morning before office hours. Office hours typically begin at 9:00 A.M. and continue to 12:00 noon. Medical offices are usually closed from 12:00 to 2:00 and open again from 2:00 to 5:00 P.M. Surgeons try to do the bulk of their surgery in the morning and reserve the afternoon for office visits by patients.

In a five-person practice, for example, the physicians' schedules will usually be arranged so that no more than three are in the office at any one time. This negates the need for each of the five to have the use of exam rooms all at the same time. By efficiently coordinating their schedules, the group can function well in less space without sacrificing income or service to patients. One doctor may have a day off while a second may be seeing patients at a satellite office, and a third may be seeing patients at the hospital, leaving the other two in our hypothetical group of five in the primary office. At a busier point in the day, schedules may be arranged to that three or four of the internists are in the primary office to see patients.

Internal medicine is a medium-volume practice. It is based on diagnosis, and that requires long history-taking interviews by the physician and sometimes a complicated battery of tests. The internist, being primarily a diagnostician, spends a good deal of time with a patient. However, follow-up visits may be considerably shorter, so overall, a well-organized, efficient practice can process a fairly high number of patients each day. Some internists prefer to do the initial interview in the consultation room, whereas others find it more efficient to do it in the exam room. If the consultation room is used, it should be large—12 x 12 feet—with comfortable seating. There is a lot of lab work associated with internal medicine and one must determine which tests are to be done within the suite and which are to be sent out. If a substantial number of tests are to be done within the suite, a 12 x 12-foot minimum size lab should be set up. The reader is referred to Chapter 5 under *Small Laboratory* for further details.

An internist needs three exam rooms or five for each two physicians. Ten exam rooms should suffice for a group of five physicians, allowing that at least one person is absent at any time and a second person may be absent for certain periods of the day. A small X-ray room should be provided for films of the chest, gallbladder, etc. Usually the more involved gastrointestinal studies are referred to a radiologist.

A large storage room should be provided for storing specialized, seldom used equipment and for storing patient's X-ray films.

Electrocardiograph (EKG) Room

A large exam room (10 x 12 or 12 x 12 feet) may be provided for EKG studies. Some physicians dedicate a special room to this function, while others feel that dedicated rooms result in a loss

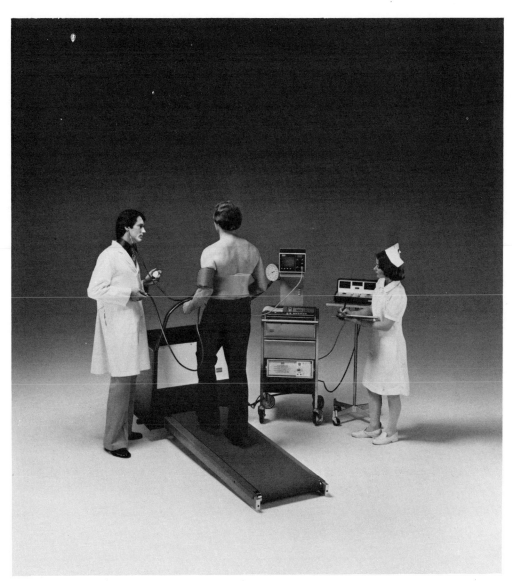

Fig. 3-21. Stress testing: Exercise tolerance system includes electrocardiograph, monitor/heart-rate meter, defibrillator, mobile blood pressure unit, and treadmill. (Courtesy The Burdick Corp., Milton, Wisconsin.)

49

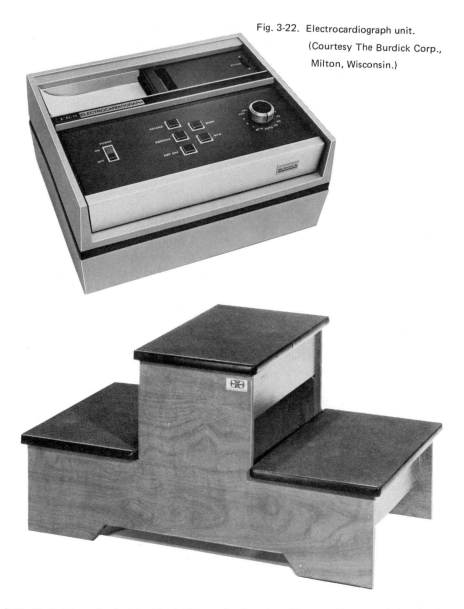

Fig. 3-22. Electrocardiograph unit.
(Courtesy The Burdick Corp.,
Milton, Wisconsin.)

Fig. 3-23. Master's two-step footstool for testing cardiac function. (Courtesy Hausmann Industries, Inc., Northvale, New Jersey.)

of flexibility. Since the equipment is fairly portable, it can be moved from room to room as needed. A monitoring unit on a mobile cart is brought to the patient and electrodes attached to wires on the machine are placed on the patient's chest, leg, and wrist. The patient will be lying on an exam table or a physical therapy table for this procedure. The instrument records the changes in electrical potential occurring during the heartbeat by photographing the vibrations and producing a printout—the electrocardiogram—which is then interpreted by the internist. The heartbeat patterns on the printout indicate either normalcy or the type of cardiovascular abnormality from which the patient suffers. This type of EKG (where the patient lies supine) is called *static*. By contrast, a *dynamic* EKG involves an active patient whose heartbeat is monitored while walking on a motorized treadmill with remote control (Fig. 3-21). The treadmill is not easy to move around, so if dynamic EKGs are done it is better to locate the equipment in one room and leave it there. An EKG room without a treadmill can be the size of a normal exam room (8 x 12 feet) with space for a 2 x 6-foot table for the patient to lie on, the monitoring equipment (Fig. 3-22), a two-step footstool apparatus (Master's Exercise Toleration Technique—see Fig. 3-23), and a 4-foot countertop area for mounting the printouts on cardboard holders. Often the mounting area is outside of the EKG room. If space permits, an alcove should be provided in which a patient can dress. A cabinet should be located in the room for storage of supplies associated with the procedure.

50

Pulmonary Function/Inhalation Therapy Lab

Persons with impaired lung function are diagnosed in the pulmonary function lab. The spirometer, an instrument for measuring the vital capacity of the lungs (Fig. 3–24), is the basic tool for pulmonary function studies. It, along with an analysis of blood gases and other clinical tests, helps the physician to evaluate the extent and nature of lung damage. Often a bronchodilator medication is administered when the spirometer studies are performed.

Once the patient has been screened, the treatment phase would be called *inhalation* or *respiratory therapy.* The treatment generally consists of breathing mechanically pressurized air with medication. The Bird positive pressure breathing machine (Fig. 3–25) is a basic piece of equipment used in this type of therapy. The treatment might also consist of chest physiotherapy, in which a patient lies on an angled bed and the gravity flow drains different lobes of the lung. The therapist, after administering bronchodilator medication, cups the patient's back and the patient coughs up the mucus.

There is not a generally accepted standard layout for a pulmonary function/inhalation therapy lab. Frequently these services are combined with cardiovascular screening in which case it is called a *cardiopulmonary* lab. One would have to allow space for two exercise bicycles, a treadmill, a body pressure booth, and the equipment for analyzing the data. A well-equipped physiology lab may have a sizable amount of sophisticated electronic machinery that must be accommodated. Sometimes pulmonary function screening is separated from respiratory therapy. With so many variables, the internists and pulmonary technicians must give

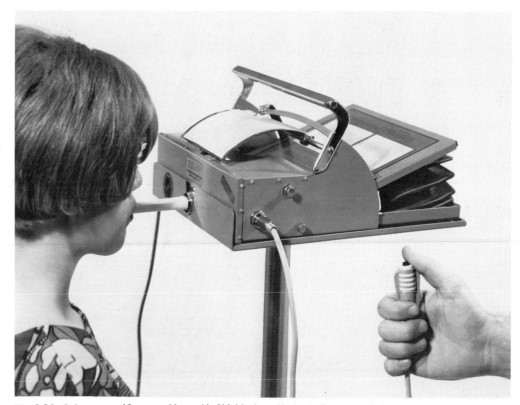

Fig. 3-24. Spirometer. (Courtesy Marco Air-Shields, Inc., Hatboro, Pennsylvania.)

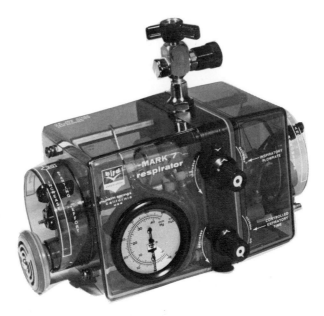

Fig. 3-25. IPPB respirator. (Courtesy Bird Corp., Palm Springs, California, 3M 1980.)

respiratory therapy unit) will determine the number of individual therapy stations required. Only one spirometer is necessary even in a multistation facility, and it requires 2 to 3 feet of counter or tabletop space along with its related apparatus, or it can be on a mobile stand. The individual IPPB (Inter Positive Pressure Breathing) unit, a small metering device pressurized by a mechanical compressor or an oxygen tank (Fig. 3-25), can be a mobile unit or can be set up at individual patient stations—a countertop area with the respirator mounted about 5 inches above the counter, concealed tubing, a waste receptacle, a tissue box dispenser, and a washable plastic laminate or vinyl wall surface.

A large facility may process 2000 inhalation therapy patients in a month with eight or ten individual stations. Or the facility may consist of just one room in an internist's office (Fig. 3-26). Regardless of size, a separate sterilization area must be provided. Cold sterilization is used for mouthpieces, valves, fittings, and other apparatus. The items are first washed in soap and water, then put in a disinfectant solution, rinsed, and air dried on a towel or a drying rack alongside the sink. A standard double-compartment sink is adequate. A small gas sterilizer unit may also be used. Today, labs use disposable supplies whenever possible, negating the need for sterilization. This volume of disposable "setups" (mouthpieces, hoses, etc.) demands a large well-designed storage/prep room with shelves and cabinets sized to accommodate the cartons in which the disposables are packed.

As with any clinical laboratory contained within an internist's suite, if it is large enough to process a high volume of patients daily, it should have its own waiting area, bathroom, supervisor's office, and storage room.

the designer the parameters of their *individual* program before the designer can determine space requirements.

Pulmonary dysfunction may be acute or chronic. A patient recovering from pneumonia, for example, may need treatment once or twice for an acute problem, or a patient with lung cancer may need therapy twice a week for the remainder of his or her life. The composition of a pulmonary specialist's practice (age of patients, volume of patients, proximity to a hospital's outpatient

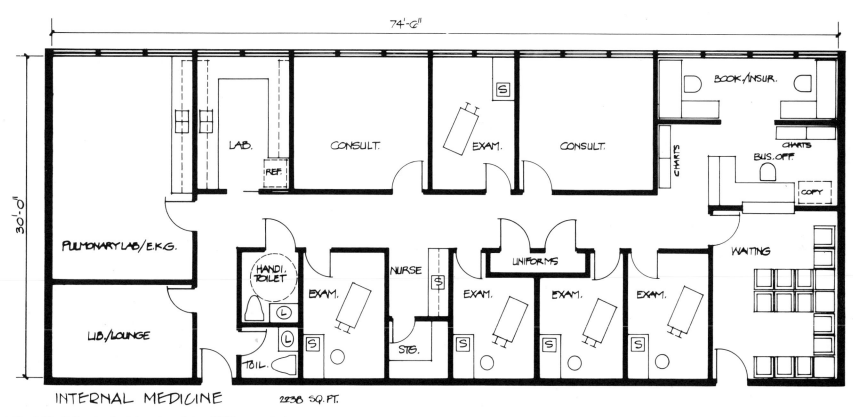

Fig. 3-26. Suite plan for internal medicine, 2238 square feet.

Proctology Room

Most internal medicine suites will have a proctology room for rectal and intestinal examinations which is approximately 10 × 12 feet, adjacent to a toilet room, and with a small area (4 × 4 feet) for preparation nearby. The examination table used for a proctoscopy procedure is larger than a standard exam table and is motorized to adjust to Trendelenberg position (Fig. 3–28).

In summary, a large internal medicine suite (5000 to 7000 square feet) will have a proctoscopy area, an EKG room and mounting area as well as a large lab with its own waiting room, blood draw, toilet with specimen pass-through, and storage. Certain types of X-rays may be done in the office and, if so, an X-ray room with adjoining darkroom and film viewing area will be included in the suite. The business office in a suite of this size will be composed of separate rooms for transcription, business manager, insurance clerk, medical records, bookkeeper, and receptionist. A staff lounge should also be included. The reader is referred to Chapter 6, *Group Practice* for aid in laying out suites of this size. .

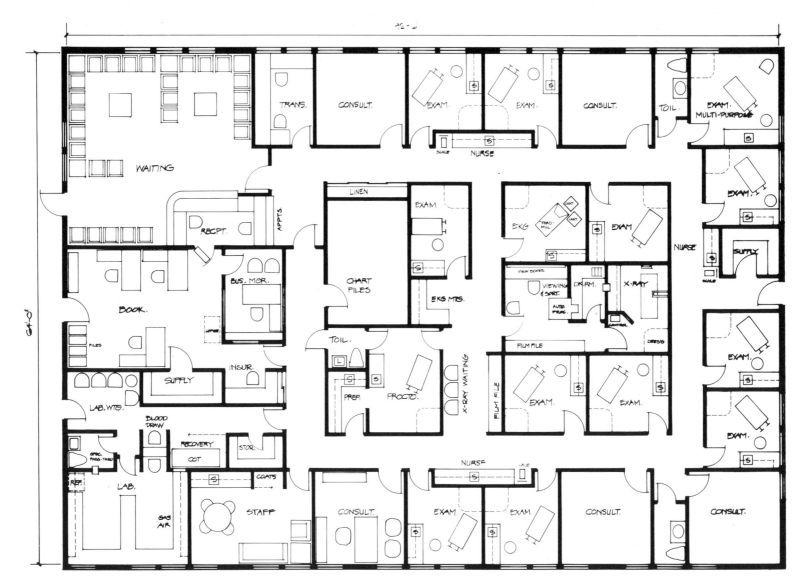

INTERNAL MEDICINE
5920 SQ. FT.

Fig. 3-27. Suite plan for internal medicine, 5920 square feet.

Table 3-2. Analysis of Program.
Internal Medicine

No. of Physicians:	2	3	4
Consultation	2 @ 12 × 12 = 288	3 @ 12 × 12 = 432	4 @ 12 × 12 = 576
Exam Rooms	5 @ 8 × 12 = 480	8 @ 8 × 12 = 768	10 @ 8 × 12 = 960
Waiting Room	14 × 18 = 252	18 × 20 = 360	23 × 24 = 552
Business Office	16 × 20 = 320	20 × 20 = 400	24 × 26 = 624
Office Manager	—	10 × 10 = 100	10 × 10 = 100
Nurse Stations	8 × 10 = 80	10 × 12 = 120	12 × 14 = 168
Toilets	2 @ 5 × 6 = 60	3 @ 5 × 6 = 90	4 @ 5 × 6 = 120
Storage	6 × 8 = 48	6 × 8 = 48	8 × 10 = 80
Proctoscopy Room[a]	12 × 15 = 180	12 × 15 = 180	12 × 15 = 180
Staff Lounge	10 × 12 = 120	10 × 12 = 120	12 × 12 = 144
Laboratory[b]	12 × 12 = 144	12 × 18 = 216	18 × 24 = 432
EKG	10 × 12 = 120	10 × 12 = 120	10 × 12 = 120
Pulmonary Function Lab	—	(optional)	14 × 16 = 224 (optional)
Radiology[c]	—	12 × 20 = 240	12 × 20 = 240
Subtotal	2092 ft^2	3194 ft^2	4520 ft^2
15% Circulation	314	479	678
Total	2406 ft^2	3673 ft^2	5198 ft^2

[a] Includes prep area and toilet.
[b] Includes lab, lab waiting, and blood draw.
[c] Includes darkroom, control, film filing, radiology room, and viewing area.

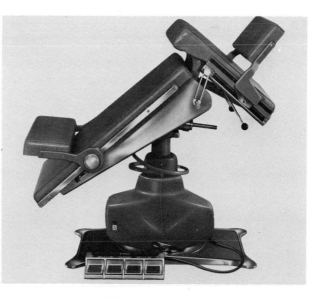

Fig. 3-28. Protoscopy table. (Ritter, Mfg. by Sybron Medical Products Div., Rochester, New York.)

PEDIATRICS

A pediatrician treats children from birth through adolescence. The office visits are frequent and are of relatively short duration in the exam room, but frequently involve a protracted period of time in the waiting room. This is a high-volume specialty and the practice is almost always composed of two or more physicians. It is rare to find more than three pediatricians working in the same office, although a busy practice may staff a second or third office. (See Fig. 3–29.)

Waiting Room

Waiting rooms must be larger than for other specialties as mothers often bring all their children and sometimes a grandmother when one child has to visit the doctor. A pediatric office should have a sick-baby or contagious waiting room and a well-baby waiting room. The basis for this is to limit contagion. Since physicians rarely make house calls, children with infectious diseases are brought into the office where they may spread their infection to well children who may be present for a routine checkup or injection. Thus any effort the designer can make to control the spread of disease is worthwhile.

If space is limited, a sick-baby waiting room can be devised by direct entry into an exam room (Fig. 3–30). One exam room would have a door to the outside or building corridor, as the case may be, and would have a buzzer or bell to summon the nurse for entry. The nurse would tell the mother over the phone to come to that door and buzz. The door would be marked *Contagious Entrance.* The sick-baby exam should be near a toilet, and the room must have a sink.

If the suite is large enough to have a contagious waiting room, one exam room in close proximity to the waiting room should be designed as a sick-baby exam room with a sink cabinet and a toilet nearby. The other exam rooms should be clustered around the nurse station (Fig. 3–31).

In this specialty it is a good idea to have a toilet accessible from the waiting room so that mothers may change diapers in advance of entering the exam room and the staff is not continually interrupted in order to direct children to the bathroom (Fig. 3–32). The bathroom should have a sink countertop large enough to change diapers on, a shelf for disposable diapers, talcum and paper towels, and a large trash receptacle. Doctors disagree on the practicality of having a child's-height drinking fountain in the waiting room. If the room is not well supervised, it can lead to problems.

The waiting room should contain some tables or flat areas built into the seating where mothers can put down an infant in a carrier without occupying an adult's seat (Fig. 3–33). A pediatric waiting room should be as large as space and budget permit. Each patient is accompanied by one to three people. Children can get pretty rowdy playing together in a pediatrician's waiting room, so an effort should be made to occupy them with something unique. A special seating unit or climbing play structure (Fig. 3–34, Plate 2) could be devised. Built of plywood and padded and upholstered with carpet, these custom-built units appeal to children's need for physical movement. Their pent-up energy can be released while climbing through tunnels and hiding in "secret" compartments. In fact, a waiting room that is designed imaginatively can be so appealing to children that it results in tantrums when it is time to leave! Custom play furniture must be designed to eliminate sharp corners and edges against which a toddler may fall and become injured.

The waiting room should also contain bins for toys and magazine racks at a height accessible to children. Pediatricians disagree in their choice of toys for this room. More conservative physicians tend to feel that toys spread infection (drooling on toys, fingers in mouth, etc.) and will limit the type of amusements they condone. Younger pediatricians seem to be more relaxed and humanistic (many refuse to wear white coats which may frighten children) and feel that germs are everywhere and inevitable. If a child is not exposed to germs in the office, he or she will surely be exposed to infection from playmates.

In a pediatric waiting room, one can break the rule about providing individual chairs. One can take liberties in furnishings here since it is a homogeneous population—mostly mothers from

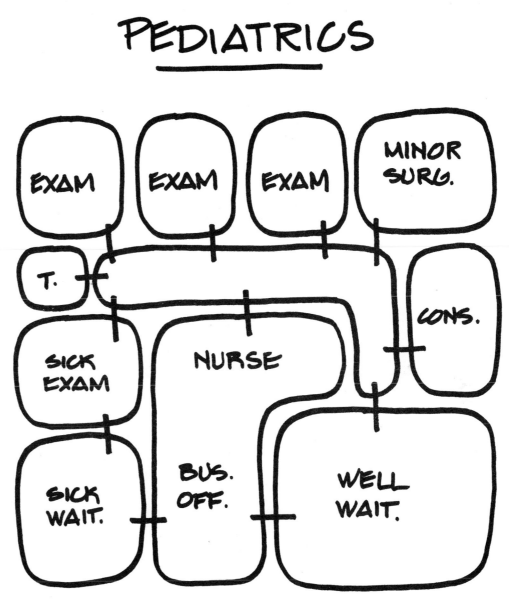

Fig. 3-29. Schematic diagram of a pediatrics suite.

57

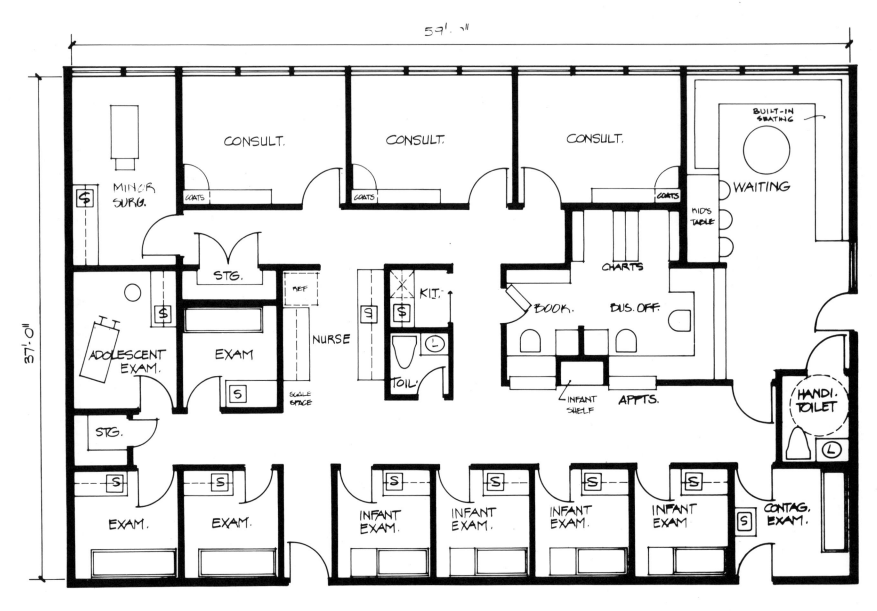

PEDIATRICS

2183 SQ. FT.

Fig. 3-30. Suite plan for pediatrics, 2183 square feet.

58

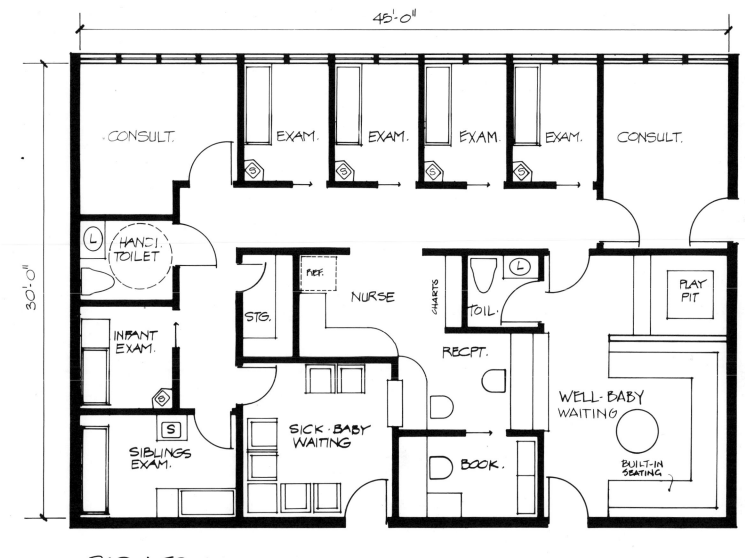

PEDIATRICS

1350 SQ. FT.

Fig. 3-31. Suite plan for pediatrics, 1350 square feet.

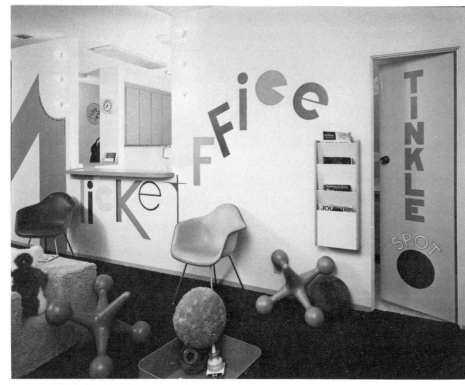

Fig. 3-32. Pediatric reception area.

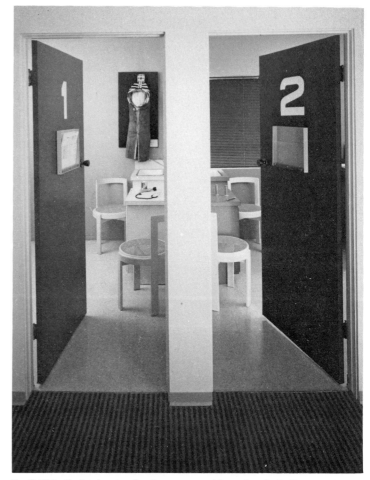

Fig. 3-32A. Pediatric examination rooms with authentic Indian papoose carriers on wall.

the same neighborhood, approximately the same age, and sharing a common interest—their children. Thus the mothers do not seem to mind sitting next to each other in continuous (common seat and back) seating. Figure 3-37 (Plate 3) shows the author's solution for adult seating which saves space and accommodates a maximum number of people in a small waiting room. Whatever the type of seating provided, one may wish to provide a few standard-height chairs with arms for pregnant women, who often find it difficult to get out of low lounge-type seating.

Other design ideas for the waiting area include a large tackboard for display of the patients' artwork, or for display of photos of the patients. Colorful wall murals of fanciful characters would be appropriate (Figs. 3-38, 3-39, and 3-40, Plate 3). A magnetized tic-tac-toe board or a chalkboard may be considered. But even with dustless chalk, the erasers make quite a mess. There is no end to the fanciful design ideas that can be implemented in a pediatric office. (See Figs. 3-41 through 3-43a.) The reader is referred to Chapter 10 for additional information on furnishings and interior finish specifications.

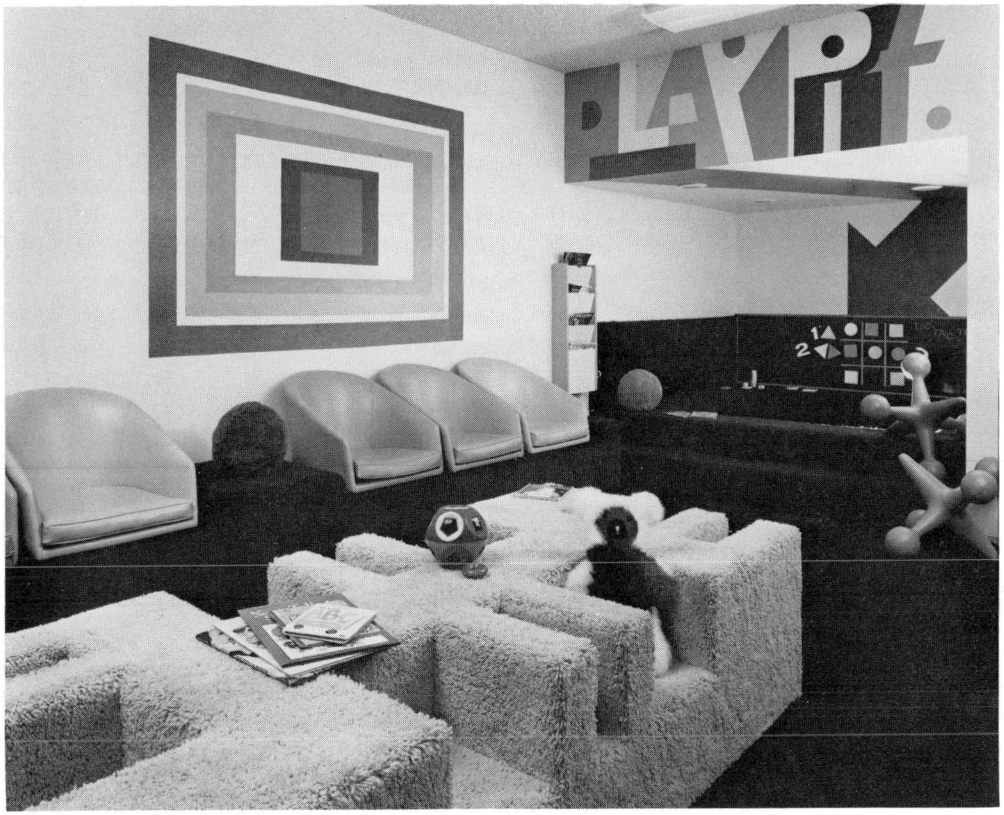

Examination Rooms

Each pediatrician should have a minimum of three exam rooms, but four is better. It is important to plan for growth. A pediatric practice grows rapidly, and before long a two-physician practice with five or six exam rooms will be able to use eight. Thus the designer should guide the client at the outset to lease a large enough space. Since examinations are short the physician can quickly move on to the next patient while the mother is

Fig. 3-33. Pediatric waiting room: Note magnetized tic-tac-toe board at rear of playpit.

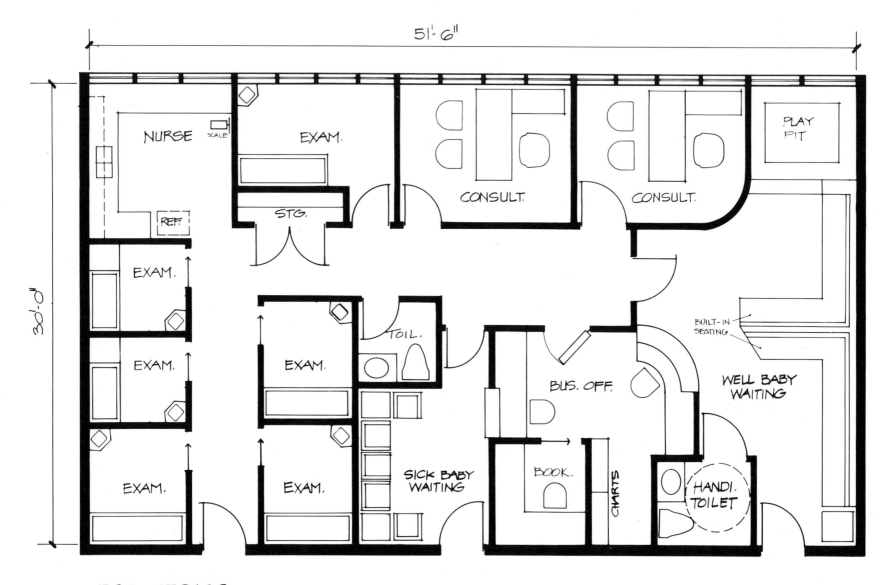

51'-6"

30'-0"

NURSE

SCALE

EXAM.

CONSULT.

CONSULT.

PLAY PIT

REF.

STG.

EXAM.

EXAM.

EXAM.

TOIL.

BUILT-IN SEATING

WELL BABY WAITING

EXAM.

BUS. OFF.

SICK BABY WAITING

BOOK.

CHARTS

HANDI. TOILET

EXAM.

EXAM.

PEDIATRICS

1545 SQ. FT.

Fig. 3-35. Suite plan for pediatrics, 1545 square feet.

dressing the child and the nurse cleaning up the last exam room. It is a good idea to make one exam room large enough to accommodate an infant exam table and a child's table, since it is more efficient to examine two siblings in the same room (Fig. 3–31). Most pediatric practices (particularly true with older physicians who have been in practice a number of years) must accommodate a number of adolescent patients. A standard-size adult exam room (8 × 12 feet) should be provided with a standard-size pelvic exam table and decor suitable to a teenager. Care must be taken in the interior design of the office not to gear it too much to infants and toddlers as it will offend the older children who are quite sensitive about being considered *children.* Rooms designed to accommodate older children should have a floor scale. Since the children may be shy or modest about being weighed at the nurse station, it is best to have a scale in the exam room.

It is not necessary to have a sink in every exam room if a sink is available nearby in the corridor outside the exam rooms. However, it is more efficient to have a sink in each exam room since children often vomit or urinate during an examination and having a sink in the room saves time by eliminating the need to leave the room in order to clean it up or wash hands.

Pediatric exam rooms may be very small, particularly an infant room. They need not have a door that opens to shield the patient. In fact, frequently the exam rooms are so small that a pocket door is the most practical solution. The room may be no more than 6 × 7 feet (Fig. 3–35). If space permits, a small writing desk for the doctor and a guest chair for the parent should be included. A 6 × 8 or 8 × 9-foot room is not as cramped, but it is preferable to make the exam

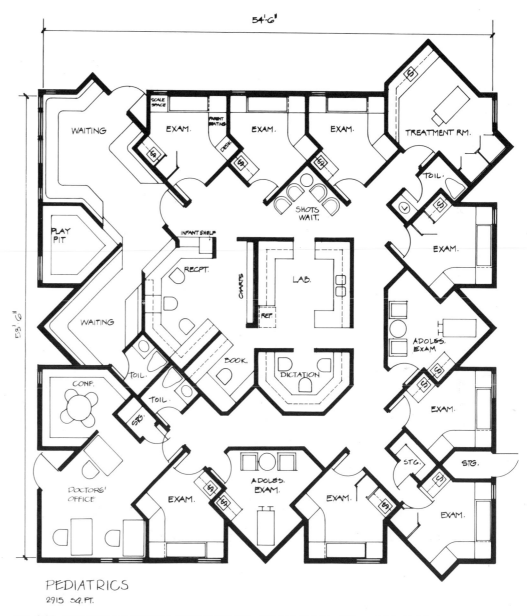

PEDIATRICS
2915 SQ. FT.

Fig. 3-36. Suite plan for pediatrics, 2915 square feet. (Gary Andresen, AIA, and Jain Malkin.)

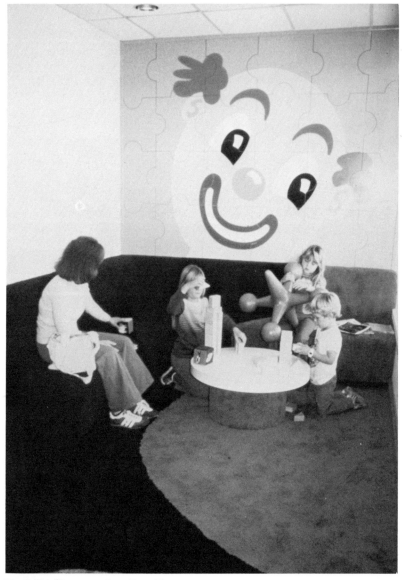

Fig. 3-38. Clown puzzle wallgraphic.

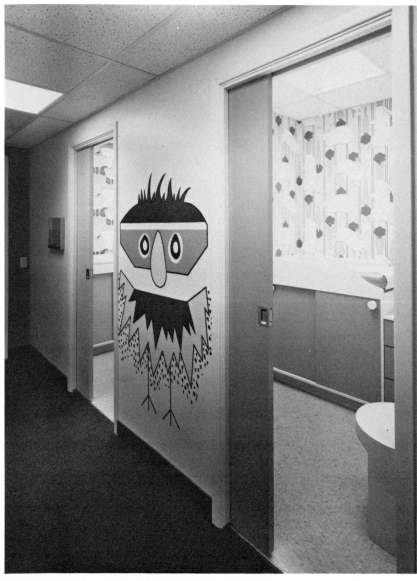

Fig. 3-39. Pediatric corridor and exam rooms.

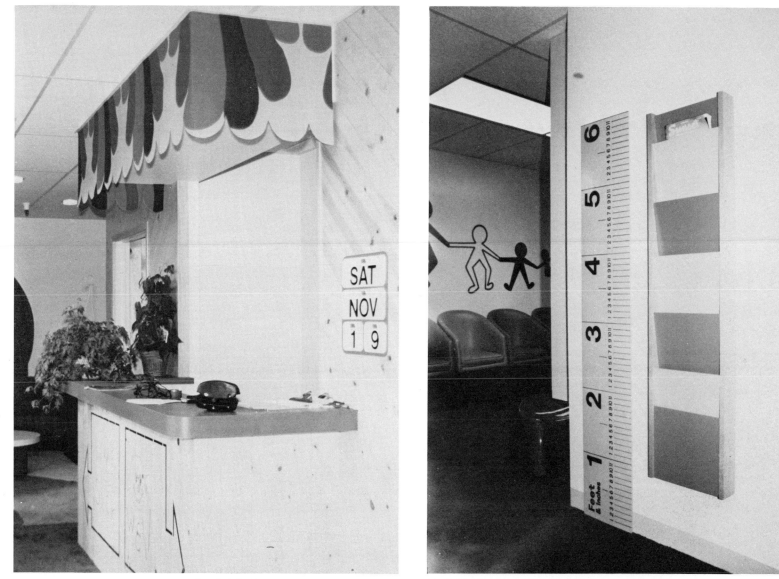

Fig. 3-41. Fabric canopy makes a reception desk festive.

Fig. 3-42. Custom yardstick lets children measure each other.

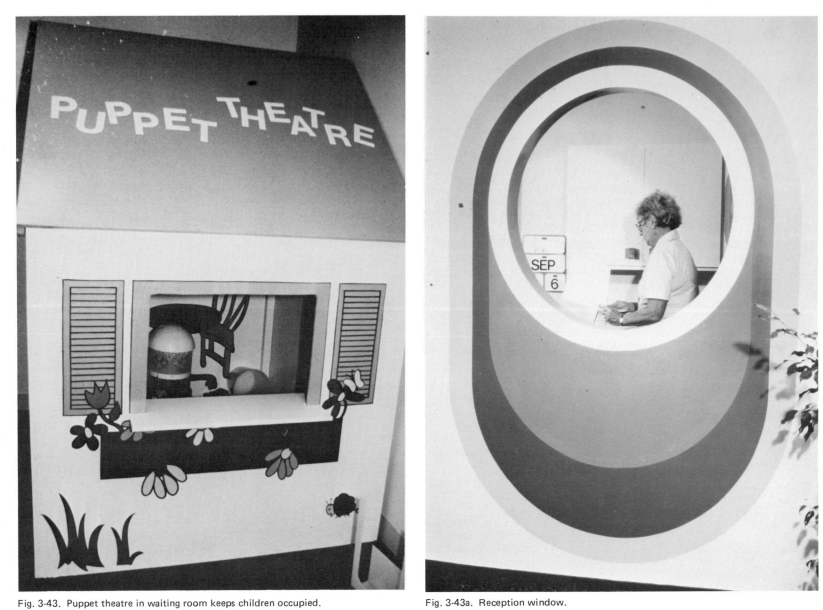

Fig. 3-43. Puppet theatre in waiting room keeps children occupied.

Fig. 3-43a. Reception window.

rooms minimum size in order to squeeze in an extra exam room. Pedo exam tables are available as manufactured items (Fig. 3–44) but often are custom built with storage underneath (Fig. 3–45). The size is 2 × 4 feet for an infant table (this increases to 6 feet if a lowered potion for a baby scale is included) or 2 × 6 feet for a child's table. The table is always placed against a wall to minimize the hazard of a child falling off. It should be positioned so that the doctor can examine from the right side of the patient, unless the doctor is left-handed and examines with the left hand. If a lowered area for a baby scale is not incorporated into the table, a portion of the sink cabinet countertop should be lowered for this purpose. It is better, however, to reserve this lowered portion of the sink cabinet for a doctor's writing desk.

Some method by which one may measure an infant's length should be incorporated into the exam table. Some pediatricians are very relaxed about this sort of measurement and others require a fairly elaborate device. The length of the table on one side can be routed with a slot for a tape measure and a sliding wooden arm may be pushed up to the baby's feet to hold the child steady and at the same time indicate on the tape the child's length. The table must also have a paper roll holder inside the cabinet with a slot in the tabletop so that a continuous roll of paper can be pulled over the vinyl-covered exam table pad and quickly changed between patients. It should be noted that the minimum-size exam room will not accommodate a sink cabinet. The sink must be wall hung—usually a corner sink works best in small rooms.

The exam rooms should be gaily decorated with one or two walls of colorful patterned wall-covering and some artwork of interest to children.

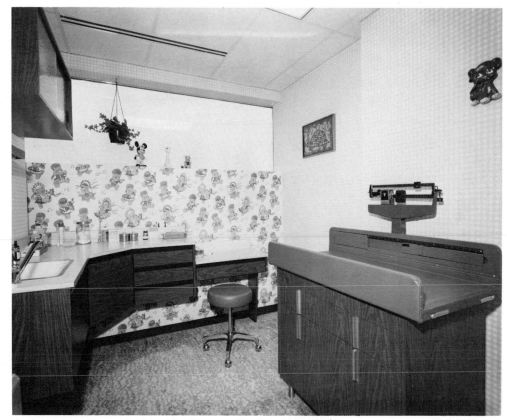

Fig. 3-44. Pediatric examination table. (Courtesy Hamilton Industries.)

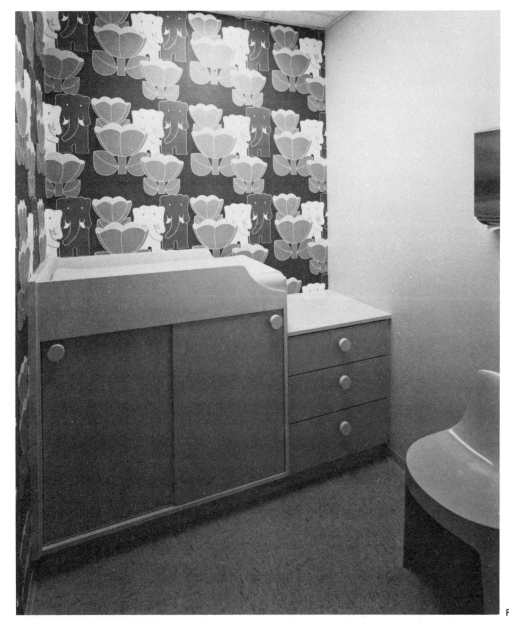

The wallcovering is of interest even to infants and serves to distract them, thus making the doctor's examination that much easier. One of the papered walls should be the long wall behind the exam table so that the children can see it while lying down.

Nurse Station

Pediatric suites require large nurse stations because the nurses administer many injections. After an injection, a patient must be observed for 10 to 15 minutes in order to note any negative reaction to the drug. A few chairs or a bench must be provided either in the corridor adjacent to the nurse station or perhaps within the nurse station. The nurse can attend to other business but still keep a watchful eye on the patient. A full-size refrigerator must be accommodated in the nurse station to store the medications. Pediatricians who administer allergy shots should have a nurse station located near the front of the suite so that patients coming just for injections can enter and leave without adding to the congestion in the examination area of the suite. The nurse station should have a knee-space area with telephone, an area for a microscope, and a double sink.

Business Office

The business office is as described in *General Practice,* although sometimes the nurse station can be combined with the business office (Fig. 3-31). This is efficient in a small office as the

Fig. 3-45. Infant exam room.

staff can substitute for each other at critical periods of the day. The pediatric business office should have a reception window facing both the sick and the well waiting rooms (Fig. 3–31). The appointment/cashier counter should have a wide shelf or a secure niche in the wall where a parent may put an infant in a carrier while he or she is writing a check or chatting with the staff (Fig. 3–36).

Consultation Room

Pediatricians spend little time in a consultation room and seldom see patients there; therefore it is not uncommon for two physicians to share a private office (Fig. 3–36). Basically, it is used for storing medical reference books and for returning phone calls. Pediatricians dispense a lot of literature and pamphlets on child care, so a wall rack should be provided for the organized storage of these materials either in the consultation room, the nurse station, or the corridor adjacent to the exam rooms.

Corridor

One corridor should be selected for a 20-foot refraction lane. An eye chart would be tacked to a door or placed on the wall at the end of the corridor for a brief eye test. A circle inset into the carpet can mark where the child's heels should be placed to assure a distance of 20 feet. The corridors should be cheerful and may have cartoon characters or colorful supergraphics.

Table 3-3. Analysis of Program. Pediatrics

No. of Physicians:	2		3	
Business Office	12 × 16 =	192	14 × 18 =	252
Examining Rooms[a]	6 @ 6 × 8 =	288	9 @ 6 × 8 =	432
Adolescent Exam	8 × 12 =	96	8 × 12 =	96
Toilets	2 @ 5 × 6 =	60	2 @ 5 × 6 =	60
Consultation Room	2 @ 10 × 12 =	240	3 @ 10 × 12 =	360
Nurse Station	8 × 12 =	96	12 × 12 =	144
Waiting Room/Sick-Baby	12 × 12 =	144	12 × 14 =	168
Well-Baby	18 × 20 =	360	22 × 26 =	572
Storage	6 × 6 =	36	6 × 6 =	36
Subtotal		1512 ft^2		2120 ft^2
15% Circulation		227		318
Total		1739 ft^2		2438 ft^2

[a] Note: Designer may wish to make one exam room 10 × 12 feet for use as a minor surgery room as well as provide a staff lounge if space permits.

Hearing Test Room

Some pediatricians like to do a preliminary hearing test to screen out patients who need to be referred to an ENT specialist. Sometimes this can be set up in a dual-purpose room. The hearing test can be performed in a consultation room or in a small 6 × 6-foot room dedicated to that purpose. One needs a table 24 × 48 inches on which to place the equipment, a chair for the patient and one for the technician. The walls of the room must have sound insulation and the inside of the walls may be covered with carpet to enhance the sound-absorbing qualities. The room should be located at the rear of the suite, away from the hectic front office.

Storage

The office should have a small storage room 6 ×6 feet for drug samples, disposable supplies, office forms and stationery, and handout pamphlets.

Interior Design

The suite should be colorful and imaginatively designed to reduce the children's anxiety and make them forget any negative associations they may have had about visiting the doctor. All rooms except exam rooms should be carpeted. Some physicians even carpet the exam rooms. Although carpeting does make the job of cleaning up vomit and urine that much harder, it has the advantage of making the room nicer for crawling infants. The reader is referred to Chapter 10 for additional information on furnishings and interior design.

Chapter 4
Medicine—Specialized Suites

The American Board of Medical Specialties recognizes, as of this writing, 23 medical specialties and about a dozen and a half subspecialties. The specialties are: Allergy and Immunology, Anesthesiology, Colon and Rectal Surgery, Dermatology, Family Practice, Internal Medicine, Neurological Surgery, Nuclear Medicine, Obstetrics and Gynecology, Ophthalmology, Orthopaedic Surgery, Otolaryngology, Pathology, Pediatrics, Physical Medicine and Rehabilitation, Plastic Surgery, Preventive Medicine, Psychiatry and Neurology, Radiology, Surgery, Thoracic Surgery, Urology, and the newest specialty, Emergency Medicine.

Subspecialties under Internal Medicine are: Cardiovascular Disease, Endocrinology and Metabolism, Gastroenterology, Hematology, Infectious Disease, Medical Oncology, Nephrology, Pulmonary Disease, and Rheumatology. Subspecialties under Pediatrics are: Pediatric Cardiology, Pediatric Endocrinology, Pediatric Hematology-Oncology, Neonatal-Perinatal Medicine, and Nephrology. There are a few other subspecialties under Psychiatry and Neurology such as Child Psychiatry and Child Neurology.

Although Family Practice, Pediatrics, and Internal Medicine are primary medical practices, they are also listed as specialties by the American Board of Medical Specialties since physicians in these specialties must take and pass specialty boards that certify their competence in their respective fields. These three "specialties," then, are primary practice entry-level physicians, whereas the other specialties listed above tend to be referral specialties—patients are referred by their primary physicians in many cases.

This chapter will discuss the requirements of the medical specialties the designer or architect is most likely to encounter in a medical office building.

OBSTETRICS AND GYNECOLOGY

This is a high-volume practice, so the patient flow must be carefully analyzed. The obstetrical patients usually make monthly visits which entail weighing and a brief examination. The gynecology patients require a more lengthy pelvic examination. This type of practice requires a large staff as each physician needs one or two nurses and often two physicians share three nurses or aides

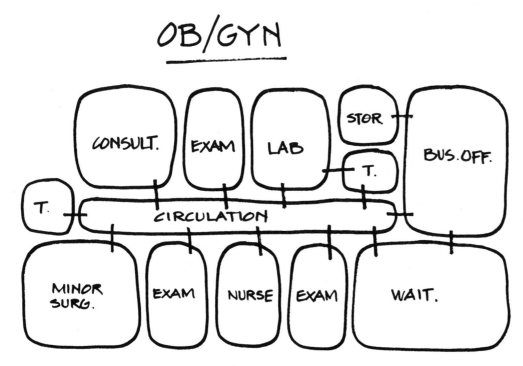

OB/GYN

Fig. 4-1. Schematic diagram of an OB-GYN suite.

in addition to the front office staff. It is customary for a nurse to be present during pelvic examinations, necessitating more staff per doctor than required with many other medical specialties.

A recent trend in this field is the use of a *nurse practitioner* to perform routine patient examinations. An RN with additional training in OB-GYN can be certified to work in this capacity. This frees the physicians from routine pelvic examinations and Pap smears on healthy patients, allowing them to concentrate on diagnosis of disease. Offices using nurse practitioners will need larger nurse stations and even a small private office for them.

There probably would not be more than three doctors working in an office at one time even if it were a four-or-five-person practice, since one or two doctors may be delivering babies at any one time, or making hospital rounds, or have the day off. There should be three to four exam rooms per physician. The patient flow is from waiting room to weighing area, to toilet (urine specimen), to exam room. A good space plan will channel patients to each area by the most direct route with no backtracking or unnecessary steps. If possible, the nurse station/sterilization/lab areas should be located toward the front of the suite (centralized) so that the staff can cover for each other and duplication of personnel is avoided.

The waiting room, as well as the rest of the suite, ought to be designed to appeal to women. This may take the form of sunny colors—greens, pinks, yellows—and a garden design with lattice trim, white rattan chairs, flowery wallpaper, and chintz upholstery fabrics. Or, it may be elegant and sophisticated (Fig. 4–2, Plate 3) perhaps a gray understated background punctuated by polished chrome and Plexiglas furniture, dramatic lighting, and an accent of violet or mauve in the upholstery. If a physician's leanings are traditional, the style could be formal with dark wood moldings, Louis XIV chairs with pettipoint upholstery, grasscloth or fabric wallcoverings, and oriental rugs on a wood floor (Fig. 4–3, Plate 4). Or, the tradititional style might be less formal—country French. The options are many. Because the patients are all women, this specialty allows the designer a great amount of freedom; obstetricians and gynecologists usually like to present a well-decorated office to their patients. Whatever the design style, chairs should not be so soft or so low that it is difficult for pregnant women to disengage themselves.

The waiting room of an OB-GYN suite should be large and comfortable. Unexpected deliveries frequently make the doctor late and necessitate a long wait for patients. The patient is apt to be more forgiving if her wait is in a well-designed room with good lighting, current magazines, comfortable seating, and interesting artwork on the walls. A play area for children would be a practical addition to the waiting room, since many of the patients are young mothers who are apt to bring their children with them (Fig. 4–4, Plate 4).

Exam rooms should have one or two walls of attractive wallcovering, carpet, and a dressing area where patients may disrobe in privacy and hang underwear out of sight, and upon dressing, may check makeup and hair in a mirror before leaving the exam room (Fig. 4–5). This dressing area may be a 3 × 3-foot corner of a room with a ceiling-mounted cubicle drape and a chair or built-in bench. Or it can be a hinged space-saver panel which opens perpendicular to the wall. The door to the exam room must open to shield the patient. The position of the sink cabinet is particularly im-

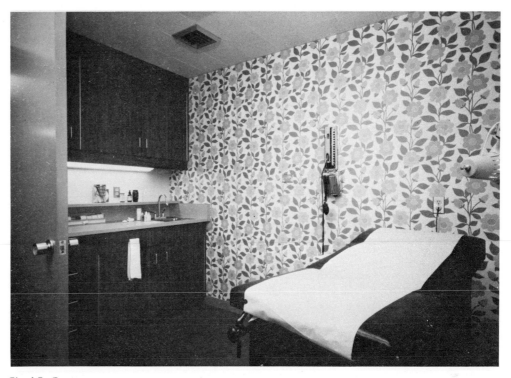

Fig. 4-5. Exam room.

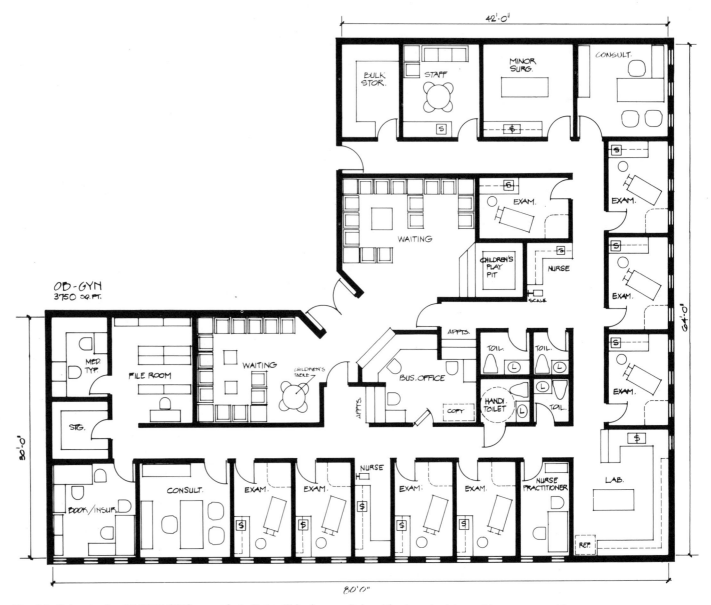

Fig. 4-6. Suite plan for OB-GYN, 3750 square feet. Note: This plan was designed for two physicians with a nurse practitioner and a part-time physician who does not have a consultation room. This suite has 20% circulation.

74

portant in an OB-GYN exam room. The physician should be able to examine the patient with the right hand and reach for instruments from the cabinet with the left hand (Fig. 4–6). The exam table used here is a pelvic table with stirrups (Fig. 4–7). More expensive tables will have a built-in speculum warmer. Or, one drawer of the sink cabinet may have an electrical outlet at the rear for warming instruments. Three electrical outlets are required: One must be located near the foot of the table for the gooseneck lamp used by many practitioners for pelvic exams, one should be located above the sink countertop, and the third should be located near the head of the table.

It is pleasant to have windows in an OB-GYN exam room. The wait is frequently very long and being able to look outside makes the wait a little more bearable. Narrow-slat metal window blinds serve exam rooms well since they permit light and view to enter the room but just a slight slant of the slats is enough to protect the occupant's privacy (Fig. 4–8).

Many physicians write a prescription in the exam room, but others ask the patient to dress and come to the consultation room. In any case, it is a good idea to provide a writing desk in the exam room so that the physician can make notations on the patient's chart and write a prescription.

Most OB-GYN suites will have a minor surgery room where a variety of procedures will be performed. Although some of these procedures used to be performed in a hospital, they can safely be handled in a well-equipped minor surgery within the physician's office. The size of the room may vary from 12 × 14 feet to 14 × 16 feet depending on the number of assistants who must be in the room and the amount of medical equipment.

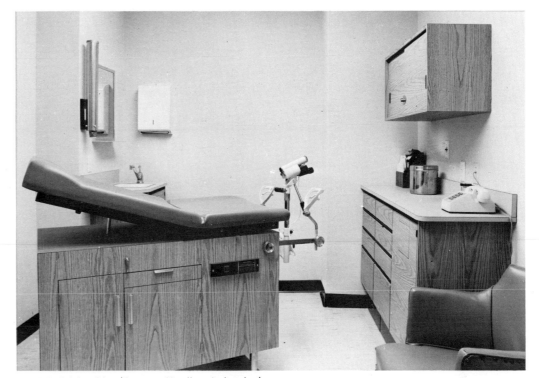

Fig. 4-7. Pelvic table. (Courtesy Hamilton Industries.)

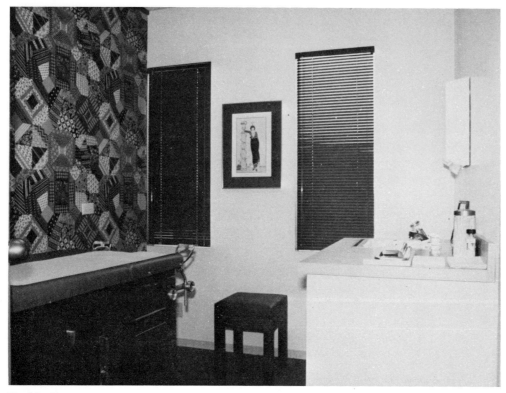

Fig. 4-8. Exam room.

Many printed pamphlets are distributed, and suitable storage racks should be provided in the waiting room or in the corridor near the nurse station. Sometimes OB-GYN physicians use visual aides for patient education. A rear projector might be located in a consultation room that is not generally used during the day. Or a niche in the corridor may be provided for audiovisual education. Videotape units (with drop-in cassettes) are more practical and easier to use than a rear projector.

A large amount of trash is generated in this practice. A disposable gown, sheet, and exam table paper must be discarded after each patient as well as paper hand towels and certain disposable instruments. Each exam room should have a large trash receptacle which may be built into the cabinet or separate.

Since each patient must empty her bladder before an examination, an OB-GYN suite needs a minimum of two toilet rooms. If it is possible to locate the toilet rooms near the nurse station or lab, a specimen pass-though (see Appendix) in the wall can eliminate the need for the patient to carry the urine specimen to the nurse station. Toilet rooms need a hook for hanging a handbag and coat, a shelf for sanitary napkins and tampons (if provided), and a receptacle for sanitary napkin disposal. It would be a nice touch to wallpaper the bathrooms. It is not necessary to provide separate toilet facilities for the staff. If they share facilities with the patients, it is certain the bathrooms will be better cared for.

The laboratory should be at least 10 × 12 feet and must include a sit-down space for a microscope and countertop space for a centrifuge and an autoclave. Space should be allotted for an under-counter refrigerator. If the physicians elect to do a good deal of the lab work in the suite, in-

Physicians in this specialty often like a well-appointed consultation room. The furnishings are usually more elegant and refined than one might find in a consultation room of a G.P., for example. The room may be designed along the lines of a residential library or den with a wood parquet floor and oriental rug, bookshelves, fabric wallcoverings, velvet or fabrics of similar texture on the seating, and a desk of unusual design. The window treatment, likewise, may be more of what one would find in a residence, rather than a medical office. Figure 4-9 (Plate 5) shows a room designed with a linen mural titled "Ladies of Elegance" on the wall, a thick white shag carpet, white Haitian cotton sofa, and cantilevered chrome and marble arc light.

In summary, the patients here—due to the nature of the specialty—are generally happy, and this upbeat mood should be enhanced by the interior design. All rooms except the laboratory, minor surgery, and toilets may be carpeted. Gynecologists rarely use gentian violet anymore, so the argument against carpeting exam rooms is no longer valid.

OTOLARYNGOLOGY

An otolaryngologist treats diseases of the ears, nose, and throat. The specialty is more commonly known as ENT (ear, nose, and throat) and its practitioners often practice facial plastic surgery as well.

A solo practitioner would need three examination rooms, a waiting room that seats 10 or 11 persons, an audio test room, a minor surgery room (of if facial plastic surgery is practiced, an outpatient surgery room and recovery room), an X-ray room and darkroom, a business office, a consultation room, and a nurse station/lab.

**Table 4-1. Analysis of Program.
Obstetrics and Gynecology**

No. of Physicians:	1			2 (Plus Nurse Practitioner)		
Exam Rooms	3 @	8 × 12 =	288	8 @	8 × 12 =	768
Consultation Rooms		12 × 12 =	144	2 @	12 × 12 =	288
Nurse Station		8 × 10 =	80[a]		10 × 12 =	120
Laboratory		—			12 × 16 =	192
Toilets	2 @	5 × 6 =	60	4 @	5 × 6 =	120
Minor Surgery		12 × 12 =	144		12 × 14 =	168
Staff Lounge		—			11 × 12 =	132
Storage		4 × 6 =	24		10 × 12 =	120
Nurse Practitioner		—			8 × 10 =	80
Business Office/Book.		12 × 16 =	192		12 × 30 =	360[b]
Medical Records		—			10 × 14 =	140
Waiting Room		12 × 20 =	240		14 × 30 =	420
Subtotal			1172 ft²			2908 ft²
15% Circulation			176			436
Total			1348 ft²			3344 ft²

[a] Combined with lab.
[b] Includes transcription, reception, bookkeeping, and insurance.

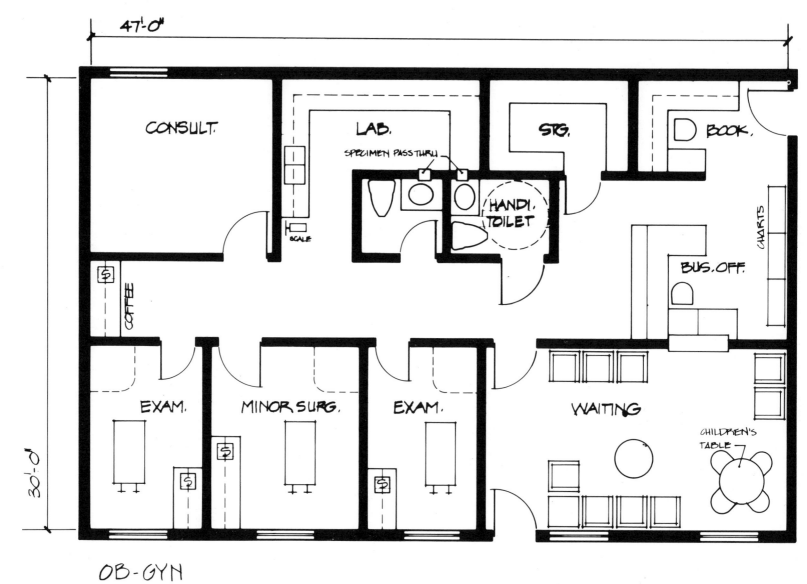

OB-GYN

1410 SQ. FT.

Fig. 4-10. Suite plan for OB—GYN, 1410 square feet.

The consultation room should be large (12 × 14 feet) since patients are often brought into this room to discuss fees for surgery or to discuss the feasibility of a particular surgical procedure. The X-ray room can be as small as 8 × 12 feet (depending on the physician's equipment) since the films are limited to the head and neck area. The reader is referred to Chapter 3 for space planning details of an X-ray room, control area, darkroom, and lead shielding. The darkroom can be small since the physician will probably have a tabletop model automatic film processor similar to the kind used by dentists. The designer must obtain the specs on the plumbing and electrical requirements from the manufacturer of the unit.

The examination rooms need be only 8 × 12 feet with the sink cabinet located on the wall with the door. A special motorized examination chair (Fig. 4–12) would be located in the center of the room on an angle with the patient facing the door and the physician working off of a cart along the wall to the right of the patient. Most of the time the physician would be seated on a stool with casters. Each exam room should have an X-ray view box recessed in the wall. The unit from which the physician works is usually a specialized manufactured stainless steel cabinet on casters (or it may be wall hung) containing a suction unit and pump, compressed air, a cautery, an electrical panel for instruments, racks for solution bottles, and a shelf and drawers for medications, cotton jars, irrigation syringes, and atomizers (Fig. 4–13). The unit also has a pull-out writing shelf. Approximately 23 inches wide × 18 inches deep × 46 inches high, it requires a grounded duplex outlet. If the unit is to be wall hung, wood blocking must be added to the wall between the studs to support 75 to 100 pounds.

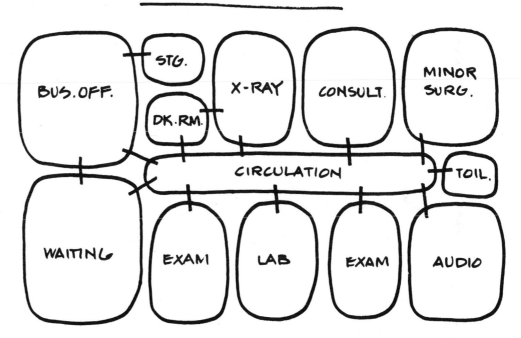

Fig. 4-11. Schematic diagram of an otolaryngology suite.

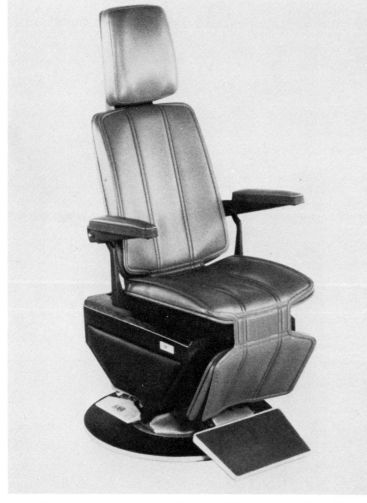

Fig. 4-12. Power examination chair. (Courtesy SMR, St. Louis, Missouri.)

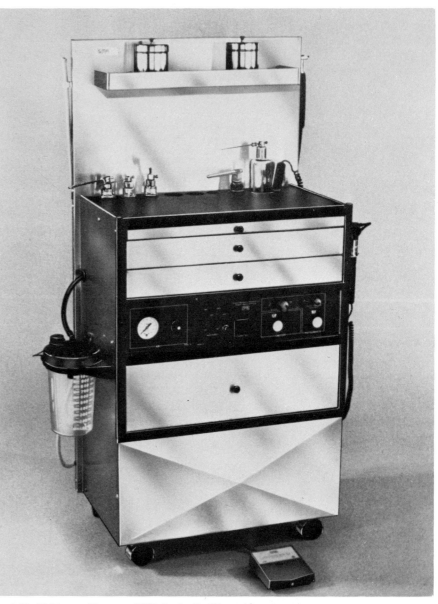

Fig. 4-13. ENT cart. (Courtesy SMR, St. Louis, Missouri.)

Sometimes the medical examination cabinet is purchased without the suction and air features, in which case the designer will need to provide a vacuum system within the suite. A small room, 4 feet 6 inches × 5 feet, should be provided close to the examination rooms to eliminate long-distance piping. Vacuum pumps and air compressors are noisy, so the walls of this room should be well insulated. Usually two 20-ampere separate circuits will be required. A local vacuum contractor will provide the designer with specs on the equipment and will usually run the plastic piping and install the system. The piping would be done after the HVAC (heating, ventilating, and air-conditioning) has been completed but before the partitions are closed up.

A nice feature in the exam rooms and recovery room would be a wall-mounted cosmetic mirror unit—perhaps a small plastic laminate cabinet with two hinged doors which, when opened, reveal a good-quality mirror and two rows of makeup lights which are electric eye operated so that opening the doors activates the lights. A dressing area is not required in ENT exam rooms.

If the physician does only ENT and no facial plastic surgery, a minor surgery room (refer to Chapter 3 under *General Practice*) would be used for special procedures and for emergency care. As the practice matures, an otolaryngologist tends toward more cosmetic and reconstructive facial plastic surgery because it is more lucrative and, perhaps, more interesting than routine ENT procedures. Procedures such as nose reconstructions, face lifts, eye tucks, repair of cleft palate and face peels may be performed in the office in a well-equipped outpatient surgery room with ancillary recovery room, scrub, and prep areas. The surgery room should contain one wall of built-in cabinets and the sink should have a plaster trap and foot lever control for hot, warm, and cold water. Scrub and prep can be done in the surgery room if the room is large enough and if the patient volume is low. An electrical outlet is required in the floor for the motorized table. Other electrical outlets and connections for suction, compressed air, and instruments should be located by the physician since this room allows for a variety of options with respect to work habits. The reader is referred to *Plastic Surgery* for a detailed discussion of an outpatient surgery room.

A basic part of an otolaryngologist's practice involves diagnosing and treating persons with a hearing loss. An audio booth is used for measuring a person's hearing. It is a soundproofed "room" approximately 5 feet wide × 6 feet 6 inches long with a door at one end. The patient sits inside and listens to test noises through earphones. The technician or audiologist sits outside the booth at a counter facing the patient and looks into the booth through a window so that the patient is always in sight (Fig. 4–14). The countertop she works at contains the audio equipment from which she controls the sounds transmitted to the patient in the booth. The patient's responses are recorded and a graph of hearing loss is produced for the physician's evaluation.

The audio booth is available as a prefabricated unit (Fig. 4–15) that breaks down into components and is assembled in the room by a skilled installation technician. The booth has an exhaust fan and various electrical requirements foremost of which is connecting it to the testing equipment (an exposed low-voltage cable is commonly used). It is mandatory that the audio testing room be located in a quiet part of the suite away from

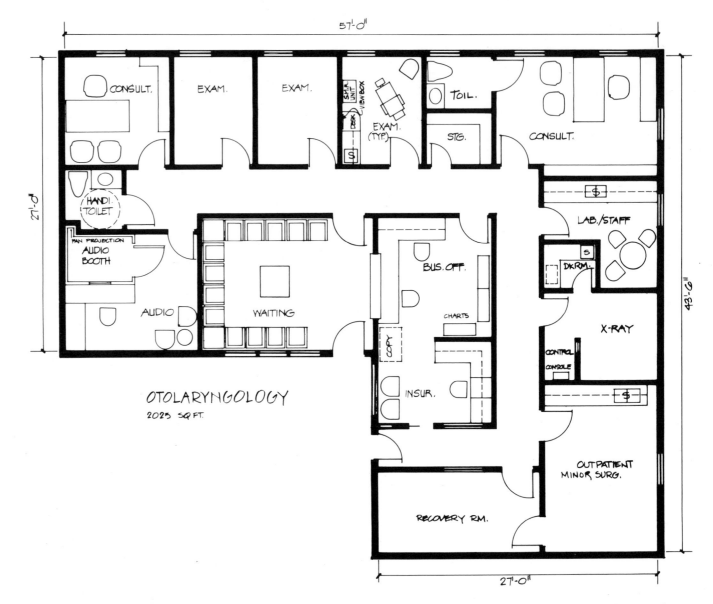

OTOLARYNGOLOGY

2025 SQ FT.

Fig. 4-14. Suite plan for otolaryngology, 2025 square feet.

82

Table 4-2. Analysis of Program.
Otolaryngology

No. of Physicians:	1			2		
Exam Rooms	3 @	8 × 12 =	288	5 @	8 × 12 =	480
Consultation Rooms		12 × 14 =	168	2 @	12 × 14 =	336
Business Office		12 × 18 =	216		12 × 18 =	216
Nurse Station/Lab		8 × 10 =	80		8 × 12 =	96
Waiting Room		14 × 16 =	224		14 × 20 =	280
Audio Room		11 × 12 =	132		11 × 12 =	132
Toilets	2 @	5 × 6 =	60	2 @	5 × 6 =	60
Minor Surgery		12 × 12 =	144		—	
Outpatient Surgery		—			12 × 16 =	192
Recovery		—			8 × 14 =	112
Storage		6 × 8 =	48		6 × 8 =	48
X-ray		9 × 12 =	108		9 × 12 =	108
Darkroom		4 × 6 =	24		4 × 6 =	24
Staff Lounge		8 × 10 =	80		10 × 12 =	120
Subtotal			1572 ft^2			2204 ft^2
15% Circulation			236			330
Total			1808 ft^2			2534 ft^2

Note: The one-physician suite outlined above would serve an otolaryngologist who does not practice facial plastic surgery; The two-physican suite is designed for practitioners who do.

the heavy traffic of the waiting room and business office.

A custom audio booth can be built on the job, but rigid construction specifications must be adhered to in order to achieve a sound transmission class of 55 to 60 decibels. Double-stud walls with several layers of sound board, insulation batting, and a solid-core door with an acoustic seal on all sides would be required (see Chapter 12).

There are no special requirements for interior design in this suite. If the practice tends toward facial plastic surgery, the office design should reinforce the image of the surgeon as a successful, skilled professional with a refined aesthetic taste. The reader is referred to *Plastic Surgery* for additional discussion on this topic.

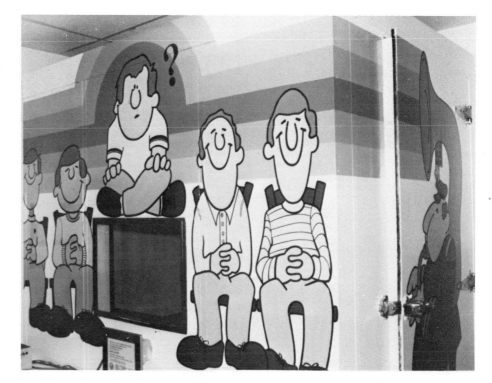

Fig. 4-15. Audio booth with cartoon design.

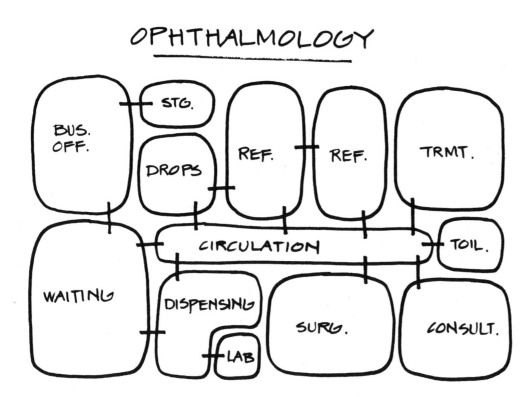

OPHTHALMOLOGY

Fig. 4-16. Schematic diagram of an ophthalmology suite.

OPHTHALMOLOGY

This specialty is characterized by a variety of options in suite design. The individual practitioner will have to make the basic decisions on his or her work habits before the designer can begin work. There seems to be an ever-increasing need for specialized eye care, which means that the ophthalmologist will attain a capacity patient load often within the first year of practice. Thus it is important to project at the outset what the ophthalmologist's space needs will be in two or three years. Too often young ophthalmologists setting up their first office will try to be too economical. They set up a minimally functional office based on their patient projection (usually underestimated) at that moment. Then, for the remainder of their lease (usually five years), they are handicapped by a small, poorly laid out office which greatly inhibits the growth of their practice.

The average ophthalmologist schedules three patients per hour for regular eye examinations. Added to that are the unscheduled patients—emergency and trauma—and the postoperative patients, and it is not unusual for an ophthalmologist to see four patients an hour. Individual practice habits may differ, with some doctors spending more time informally chatting with patients than those who choose to work in a more restricted, tightly scheduled manner. The more relaxed ophthalmologist may see only two patients per hour, particularly if he or she does all the testing himself or herself with little assistance from aides.

It is quite common for ophthalmologists to practice as solo practitioners with the help of an assistant or technician and frequently with an optometrist. An optician may also be part of the practice, in which case an area approximately 10 × 24 feet will be needed, divided into a lab (see Fig. 4-30, Plate 6), a contact lens area (see Fig. 4-31, Plate 7), and a fitting area. The lab would have walls lined with cabinets and work counters and shadow-free lighting. The contact lens area would have a small fitting table 2 × 4 feet that may have a mirrored top. The patient sits on one side and the optician on the other. The room may also have a storage cabinet and a small sink. The fitting area would have a long table divided into three fitting stations each with a mirror and panels of eyeglass frames (frame bars) located on either side of the patient (see Fig. 4-32, Plate 7). The optician sits on a stool behind the table and works off of drawers and cabinets to the side and behind him or her. Attractive wall frame bars can be purchased ready-made, or they may be designed and custom fabricated to hold the multitude of eyeglass frames and displays.

Ophthalmologists used to arrange their offices so that different tests were performed in different rooms. And some ophthalmologists may still practice that·way. It is far more efficient for the patient to remain in one room. Each time the patient has to gather up a sweater, eyeglasses and handbag, and move to another room, then again get comfortable, valuable time (and money) is lost. For the composition of the average ophthalmology practice, with the modern instrumentation now available, a complete examination and treatment can be done in the same room with the patient in the same chair.

The most important room is the refraction room, a multipurpose examination room with equipment and instruments grouped around the patient and the doctor sitting either in front of the patient or just to one side. Right-handed physi-cians will prefer to examine from the patient's right side. The dimensions of this room are crucial, and both the ophthalmologist's work habits and the instruments will dictate the critical distances that must be observed. Refraction rooms have two basic sizes, although their shapes may vary considerably. Since a standard eye chart is designed for a distance of 20 feet from chart to patient's eye, the traditional refraction room is approximately 24 feet long (20 feet for the refraction lane plus 4 feet for the examining chair and space to walk around it) as in Figs. 4-17 and 4-18. More recently, with the aid of projectors and mirrors, ophthalmologists have been able to cut the room length to 10 or 12 feet. A 10-foot-wide × 12-foot-long room would be suitable.

To compensate for a room length of less than 24 feet, two mirrors are placed on the wall in front of the patient and a screen is placed on the wall behind the patient (Fig. 4-19). A projector projects the text characters onto one of the front mirrors, which in turn projects it back to the screen behind the patient. The second mirror in front of the patient reflects the image from the rear screen. The refracting lane in this case is the distance measured between the second mirror and the screen plus the distance between the mirror and the patient. The letters of the eye chart can be adjusted in size by the projector so that correct visual acuities can always be maintained.

There are several types of procedures performed in the refracting room, but the primary task is to determine the refractive power of the eye. To do this the doctor selects various lenses from a partitioned rack (Fig. 4-20), a *trial lens box* (approximate size 12 1/2 × 20 1/2 × 20 1/2 inches), and places them in a holder through which the patient looks, and he or she is asked to read the test letters to determine which lens is best. Sometimes a *refractor,* an instrument containing lenses, is used. The interior of the eye, the *fundus,* is examined by an ophthalmoscope, a hand-held light source, while the conjunctiva, lens, iris, and cornea (the front portions of the eye) are examined by a *slit lamp,* an illuminated microscope (Fig. 4–21), which may be mounted on a shelf of the instrument stand (Fig. 4–22, Plate 5) or may be on a mobile instrument table (see also Figs. 4–34, 4–35, 4–36).

It should be mentioned that an automated refractor (Fig. 4–23) is now available. This microcomputer tabletop unit permits an assistant to check the patient's visual acuity, thereby reducing the number of practitioner-performed refractions and streamlining those that are necessary. The great advantage of this unit, in addition to the time it saves over the conventional method of refraction, is that it does not rely upon the patient's subjective comparison: *Is this clearer than that?* The patient merely looks into the viewing window of unit and adjusts a knob until the image is in focus. The machine automatically gives a digital readout of the patient's visual acuity. This unit can also compare the patient's current prescription with the new one. Used as a general screening device, this machine would be located in the *data collection room* along with other instruments used by the aides (see Fig. 4–33, Plate 7). After a patient has been refracted on the machine, he or she would move to an examination room where the ophthalmologist would review the findings and study the patient history. If the difference between the old and the new prescription is not great and the patient has no complaints, a conventional examination by the practitioner may not be necessary.

Examining chairs are available in tilt or nontilt models. In a room for a right-handed physician, the chair would be positioned with the instrument stand console to the patient's left. The chair should be positioned in the room so that the physician can walk behind it (allow 3 to 4 feet behind it) even when the chair is in reclined position. The chair and attached instrument stand console together are approximately 4 feet wide (Fig. 4–24). A clear space of 24 to 30 inches to the left side of the patient (in a right-handed room) and 5 to 6 feet to the right is desirable. As with any medical equipment, the designer must verify the dimensions and critical spatial relationships of the physician's specific equipment. This chapter states general dimensions, but each manufacturer's literature must be consulted for specifics.

The doctor may work off of the instrument stand as well as the sink cabinet located to the

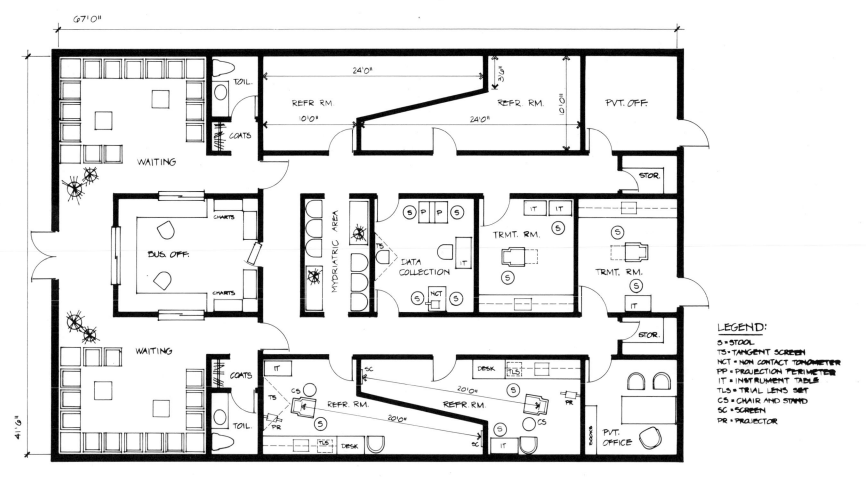

OPHTHALMOLOGY (NON-DISPENSING PHYSICIAN)
2780 SQ. FT.

Fig. 4-17. Suite plan for ophthalmology, 2780 square feet. (Nondispensing physician.)

LEGEND:

S = STOOL
TS = TANGENT SCREEN
NCT = NON CONTACT TONOMETER
PP = PROJECTION PERIMETER
IT = INSTRUMENT TABLE
TLS = TRIAL LENS SET
CS = CHAIR AND STAND
SC = SCREEN
PR = PROJECTOR

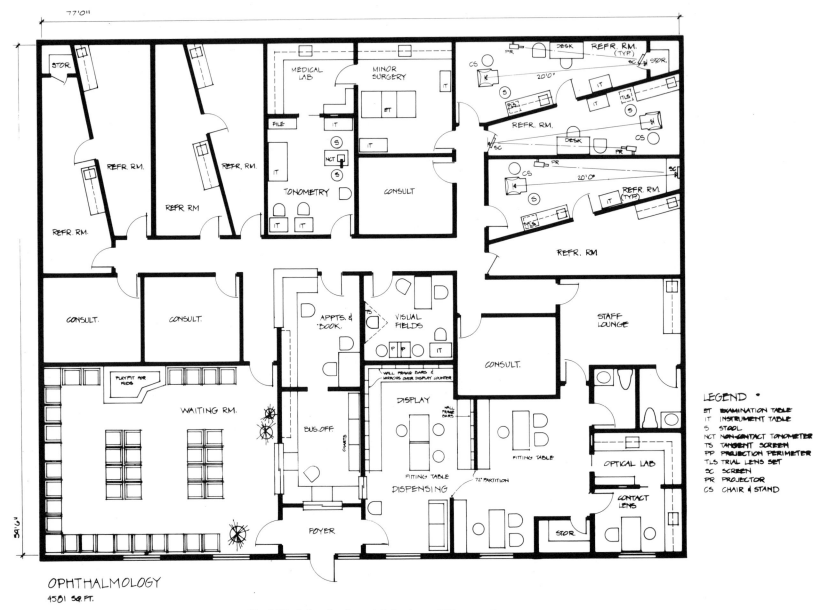

OPHTHALMOLOGY
4581 SQ. FT.

Fig. 4-18. Suite plan for ophthalmology, 4581 square feet.

88

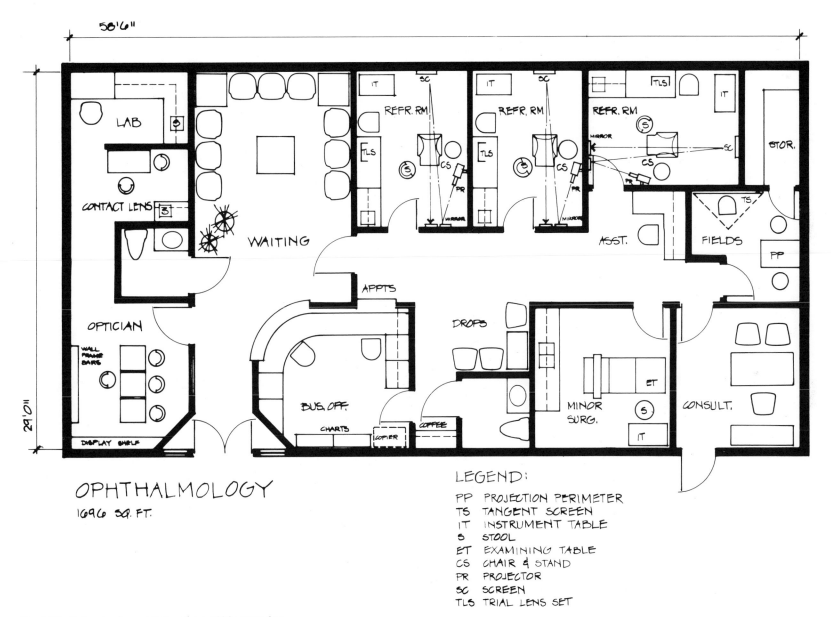

OPHTHALMOLOGY

1696 SQ. FT.

LEGEND:

PP PROJECTION PERIMETER
TS TANGENT SCREEN
IT INSTRUMENT TABLE
S   STOOL
ET EXAMINING TABLE
CS CHAIR & STAND
PR PROJECTOR
SC SCREEN
TLS TRIAL LENS SET

Fig. 4-19. Suite plan for ophthalmology, 1696 square feet.

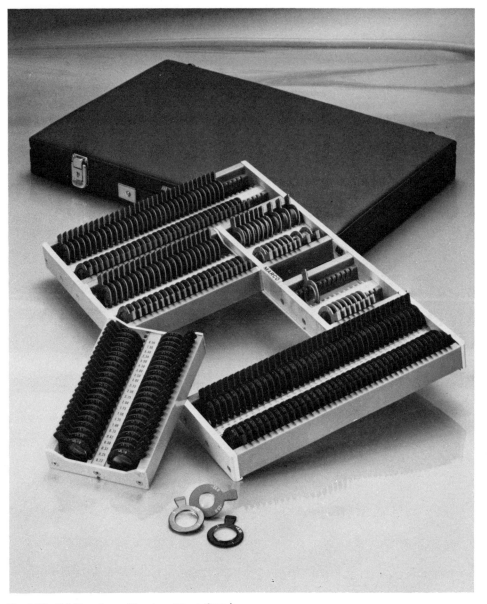

Fig. 4-20. Trial lens box. (Courtesy Marco Corp.)

right of the patient. The instrument stand console may be specially wired so that the physician may control the room lights, fixation light, projection chart, and other instruments from it. Or, the sink cabinet may be extended to include a knee space (see Fig. 4–19) with an electrical panel for remote control of the room's overhead lights, the projector, the fixation light, and a nurse call buzzer. (The switches and controls should be located on the face of the cabinet or in the knee-space opening so that they are within easy reach of the ophthalmologist during the examination.) Thus the ophthalmologist, from a seated position alongside the patient, may control illumination and instrumentation from either the instrument stand or the wall cabinet, or both. The room's lights should have a three-way switch so that they may be controlled from the door and the console, and they should have a dimmer control. Local codes must be checked with reference to controlling the room's lights from the instrument stand. Low-voltage wiring is usually required. Lighting that works well in an ophthalmology exam room is fluorescent lamps around the perimeter of the room, concealed by a wood valance (Fig. 4–25). It is less glaring than standard overhead fixtures.

Other electrical requirements for the room are: an outlet for a *fixation light* mounted on the wall at approximately a 72-inch height directly behind the patient; an outlet for the *projector,* usually at a 60-inch height on the wall to the left of the patient, or behind the patient (the designer must specify wood blocking in the wall to support the weight of the projector); a duplex outlet above the countertop for miscellaneous instruments and recharger modules for the cordless hand instruments; and a floor outlet (15-ampere circuit) for the instrument stand console. One duplex outlet should be located at a 12-inch height on the wall to the left of the examining chair, and all outlets should be grounded. The electrical requirements of ophthalmic equipment are highly specialized. A thorough review of the practitioner's practice habits and specific instrumentation is necessary before planning the electrical layout.

The trial lens case may be placed on a countertop (see Fig. 4-21), or it may fit in a drawer or be built into a mobile cart designed for that purpose (Fig. 4-26). If it is to fit in a drawer, the designer must determine if the rack should be tilted for easier visibility, in which case the drawer must be deeper.

All refracting rooms should be exactly alike in layout, arrangement of instruments, and quality of equipment. If one room has a better slit lamp than another, the rooms will not get equal usage. Patients will be shifted around in order to utilize favored equipment thus defeating the basic efficiency of the suite.

The distance the doctor must walk between refraction rooms should be minimal. To this end some ophthalmologists request connecting doors between two refraction rooms (see Fig. 4-18). Although it saves steps it creates an acoustics problem. And since many persons with poor eyesight happen to be elderly, they may also suffer from a hearing loss which means the doctor may have to shout to be understood. All the more reason to provide good sound insulation around these rooms.

Toward the end of an eye examination the patient may receive eye drops to dilate the pupil. Then the patient is asked to return to the waiting room or a secondary waiting area adjacent to the

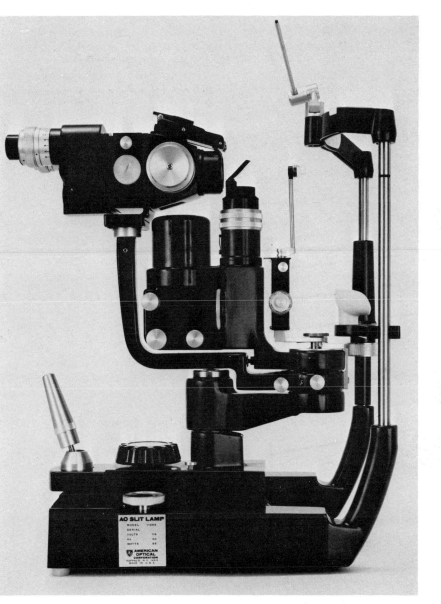

Fig. 4-21. Slit lamp. (Courtesy American Optical, Southbridge, Massachusetts.)

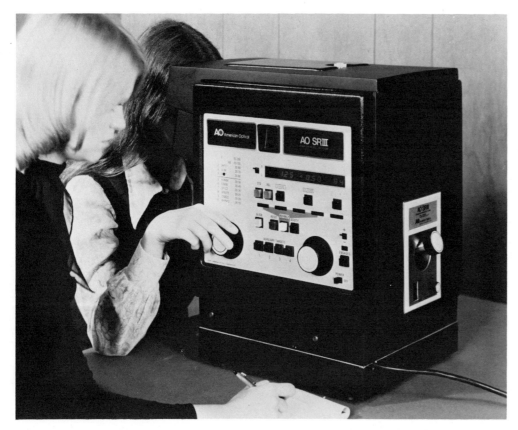

Fig. 4-23. Automated refractor. (Courtesy American Optical, Southbridge, Massachusetts.)

refraction rooms called a *drop* or *mydriatric room* to wait 15 to 20 minutes before being readmitted to the refraction room to conclude the examination.

A solo practitioner needs at least two refraction rooms plus a third multipurpose or minor surgery room/treatment room (see Fig. 4-29, Plate 6). While a patient whose examination has been concluded is gathering up possessions and receiving medications and instructions from the nurse or aide, the doctor has already stepped into the next refraction room and has begun to examine the patient with no loss of time. The minor surgery room can be used for removing a foreign body from the eye or for other emergency visits, or the doctor may see an unscheduled patient "between patients" without interrupting the scheduled patients in the refraction rooms. The minor surgery room can also be utilized as a photography room or for visual fields testing or orthoptic evaluations. Certain surgical procedures may be done in a large, well-equipped minor surgery room such as surgical implants of synthetic lenses (done with a local anesthetic) and the new radial keratotomy—the surgical correction of myopia. This room should have at least 8 lineal feet of built-in cabinets and countertops.

An ophthalmologist does not need a nurse station or lab as such, but it may be advisable to provide a work space in a niche off the corridor (Fig. 4-19) for an assistant or aide. This is where phone calls can be received or made to reschedule patients, or prescriptions can be authorized and medications dispensed. Ophthalmologists dispense a number of eye drops and medications. These samples may be stored in a rack in each examining room or else at the assistant's work area if she dispenses them.

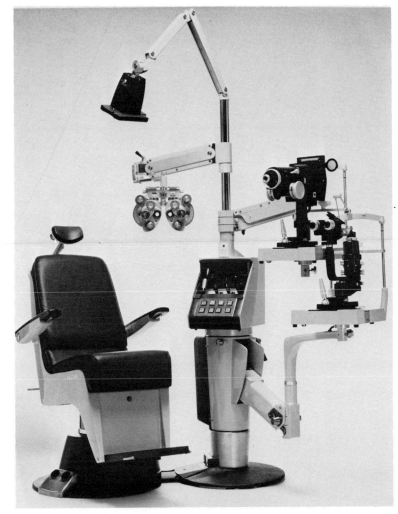

Fig. 4-24. Chair and instrument stand. (Courtesy American Optical, Southbridge, Massachusetts.)

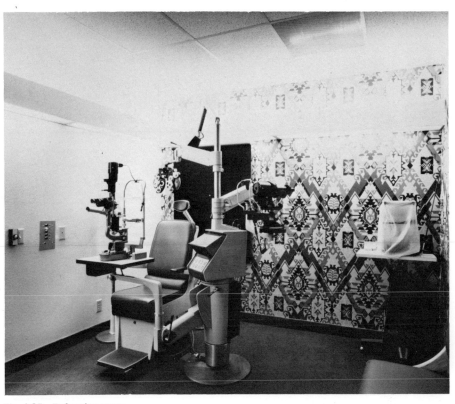

Fig. 4-25. Refracting room.

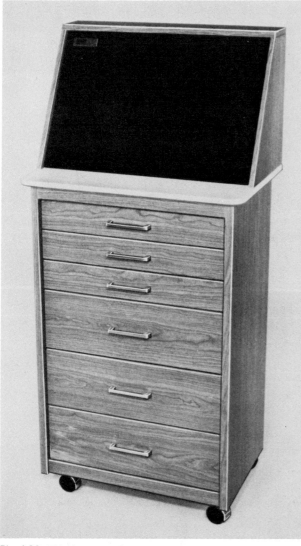

Fig. 4-26. Trial lens cart. (Courtesy SMR, St. Louis, Missouri.)

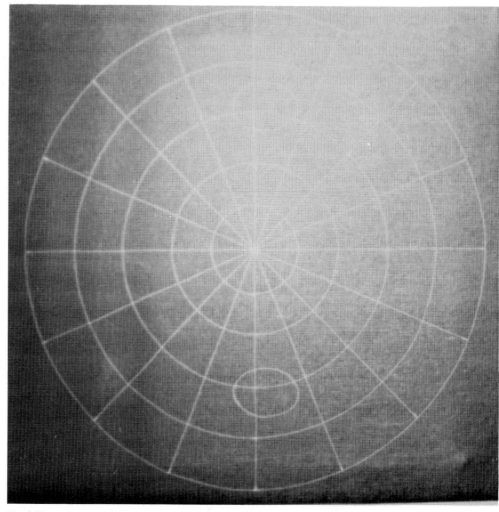

Fig. 4-27. Tangent screen. (Courtesy Richmond Products.)

Visual Fields

The charting of visual fields is commonly done with a *tangent screen,* which is a piece of black felt with meridians marked off (Fig. 4–27). Tangent screens may be rigid or roll-up, the former being preferred because they permit greater accuracy; and they are available in four sizes ranging from 1 to 2 meters, the smaller screen giving the smallest amount of information. A 1 1/2-meter screen is the average used and if placed in a dedicated room, the room need be only 8 × 8 feet. A 1-meter screen needs a room only 6 × 6 feet in size. The tangent screen may be in the data collection room, in a refracting room, or in a visual fields room, depending upon the practitioner's preference and the composition of the practice. A glaucoma specialist may have one in each refracting room. Others may have only one screen in the data collection room. The patient sits at a specified distance from the screen (which resembles a target) and pins are placed in the felt to chart the limits of the patient's visual field. If the screen is placed in the refraction room, it is convenient to locate it on the wall behind the patient. Thus the physician can spin the patient's chair around to face it. The chair must be 1 1/2 meters (60 inches) away from the screen (with a 1 1/2-meter screen).

However, the tangent screen is a *basic* screening device and not terribly accurate since one has no control over the movement of the patient's head. Perimetry is a more advanced method of doing peripheral and central fields. An *automated projection perimeter* is a computerized piece of equipment that sits on a 30 × 30 inch stand (Fig. 4–28). The patient sits on one side and the assistant on the other. The patient's visual field is

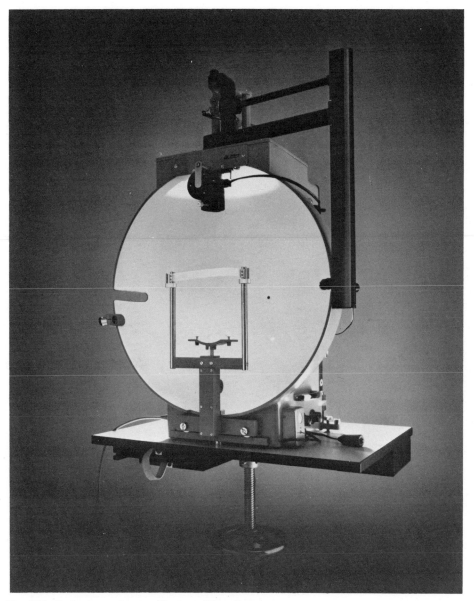

Fig. 4-28. Projection perimeter. (Courtesy Marco Corp.)

95

charted automatically and accurately since the patient's head is held firmly. The instrument will fit in a room as small as 6 × 6 feet. It may be placed in a visual fields room or in a data collection room, but the room's illumination must be controlled by a dimmer, since the procedure is done in a dark room. Since this is an expensive piece of equipment, one will not find it commonly used.

An ophthalmologist may accumulate 11 to 12 lineal feet of medical charts in a year, so the file area should accommodate about 48 lineal feet per doctor. Inactive charts can be stored in file transfer boxes in the storage room or at another location near the suite.

The consultation room will function as a private office, a place to relax between patients, to read one's mail, or to make phone calls. It is rarely used for consulting with patients; thus it can be small.

The interior design of this suite should be cheerful, and lighting is of critical importance. The waiting room should have good illumination for reading (see Fig. 4–37, Plate 8.) It would be thoughtful to provide large-print magazines for patients who do not see well. The drop room needs subdued lighting. The refraction rooms ought to be fairly neutral in color and without much pattern which might interfere with the examination.

Table 4-3. Analysis of Program.
Ophthalmology

No. of Physicians:	1	2	3
Refracting Rooms	3 @ 10 × 12 = 360[a]	4 total = 700[b]	8 total = 1400[b]
Minor Surgery	11 × 12 = 132	2 @ 12 × 12 = 288	12 × 22 = 264
Consultation	10 × 12 = 120	2 @ 12 × 12 = 288	4 @ 10 × 11 = 440
Fields Room	8 × 8 = 64	—	10 × 11 = 110
Data Collection	—	11 × 12 = 132	10 × 14 = 140
Waiting Room	12 × 18 = 216	16 × 28 = 448	22 × 26 = 572
Drops	6 × 6 = 36	8 × 12 = 96	Use waiting room
Toilets	2 @ 5 × 6 = 60	2 @ 5 × 6 = 60	2 @ 5 × 6 = 60
Business Office	12 × 14 = 168	12 × 16 = 192	12 × 20 = 240
Storage	4 × 6 = 24	6 × 8 = 48	6 × 8 = 48
Optician, Lab, and Contact Lens	10 × 24 = 240	(Non dispensing physician)	18 × 30 = 540
Staff Lounge	—	8 × 10 = 80	12 × 12 = 144
Subtotal	1420 ft^2	2332 ft^2	3958 ft^2
15% Circulation	213	350	594
Total	1633 ft^2	2682 ft^2	4552 ft^2

[a] Using mirrors
[b] Twenty-four foot refracting rooms (two "interlocking" together occupy approximately 10 × 35 ft.)

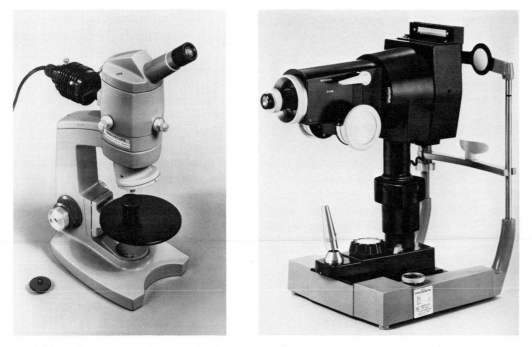

Fig. 4-34. Radiuscope: used for measuring the curvature of a contact lens. (Courtesy American Optical, Southbridge, Massachusetts.)

Fig. 4-35. Ophthalmometer: Used for examining, measuring, and fitting contact lenses, and for other diagnostic purposes. (Courtesy American Optical, Southbridge, Massachusetts.)

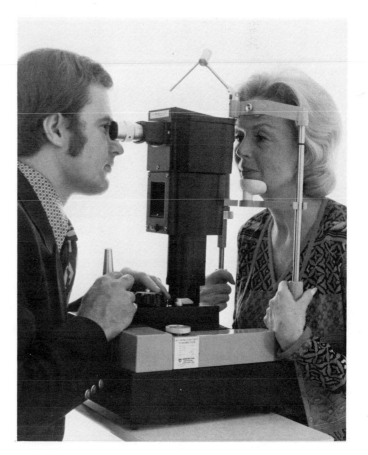

Fig. 4-36. Non-Contact Tonometer: used for measuring intraocular pressure or tension. (Courtesy American Optical, Southbridge, Massachusetts.)

97

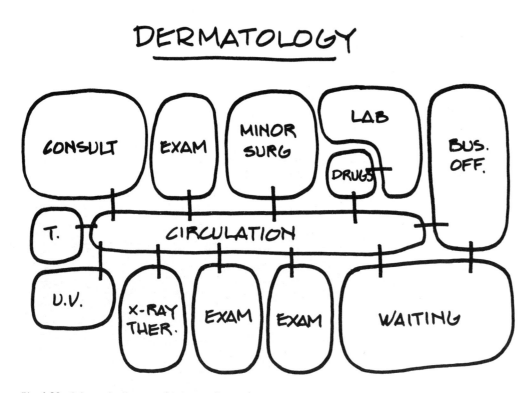

DERMATOLOGY

Fig. 4-38. Schematic diagram of a dermatology suite.

DERMATOLOGY

A dermatologist treats diseases of the skin. It is not uncommon to find a one-person practice. Since dermatologists rarely make hospital rounds or emergency house calls, their appointment schedule is strictly adhered to without the sort of interruption that plagues many other physicians. A one-physician suite would be composed of three small examination or treatment rooms, a waiting room to accommodate eight to ten persons, a small lab, a toilet room, a business office, a consultation room, a small ultraviolet therapy room (offices in warm sunny climates usually do not need a U.V. room), a minor surgery, and a large storage closet for drug samples.

The exam room can be 8 × 10 feet instead of the standard 8 × 12 feet. The exam table used is actually a flat physical therapy table, 24 × 72 inches × 36 inches high, which is usually placed against the wall. It is an advantage if both natural light (a window) and artificial light are available in the room. The room should have a sink cabinet and a dressing area and it should have a high level of illumination free of shadows (Fig. 4–39).

The ultraviolet room may be as small as 4 × 5 feet. A prefabricated silver-foil-lined box will be placed in the room to surround the patient. Some dermatologists use a portable Hanovia hot quartz lamp on casters, which they move from room to room if they need it, rather than dedicate a special room to ultraviolet. X-ray therapy is not used much anymore because the liability and subsequent malpractice insurance rates are too costly, but some dermatologists may want a small room (8 × 8 or 8 × 10 feet) set aside for this purpose. The walls may have to be lead shielded.

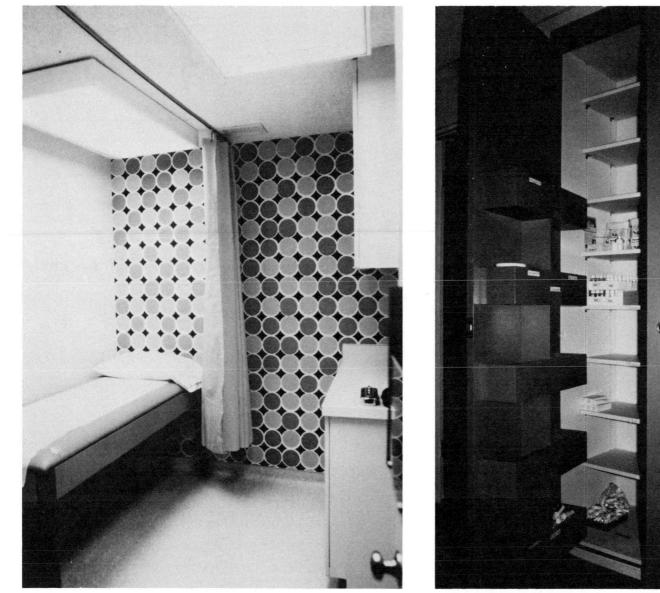

Fig. 4-39. Dermatology exam room.

Fig. 4-40. Drug sample cabinet.

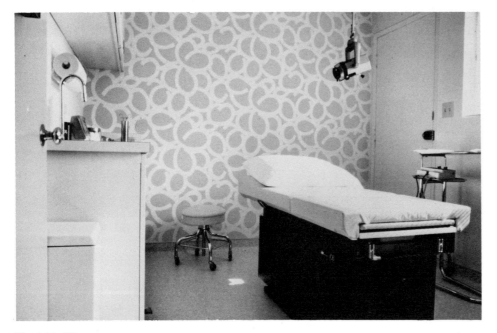

Fig. 4-41. Minor surgery.

Dermatologists dispense a lot of drug samples, salves, ointments, and so forth. A specialized closet should be provided in a convenient location in the corridor for storage of drug samples. The closet should have doors fitted with compartments or bins that sort and make accessible the frequently used products (Fig. 4–40).

The minor surgery room should be 12 × 12 feet with a long sink cabinet along one wall and a standard exam table or a motorized operating table in the center of the room (Fig. 4–41). A surgical light would be ceiling mounted over the table. The medical equipment that needs to be accommodated in this room would depend on the scope of the procedures.

The reader is referred to Chapter 6 for a suite plan of a group practice dermatology suite and to Chapter 11 for an electrical and a reflected ceiling plan for the suite shown in Fig. 4–43.

Table 4-4. Analysis of Program.
Dermatology

No. of Physicians:	1		2	
Exam Rooms	3 @ 8 × 10 =	240	6 @ 8 × 10 =	480
Minor Surgery	12 × 12 =	144	12 × 12 =	144
Toilets	5 × 6 =	30	2 @ 5 × 6 =	60
Business Office	12 × 14 =	168	16 × 18 =	288
Waiting Room	12 × 16 =	192	14 × 18 =	252
Consultation Room	12 × 12 =	144	12 × 12 =	144
Laboratory	8 × 10 =	80	10 × 10 =	100
Ultraviolet Therapy	4 × 5 =	20	4 × 5 =	20
Storage	5 × 6 =	30	5 × 6 =	30
Subtotal		1048 ft^2		1662 ft^2
15% Circulation		157		249
Total		1205 ft^2		1911 ft^2

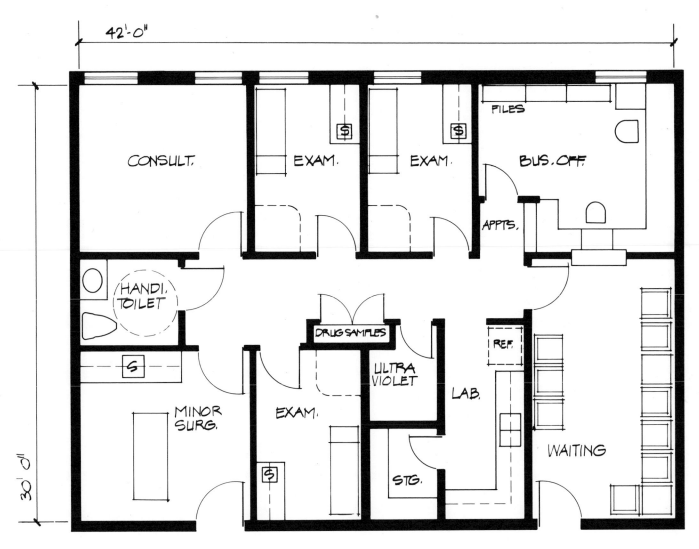

42'-0"

30'-0"

CONSULT.

EXAM.

EXAM.

FILES

BUS. OFF.

APPTS.

HANDI.
TOILET

DRUG SAMPLES

ULTRA
VIOLET

LAB.

REF.

MINOR
SURG.

EXAM.

STG.

WAITING

DERMATOLOGY
1260 SQ. FT.

Fig. 4-42. Suite plan for dermatology, 1260 square feet.

101

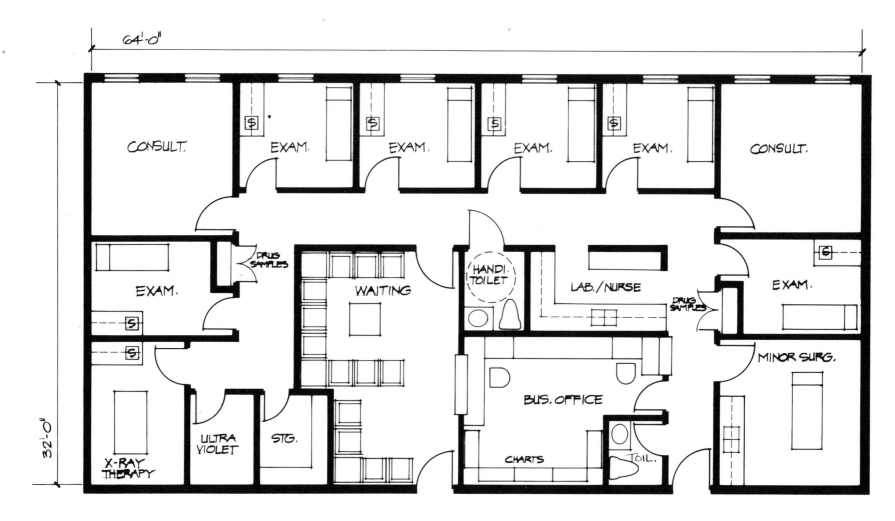

64'-0"

32'-0"

CONSULT. EXAM. EXAM. EXAM. EXAM. CONSULT.

DRUG SAMPLES

EXAM. WAITING HANDI. TOILET LAB./NURSE DRUG SAMPLES EXAM.

MINOR SURG.

BUS. OFFICE

X-RAY THERAPY ULTRA VIOLET STG. CHARTS TOIL.

DERMATOLOGY

2048 SQ. FT

Fig. 4-43. Suite plan for dermatology, 2048 square feet.

102

PLASTIC SURGERY

This suite is similar to a general surgery suite except it is usually larger and it often has an outpatient surgery room in which healthy, low-risk patients might obtain face lifts, breast implants, rhinoplasty (reconstruction of the nose), hair transplants, hand surgery, and other cosmetic or reconstructive procedures.

The trend toward performing plastic surgery on an outpatient basis in the surgeon's office is based on several factors. It lowers the costs for the patient and it permits the physician to make an extra fee rather than have it go to the hospital. The surgeon has more control over scheduling when the procedures are in his or her own office, and the patient avoids the frightening experience of entering the hospital milieu with its accompanying mountain of paperwork, the impersonal encounters with staff, and the lack of privacy. Surgery itself causes enough anxiety for a patient; anything that can reduce the stress is certainly worthwhile.

The operating room should be a minimum of 14 × 16 feet, with one wall of built-in cabinets containing a scrub sink with foot lever control and gooseneck spout; storage for linens, gowns, caps, disposable supplies, and surgical dressings; drawers for surgical instruments; and a sterilization area. If space permits, the scrub, prep, and cleanup should be a separate room off the operating room. Similar to a large nurse station, the room should be about 8 × 12 feet lined with cabinets and work surfaces. Instruments will be sterilized and wrapped here; dressings and medications are prepared. Sinks in the operating room and prep area should have plaster traps.

**Table 4-5. Analysis of Program.
Plastic Surgery**

No. of Physicians:	1	2
Consultation Room	12 × 16 = 192	2 @ 12 × 16 = 384
Exam Rooms	3 @ 8 × 12 = 288	5 @ 8 × 12 = 480
Operating Suite[a]	22 × 24 = 528	22 × 30 = 660
Waiting Room	14 × 16 = 224	16 × 18 = 288
Business Office	14 × 16 = 224	16 × 16 = 256
Toilets	2 @ 6 × 8 = 96	2 @ 6 × 8 = 96
Storage	6 × 6 = 36	6 × 8 = 48
Shampoo/Makeup	—	10 × 10 = 100
Staff Lounge	10 × 12 = 120	10 × 12 = 120
Subtotal	1708 ft²	2431 ft²
15% Circulation	256	365
Total	1964 ft²	2797 ft²

[a] Includes prep room and recovery.
Note: The above is merely an approximation, since plastic surgery suites can vary considerably in size and number of rooms, depending on the physician's scope of procedures and practice philosophy.

PLASTIC SURGERY

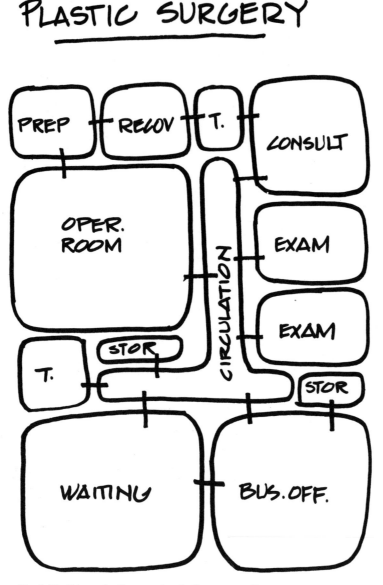

Fig. 4-44. Schematic diagram of a plastic surgery suite.

A motorized operating table (Fig. 4–45) will be located in the center of the room with a ceiling-mounted surgical light (provide wood blocking in the ceiling to support it) overhead. A crash cart (Fig. 4–46) containing emergency equipment (should a patient's heart fail) is nearby. Oxygen and suction (vacuum) either can be piped into the room or can be portable on mobile stands. The designer should check local fire code requirements for storage of anesthetic gases. (See Chapter 8 for discussion of this topic.)

The operating room must be easy to clean. Walls should have either a ceramic tile wainscot, a semigloss enamel paint finish, or a commercial vinyl wallcovering. A floor with a minimum of joints is desirable—a commercial-quality sheet vinyl with self-coved base, terrazzo, or a sheet vinyl with heat-welded seams.

A dressing room with lockers for valuables should be provided for patients. Sometimes the dressing area can be combined with the recovery room. A recovery room should be located near the operating room and nurse station so that the staff, while cleaning up the operating room and preparing it for the next procedure, can keep a watchful eye on the recovering patient. A closed circuit television is put to good use in this situation.

Typically the recovery "beds" are actually wheeled gurneys, 2 × 6 feet. A patient would be moved off the operating table onto a gurney and wheeled into the recovery room, so room layouts must allow for easy maneuvering of gurney carts without bumping into walls.

Approximately two-thirds of a plastic surgeon's cases can be done in a properly equipped operating room in the surgeon's office. The remainder will be performed in the hospital.

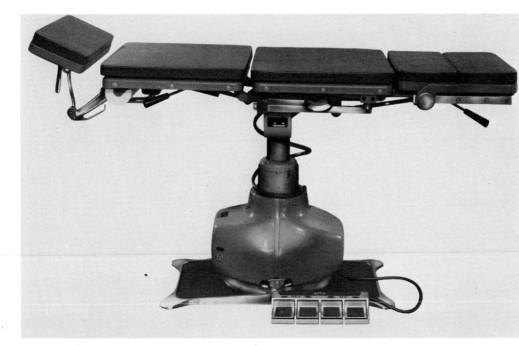

Fig. 4-45. Motorized operating table. (Ritter, Mfg. by Sybron Medical Products Div., Rochester, New York.)

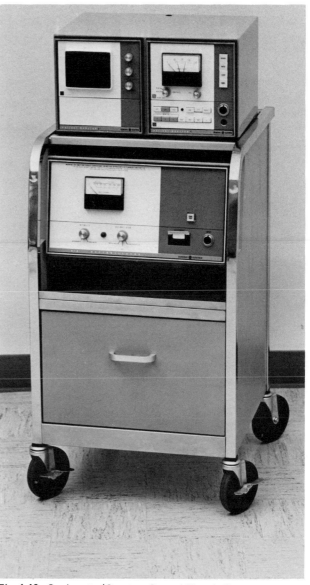

Fig. 4-46. Crash cart. (Courtesy General Electric Co., Medical Systems Div.)

The plastic surgeon takes "before" and "after" photos of patients. These photos can be taken in the examination room (where a pull-down solid-colored panel of fabric should be mounted to the wall as a background) or in a small 6 × 8-foot room designed for that purpose. A darkroom is usually not required unless the physician prefers to do his or her own film processing.

Often a practice may become known for its success with one particular procedure such as reconstruction of the nose. In such a case, a busy practice with several surgeons may perform these operations in such volume as to necessitate an operating room large enough to accommodate three patients simultaneously with just a cubicle drape on a ceiling-mounted track separating the patients. While the nurse is prepping one patient, the surgeon may be completing surgery on the next and a nurse may be applying a dressing on the third before removing the patient to a nearby recovery room. So it is not difficult to see that three operating tables can be busy simultaneously.

With procedures such as nose reconstructions, breast implants, and sometimes hand surgery, the patient is operated on in the morning, spends 2 to 4 hours in the recovery room, and goes home that afternoon. The doctor's afternoons would be spent visiting hospitalized patients, conducting office interviews with prospective patients who seek consultation about a reconstructive or cosmetic procedure, and seeing postoperative patients to change dressings or remove sutures.

The composition of the plastic surgeon's practice will dictate the design features that need to be incorporated. A practice composed largely of cosmetic surgery may cater to a wealthy clientele who will expect a posh, luxurious office. Of par-

ticular importance will be secluded entrance so that clients may park their cars and conveniently enter the office without being seen. After the procedure they can slip out the same door and elude others in the waiting room—lest they meet someone who might recognize them.

For this reason plastic surgeons who specialize in cosmetic surgery frequently prefer a ground floor location in a medical building with a private driveway or turn-around so that their patients need not walk through the lobby or public areas of the medical building (Fig. 4–47). This is valid even when the practice is composed of a less wealthy clientele: Patients who elect to have cosmetic surgery tend to be sensitive about it and prefer privacy. To that end, most plastic surgeons prefer a low level of illumination in the waiting room. If softens the appearance of bruises left by surgery and permits patients to "hide."

A busy plastic surgeon who specializes in cosmetic procedures may even have separate waiting rooms for male and female patients (see Fig. 4–51, Plate 9). A hair stylist may be on hand several afternoons a week to shampoo and style the hair of patients who have just had bandages removed after a facelift. Such patients will, understandably, be timid about visiting their own stylist in public until the bruises subside. A small room should be set aside for this purpose with a standard beautician's shampoo chair, professional hair dryer, and good-quality tinted mirrors. A gray-tinted mirror will downplay the bruises yet still provide enough reflection. The room should have colorful wallpaper and accessories to raise the patient's spirit.

A lucrative plastic surgery practice may even offer the services of a professional makeup artist for patients recovering from facial plastic surgery.

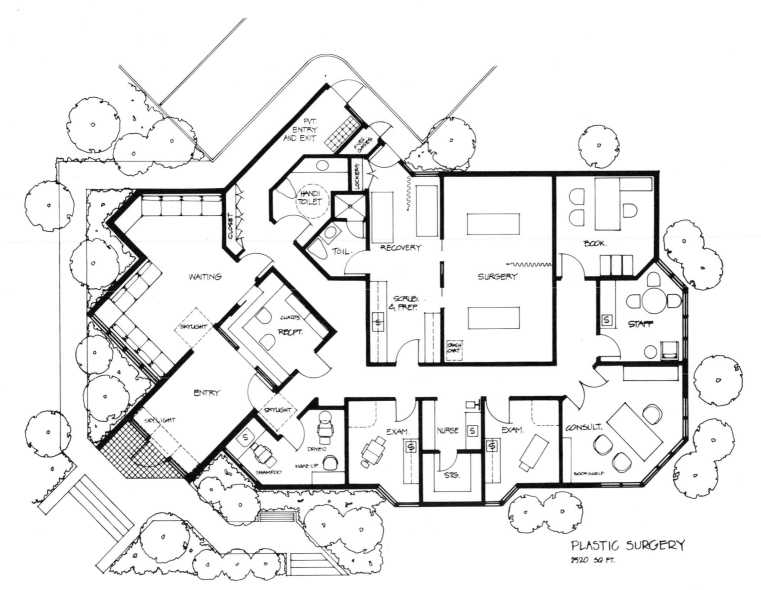

PVT. ENTRY AND EXIT

ANES. GASES

LOCKERS

CLOSET

HANDI TOILET

TOIL.

RECOVERY

BOOK.

WAITING

SURGERY

SCRUB. & PREP.

CHARTS

SKYLIGHT

RECPT.

STAFF

CRASH CART

ENTRY

SKYLIGHT

SKYLIGHT

SHAMPOO

DRYER

MAKE-UP

EXAM.

NURSE

STG.

EXAM.

CONSULT.

BOOKSHELF

PLASTIC SURGERY
2520 SQ. FT.

Fig. 4-47. Suite plan for plastic surgery, 2520 square feet.

107

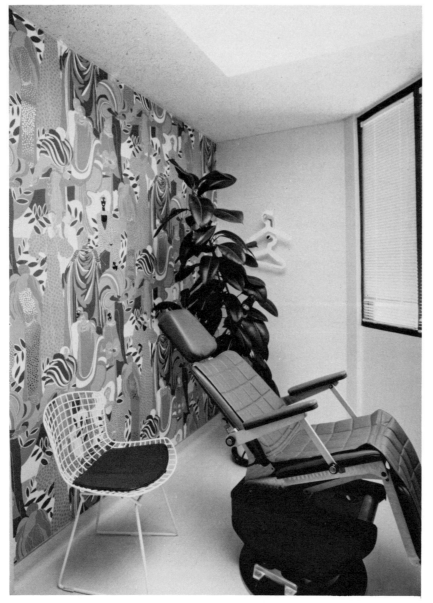

Fig. 4-50. Examination room with motorized examination chair.

Those who specialize more in reconstructive surgery—skin grafts for burn victims, surgery of the hand, repair of cleft palate, trauma, etc.— usually do not have strong sentiments about providing privacy and anonymity for their patients and are less interested in the appearance of their office.

Since this is a low-volume medical practice, the interior design can be fairly plush and residential in character. The plastic surgeon is trading in cosmetics and vanity. The image the surgeon projects is very important. People want to deal with a surgeon who appears to be successful—this amounts to a third-party endorsement of the plastic surgeon's skills. The practitioner who spends a considerable amount of money on office design and furnishings will reap the rewards tenfold. No medical specialty can benefit more from a good visual image. The plastic surgeon's letterhead and business card should also be striking and imaginative. The day has passed when serious physicians felt they had to have black engraving on white linen stock to appear professional.

All rooms of this suite may be carpeted except for the surgery and ancillary rooms. The office design should project warmth and comfort, and the lighting should be soft and flattering in all rooms except the exam rooms and operating suite. Incandescent light is preferable to fluorescent in the waiting room, corridors, and consultation room. Fabric upholstery in rich textures should be used throughout. Bathrooms are of prime importance in terms of design. Large gray-tinted mirrors and interesting lighting may be incorporated into the vanity cabinet design. Walls and ceiling should carry an attractive decorative wallpaper, and bathroom accessories such as tissue boxes, paper towelettes holder, soap dish, etc., should be residential in character. Other items a patients might use in light grooming before or after medical consultation ought to be provided.

The consultation room should convey a solid, successful image but should not be flamboyant or trendy (Fig. 4–48, Plate 9). After all, one does not want a surgeon who makes impulsive decisions. This room might be styled more conservatively than the rest of the suite. The surgeon's diplomas and awards should be displayed here in elegant frames and mats. A desk where a patient may sit and watch a video cassette tape on a particular surgical procedure may be provided in the consultation room. Also, an X-ray view box should be located convenient to the doctor's desk.

More and more persons are considering plastic surgery to correct physical imperfections. Taboos about vanity are waning, and society is placing a greater emphasis on self-expression and personal fulfillment. There is greater exposure to the benefits of plastic surgery in the media, and this has given more people the confidence to obtain treatment. Plastic surgery is no longer just an option of the rich. Many persons of modest income currently see it as a viable option. Plastic surgery is a very lucrative type of surgery, and therefore a physician who specializes in it may wish to enhance his or her image and practice in any way possible—by having a luxurious office, by providing a secluded surgery and recovery facility, and by offering amenities that leave the competition a mile behind.

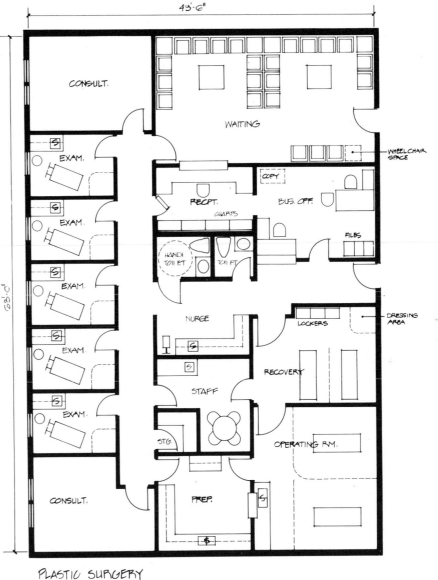

PLASTIC SURGERY
2750 SQ. FT.

Fig. 4-52. Suite plan for plastic surgery, 2750 square feet.

109

ALLERGY

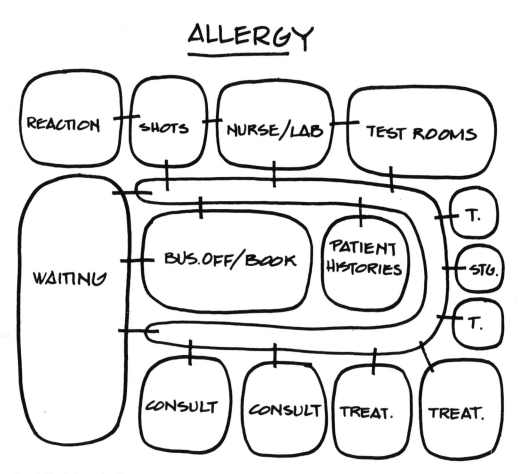

Fig. 4-53. Schematic diagram of an allergy suite.

ALLERGY

Allergy is defined as an altered reaction of the tissues to agents or allergens. Because these allergens cause a reaction in some persons but, in similar amounts, are harmless to others, allergies are often difficult to diagnose. A methodically detailed patient history is a part of any preliminary examination or interview. Some allergists have a printed questionnaire that a patient may fill out by himself or herself and, if this is the case, a desk or several alcoves with countertop writing surface, chair, and light should be included in or near the waiting room (Fig. 4–54). Other allergists prefer that the patient history be taken by the staff, and in this case, small rooms (6 × 6 feet) should be provided with a small desk (2 × 4 feet is adequate) and a chair for the patient, for the interviewer, and perhaps for a guest (a relative of the patient). (See Fig. 4–55.)

In a large practice a combination of staff interview and a printed questionnaire that the patient fills out by himself or herself may be used. In this situation an alcove may be created off the corridor for a number of tablet arm chairs. If the practice includes a large number of pediatric cases, the interview room will have to accommodate a parent, the child, and the interviewer, since the parent must usually answer the questions for the child.

There are, in fact, pediatric allergists whose entire practice focuses on children. These offices should be designed according to the needs of an allergist but with the decor and colorful vitality of a pediatrician's office (Figs. 4–56 and 4–57). In fact, the treatment or test rooms, instead of having number designations, may have large animals or cartoons painted alongside them, so that the staff can tell the child to go to the "butterfly" or the "frog" room (Fig. 4–58). One must be mindful, however, that heavy textures, shag carpeting, and many fibers (wool, in particular) cause problems for those with allergies and are to be avoided in the office. Similarly, draperies, because they collect dust, are to be avoided in favor of metal window blinds. All materials in this suite must be easy to sanitize and be as hypoallergenic as possible.

An allergy practice has a high volume of patients (as high as 50 to 60 per doctor per day) which fall into two categories: short-visit (to receive an injection) and long-visit (patient interview, skin tests). Due to the high volume of patients, an efficient layout is of the utmost importance. A large number of patients come two or three times a week, and others just weekly, to receive allergy shots. Thus the nurse station where injections are given should be located off the waiting room or just inside the suite near the waiting room so that these patients do not have to mingle with the long-visit patients.

After receiving the injection the patient will return to the waiting room and sit for 10 to 15 minutes to check any adverse reaction he or she may have had to the desensitization shot. The waiting room should be large enough to accommodate the high volume of patients. Some offices

Table 4-6. Analysis of Program.
Allergy

No. of Physicians:	1	2	3
Exam/Treatment Rooms	2 @ 8 × 12 = 192	4 @ 8 × 12 = 384	7 @ 8 × 12 = 672
Consultation Rooms	11 × 12 = 132	2 @ 11 × 12 = 264	3 @ 11 × 12 = 396
Waiting Room	16 × 16 = 256	16 × 26 = 416	20 × 30 = 600
Storage	6 × 8 = 48	6 × 8 = 48	8 × 8 = 64
Nurse Station/Lab	12 × 14 = 168	12 × 14 = 168	14 × 16 = 224
Toilets	2 @ 5 × 6 = 60	2 @ 5 × 6 = 60	3 @ 5 × 6 = 90
Shots	(Combine w/lab)	6 × 8 = 48	8 × 8 = 64
Recovery/Reaction	6 × 8 = 48	8 × 10 = 80	8 × 10 = 80
History Alcoves	—[a]	8 × 10 = 80	8 × 10 = 80
Test Rooms[b]	(2 persons) 96	(3 persons) 144	(4 persons) 192
Staff Lounge	8 × 10 = 80	10 × 12 = 120	12 × 14 = 168
Business Office	12 × 16 = 192	12 × 16 = 192	14 × 18 = 252
Subtotal	1272 ft²	2004 ft²	2882 ft²
15% Circulation	191	300	432
Total	1463 ft²	2304 ft²	3314 ft²

[a] History-taking alcoves may be worked into the circulation area or waiting room.
[b] May be one room with cubicle drape separation.
Note: The above spaces may vary greatly depending on the location of shot, test, and recovery/reaction rooms and how they are combined.

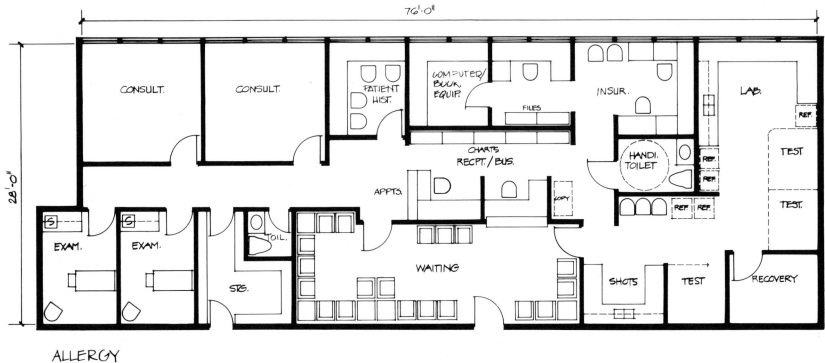

CONSULT.

CONSULT.

PATIENT HIST.

COMPUTER/
BOOK.
EQUIP.

FILES

INSUR.

LAB.

REF.

CHARTS
RECPT. / BUS.

HANDI.
TOILET

REF.

REF.

TEST

APPTS.

KOPY

REF.

REF.

TEST.

EXAM.

EXAM.

TOIL.

WAITING

SHOTS

TEST

RECOVERY

STG.

ALLERGY

2172 SQ. FT.

Fig. 4-54. Suite plan for allergy, 2172 square feet.

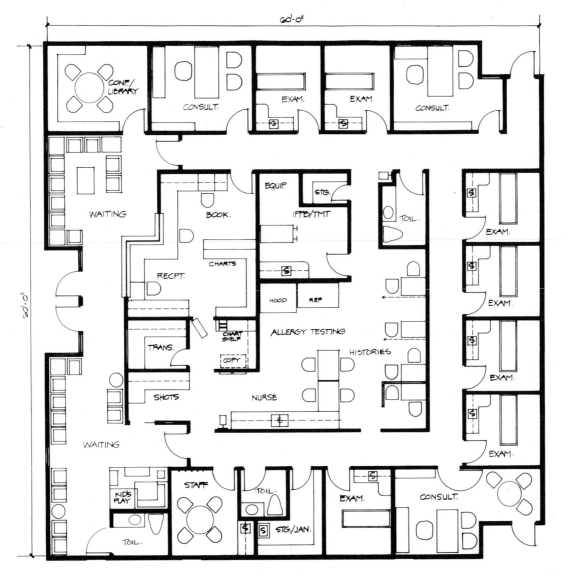

CONF./LIBRARY

CONSULT.

EXAM.

EXAM.

CONSULT.

WAITING

BOOK.

EQUIP

STG.

IPPB/TMT

TOIL.

EXAM.

CHARTS

RECPT.

HOOD

REF

EXAM.

CHART SHELF

ALLERGY TESTING

EXAM.

TRANS.

COPY

HISTORIES

SHOTS

NURSE

EXAM.

WAITING

EXAM.

KID'S PLAY

STAFF

TOIL.

EXAM.

CONSULT.

STG./JAN.

TOIL.

60'-0"

60'-0"

ALLERGY
3600 SQ. FT.

Fig. 4-55. Suite plan for allergy, 3600 square feet.

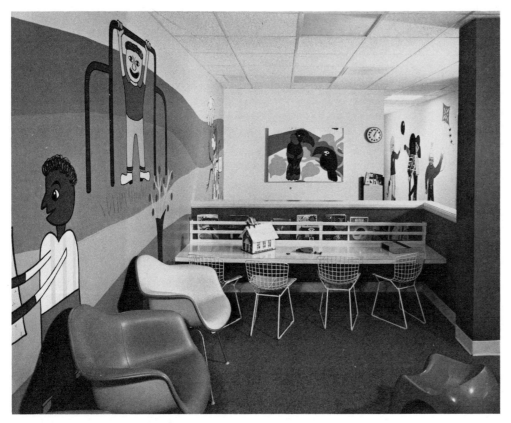

Fig. 4-56. Waiting room for pediatric allergist.

have a small secondary waiting room within the suite where patients may sit awaiting a negative reaction to an injection (Figs. 4–59 and 4–60). Other suites may actually have small reaction rooms furnished with a cot and a chair so that a patient, after receiving a desensitization injection, may lie down for 15 to 20 minutes. If reaction rooms are provided, they should be located adjacent to the patient interview area or the injections area so that staff are always nearby to watch patients who may suffer adverse reactions.

After the minutely detailed patient history is taken, a patient will be subjected to skin tests in which he or she lies on a flat table, on his or her stomach, while the nurse or aide makes rows of small scratches on the patient's back and an allergen is touched to each scratch. Intradermal tests, where a small amount of an allergen is injected just under the skin, are another type of skin test. The skin tests may be performed in small rooms 6 × 8 or 8 × 8 feet, or in a large room that has been divided into 6 × 6-foot or 8 × 8-foot areas via a ceiling-mounted cubicle drape. The patient lies on a physical therapy table (Figure 7–9) that is often placed against a wall. The technician sits alongside the patient working off

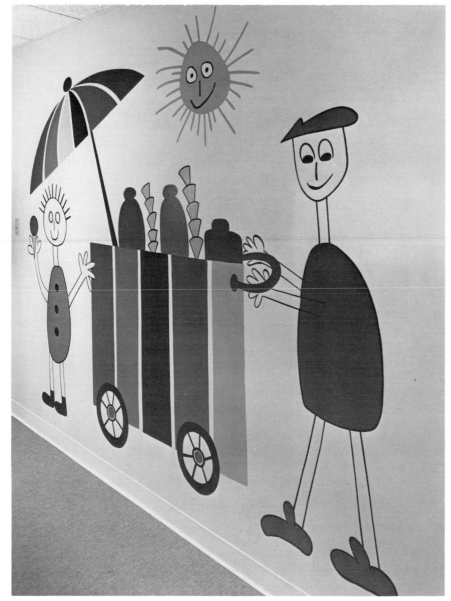

Fig. 4-57. Wallgraphic for pediatric allergy.

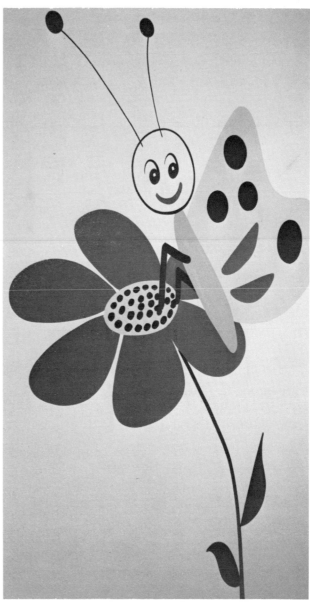

Fig. 4-58. Butterfly graphic, pediatric allergy.

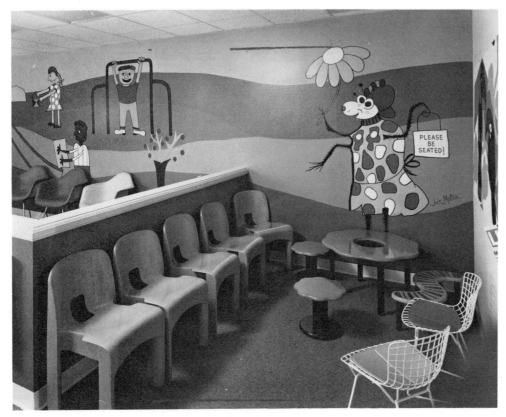

Fig. 4-59. Secondary waiting room, pediatric allergy.

of a cabinet or a mobile cart. A rack of small vials containing allergens is carried from room to room and placed on the cart next to the patient.

Healthy patients, so to speak, are seen in the test rooms, but patients who are experiencing severe symptoms such as asthma or vomiting will be examined in a standard exam room or a treatment room where the staff has access to water and respiratory equipment (IPPB Inter-Positive Pressure Breathing apparatus).

After a diagnosis has determined to which agents the patient is sensitive, a desensitization treatment program is begun in which small doses of the allergen are injected in a series of gradually increasing amounts over a period of months or, in some cases, years. Therefore this practice is characterized by many short-visit patients each day. The injections and tests are done by nurses and aides, so one doctor may have several aides.

The physician should have a large consultation room since the results of the testing and the prescribed treatment are discussed there. The nurse station/lab in this suite should be large and have space for two or more full-size refrigerators for storage of injectibles.

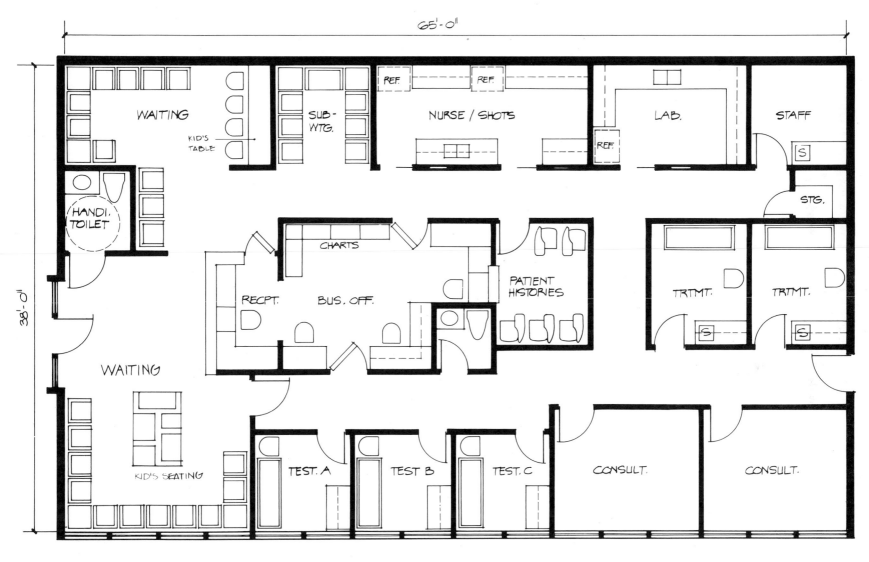

PEDIATRIC ALLERGY
2470 SQ. FT.

Fig. 4-60. Suite plan for allergy, 2470 square feet.

PSYCHIATRY

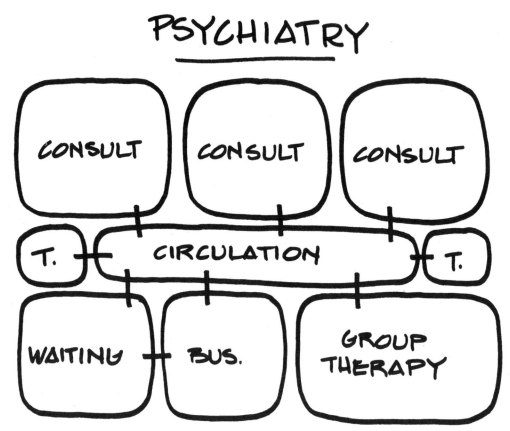

Fig. 4-61. Schematic diagram of a psychiatry suite.

This is the easiest medical suite to design. The consultation room is the key element in this suite. Each psychiatrist will have a preferred method of working depending on his or her counseling philosophy. Some prefer a casual living room decor where doctor and patient sit next to each other in lounge chairs. Others offer the patient a sofa to lie upon. Still others prefer a formal directive approach with the doctor behind the desk and the patient across from it. Those who practice hypnosis often choose to have the patient relax in a recliner chair that rocks back to elevate the patient's feet.

Regardless of counseling style, the consultation room should be a minimum of 12 × 14 feet and preferably 14 × 16 feet. Psychiatrists usually house their professional library in the consultation room, so adequate bookshelf storage should be planned. Diplomas can be framed creatively and hung as artwork in the room (Fig. 4-62, Plate 10). They may be framed with mats and frames to accent the colors of the furnishings, all frames need not match—it is more interesting if they do not.

Table 4-7. Analysis of Program.
Psychiatry

No. of Physicians:	1	2	3
Consultation Rooms	14 × 16 = 224	2 @ 14 × 16 = 448	3 @ 14 × 16 = 672
Toilets	5 × 6 = 30	5 × 6 = 30	2 @ 5 × 6 = 60
Group Therapy	16 × 18 = 288	16 × 18 = 288	16 × 18 = 288
Business Office	12 × 14 = 168	12 × 14 = 168	14 × 16 = 224
Waiting Room	12 × 10 = 120	12 × 10 = 120	12 × 16 = 192
Storage	4 × 6 = 24	4 × 6 = 24	6 × 8 = 48
Subtotal	854 ft²	1078 ft²	1564 ft²
15% Circulation	128	161	234
Total	982 ft²	1239 ft²	1798 ft²

Some psychiatrists prefer a consultation room with a window, others find it distracting to the patient's concentration. The illumination in the room should be rheostatically controlled so that it can be dimmed.

Sometimes solo practitioners share an office. Each would need a consultation room, but the business office, waiting room, and group therapy room would be shared. There should be two or three seats per doctor in the waiting room. Since each psychiatrist can see only one patient per hour, this is a very low volume specialty. The group therapy room should accommodate about 12 persons. Chairs that stack are best. The room should have a sink cabinet for preparation of coffee and perhaps a coat closet.

The waiting room should be residential in character. Patients may be nervous before therapy, so the waiting room ought to have a soothing color scheme and feel comfortable yet afford individuals some degree of privacy. Sound control is very important in this suite. All walls of the consultation rooms and group therapy room should have sound-attenuating construction (see Chapter 12).

The ambience of this suite is of utmost importance. Colors should be tranquil and serve as a background rather than be so trend-setting or interesting as to be distracting. Sharp contrasts in color or pattern should be avoided in favor or mellowness.

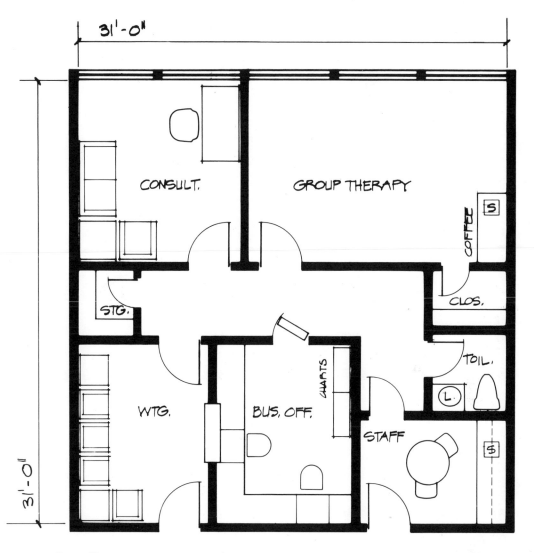

PSYCHIATRY
961 SQ. FT.

Fig. 4-63. Suite plan for psychiatry, 961 square feet.

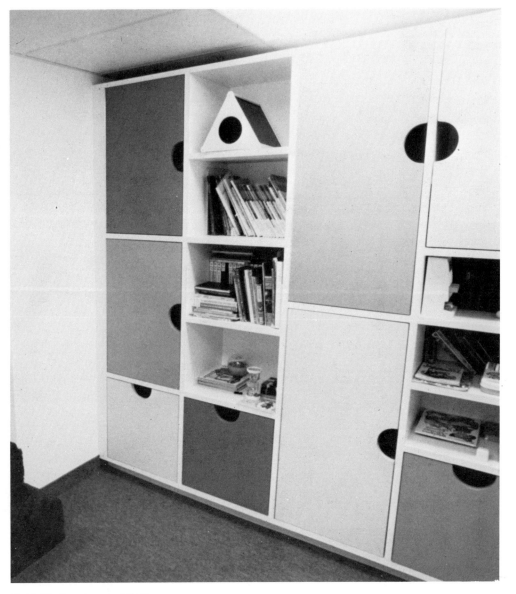

Fig. 4-64. Toy storage cabinet.

CHILD PSYCHIATRY

A child psychiatrist has the additional requirement of a room for play therapy. Typically, this room would have a one-way glass observation window, a play table with chair, and an assortment of dolls, games, and toys. Sometimes an easel and paints are provided so a sink should be included in the room if possible. An attractive cabinet should be designed to house all the toys in an orderly fashion (Fig. 4-64). If appropriate space is available, a secured outdoor play area can be developed so that the psychiatrist may study children playing naturally without their realizing that they are being observed.

NEUROLOGY

A neurologist diagnoses diseases of the nervous system and brain. His or her patients are always referred by other physicians. The patients may complain of headaches, epileptic seizures, damage suffered as a result of a stroke, or perhaps a cerebral palsy condition that has resulted in a facial distortion—a distended jaw or a drooping mouth.

This is a low patient volume specialty, and the preliminary history taking and interview in the physician's consultation room requires about 45 to 50 minutes. It is not uncommon in this specialty to have a small exam room opening off of the consultation room (Fig. 4-66).

After the interview a series of tests is performed. The most common test is the *electroen-*

cephalogram (charting of brain waves)—commonly known as EEG. This can be performed in a room as small as 5 × 8 feet if the technician does not remain in the room with the patient but sits in an adjoining control room. There are two schools of thought on this point. Some neurologists feel that the patient is comforted by the technician being in the same room; others feel that it is distracting to the patient. In either case, the patient would sit in a comfortable reclining chair since this seems to make the patient less apprehensive and more relaxed than lying flat on an exam table.

If the technician is to remain in the room with the patient, the room should be about 8 × 10 feet. If the technician is to work from a control room, the room for the patient can be as small as 5 × 8 feet and the adjoining control room (with a window into the patient's room so that the patient is always in sight) should be about 5 × 8 feet. The control area would have a small sink, a cabinet with lock for storage of drugs used to sedate patients, and open shelves for storage of EEG records which fit into containers that resemble little books. The EEG and other equipment used in this room will fit on a portable stand or a built-in shelf 42 inches wide × 24 inches deep. Since the EEG printout is prefolded when released from the machine, there is no need to provide a mounting area as is true with EKG (electrocardiogram) printouts.

Frequently a neurologist will perform EEGs for other physicians but have no personal consultation with the patient. The EEG technician would perform the test and the printout would be read or interpreted by the neurologist with a report

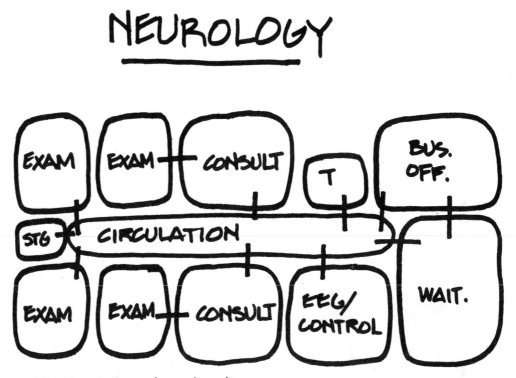

Fig. 4-65. Schematic diagram of a neurology suite.

Table 4-8. Analysis of Program. Neurology

No. of Physicians:	1	2
Consultation Rooms	12 × 14 = 168	2 @ 12 × 14 = 336
Exam Rooms	2 @ 8 × 10 = 160	4 @ 8 × 10 = 320
Business Office	12 × 14 = 168	14 × 16 = 224
Waiting Room	10 × 12 = 120	12 × 14 = 168
Toilets	5 × 6 = 30	2 @ 5 × 6 = 60
EEG/Control	8 × 12 = 96	8 × 12 = 96
Nurse Station/Lab	6 × 8 = 48	6 × 8 = 48
Storage	4 × 6 = 24	4 × 6 = 24
Subtotal	814 ft²	1276 ft²
15% Circulation	122	191
Total	936 ft²	1467 ft²

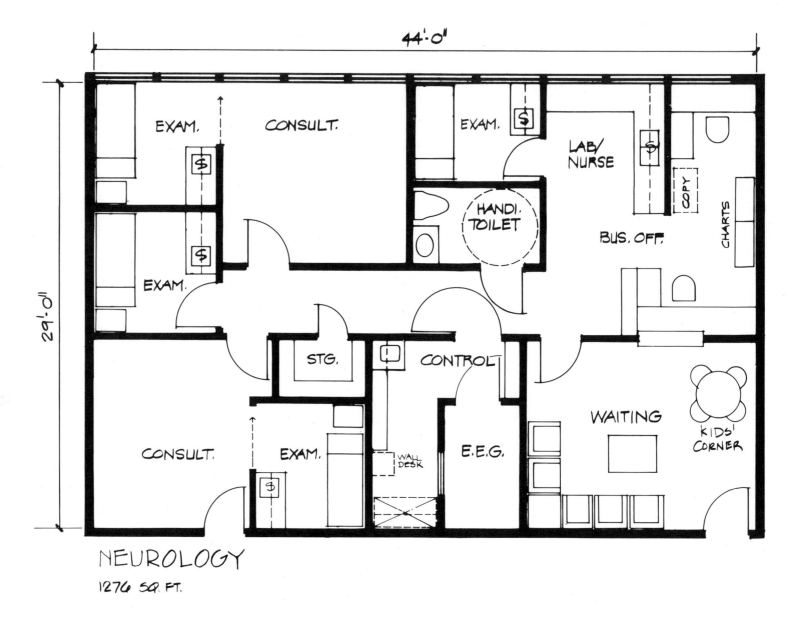

NEUROLOGY

1276 SQ. FT.

Fig. 4-66. Suite plan for neurology, 1276 square feet.

mailed to the patient's physician. But the neurologist would not consult with the patient unless the physician, after receiving the report, felt the referral was necessary for proper treatment of the patient's condition. Therefore a good location for the EEG room is near the front of the suite so that these patients do not have to pass the consulting rooms or exam rooms in order to reach the test room.

There are two ways to administer the EEG. One way requires the application of conductive paste at the temples before the leads are attached. The paste is messy and the patient must have access to a sink or bathroom to wipe it out of his or her hair afterwards. A thoughtful designer would provide a vanity counter in the bathroom with a receptacle for paper towels, a soap dispenser, and a place to hang a coat or handbag. While one does not wish to encourage the patient to shampoo his or her hair in the office, it is advisable to facilitate at least partial removal of the paste.

Another method of performing EEGs eliminates the paste and instead involves the insertion of small needles. This method, however, cannot be used with children.

A neurologist may also perform a spinal tap (to drain off fluid) in the office. For this procedure the neurologist would use an exam room with the patient lying on a exam table which is usually placed against a wall.

Another office procedure is the *electromyogram,* which shows if a muscle is deteriorating or can be rehabilitated. It measures the strength of a muscle and indicates if the nerve has been affected. Normally this test is performed in a special room with a table placed against a wall. The small machine used for this procedure should be placed on a mobile stand so that the physician can move around the patient.

The consultation room should be large and comfortably furnished since most patients will be interviewed here. Furnishings in this room and the remainder of the office should be tasteful but quiet. All colors and patterns should be selected for their restful quality—anything bold should be avoided. One must be particularly cognizant of patterns that have a figure-ground reversal and pick up a visual rhythm. Such patterns may cause a seizure in persons with certain types of neurological disorders.

All rooms may be carpeted in this suite. Carpet should have an antistatic wire woven into it or one might pick up interference from static electricity on the electronic equipment. Lighting should be rheostatically controlled so that it can be dimmed when patients are relaxing and being tested.

NEUROSURGERY

A neurosurgeon's office is often smaller than a neurologist's office and usually does not include EEG testing equipment. All of the tests would be performed in the neurologist's office and the neurosurgeon would mainly see patients for preoperative and postoperative consultations. Therefore a small number of examination rooms is necessary, in addition to a business office, a bookkeeping area, and a consultation room for each physician. One exam room per physician is usually adequate since the surgery schedule rarely permits all physicians to be there at the same time.

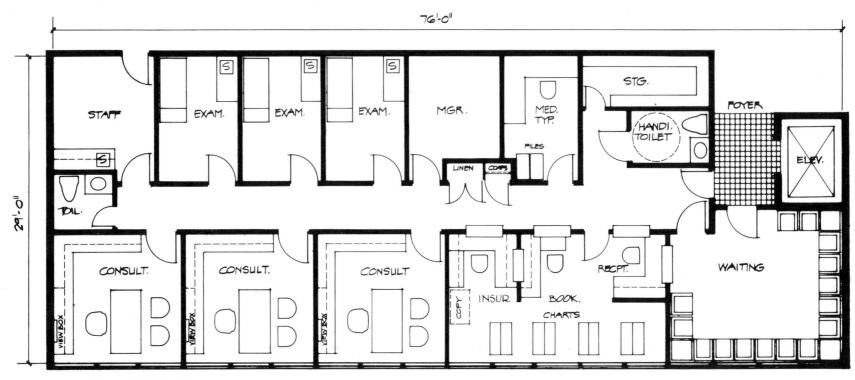

NEUROSURGERY

2024 SQ. FT.

Fig. 4-67. Suite plan for neurosurgery, 2024 square feet.

GENERAL SURGERY

This is a low-volume practice in large part dependent upon referrals from primary care physicians. The suite can be small because most of a surgeon's work is done in a hospital. Patients are examined and interviewed preoperatively and postoperatively in the office, and sutures may be removed or dressings changed in the office.

A surgeon's office will usually contain two standard-size exam rooms, a large consultation room (12 × 12 or 12 × 14 feet), a small business office, a waiting room, and a toilet room. A small nurse station, a niche in the corridor, will suffice for the sterilization of instruments and storage of dressings and supplies. An under-counter refrigerator should be built into the cabinet.

The waiting room need not accommodate more than six chairs since patients are well scheduled and usually do not have to wait a long time. Surgeons usually perform surgery in the morning and see patients in the office during the afternoon. The consultation room is larger than for many medical specialties because it is used for consulting with patients. A double-panel X-ray view box should be located near the desk.

In a one-physician practice, one employee can usually run the business office—answering the phone, booking appointments, handling insurance, and billing patients. A three or four-person practice will have an expanded business office with two or more staff performing the tasks of reception, bookkeeping, and insurance.

All rooms of this suite may be carpeted. The decor should be cheerful with warm colors but, above all, it must convey a solid, conservative image due to the nature of the specialty. A patient wants to feel that his or her surgeon is a serious person not subject to frivolities and trendy decor.

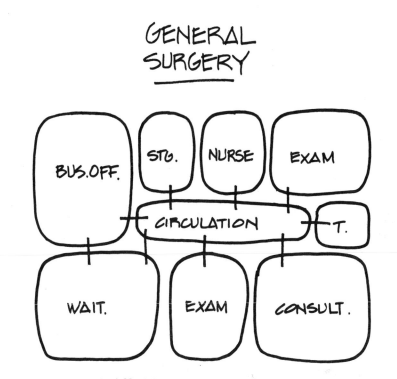

Fig. 4-68. Schematic diagram of a general surgery suite.

Table 4–9. Analysis of Program.
General Surgery

No. of Physicians:	1	2	3
Exam Rooms	2 @ 8 × 12 = 96	3 @ 8 × 12 = 288	5 @ 8 × 12 = 480
Waiting Room	12 × 12 = 144	14 × 14 = 196	14 × 18 = 252
Business Office	12 × 12 = 144	12 × 14 = 168	14 × 18 = 252
Nurse Station	4 × 6 = 24	4 × 6 = 24	6 × 8 = 48
Consultation Rooms	12 × 12 = 144	2 @ 12 × 12 = 288	3 @ 12 × 12 = 432
Toilets	5 × 6 = 30	2 @ 5 × 6 = 60	2 @ 5 × 6 = 60
Storage	4 × 6 = 24	4 × 6 = 24	6 × 8 = 48
Staff Lounge	—	—	10 × 10 = 100
Subtotal	702 ft²	1048 ft²	1672 ft²
15% Circulation	105	157	251
Total	807 ft²	1205 ft²	1923 ft²

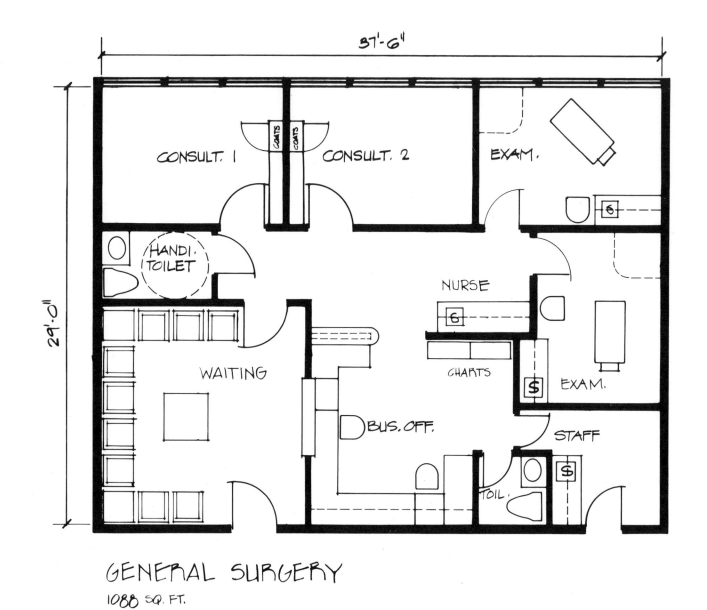

GENERAL SURGERY

1088 SQ. FT.

Fig. 4-69. Suite plan for general surgery, 1088 square feet.

126

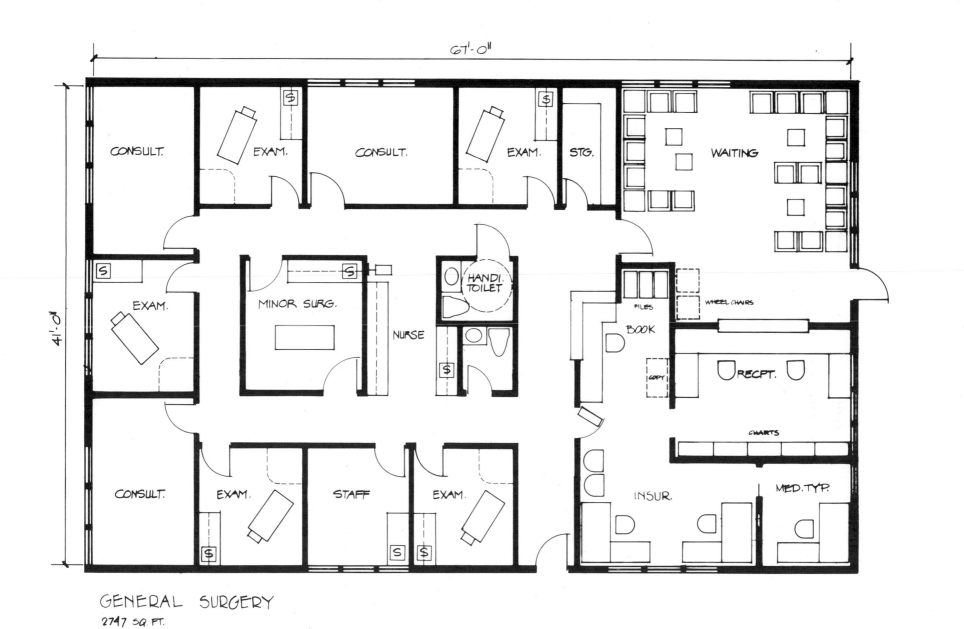

GENERAL SURGERY
2747 SQ. FT.

Fig. 4-70. Suite plan for general surgery, 2747 square feet.

UROLOGY

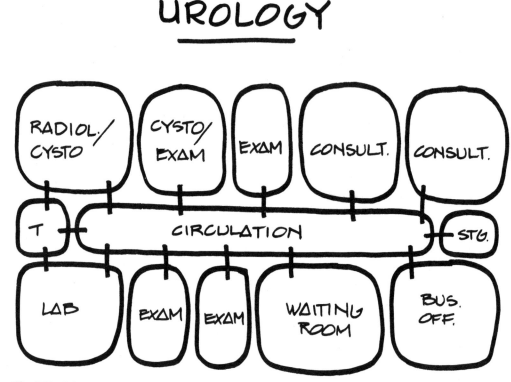

Fig. 4-71. Schematic diagram of a urology suite

A urologist treats diseases of the genitourinary tract. Thus each patient must submit a urine specimen before being examined. The toilet room should be located close to the laboratory and have a *specimen pass-through* (see Chapter 12) to the laboratory. Sometimes a toilet room is located between two exam rooms. Urologists perform most of their own lab work in the suite, and a minimum of 12 lineal feet of countertop should be provided in the laboratory. In addition, a solo practitioner would need two examination rooms, a cystoscopy room, a business office, a waiting room, and a consultation room.

Patient flow is from the waiting room to the bathroom to the exam room, and then to the cysto room if necessary. The components of this suite are standard with the exception of the cystoscopy room. A patient with an inflammation of the urinary bladder would be diagnosed by a cystoscopic procedure to determine the presence of an obstruction or an infection in the urinary tract. The cysto room is often designed as an X-ray room with darkroom, control area, and lead-shielded walls. If the urologist does retrograde cystoscopic examinations he or she will need a room that is equipped for radiography. The reader is referred to Chapter 3 under *General Practice* for details of a X-ray room.

The cysto room should have a ceramic tile floor pitched to a floor drain. If the budget does not permit a ceramic tile floor, a good-quality sheet vinyl flooring with a self-coved base is recommended, pitched to a floor drain. A cysto room not equipped with X-ray may be as small as 11 × 12 or 12 × 12 feet. With X-ray, it will be about 12 × 18 feet including the darkroom, and the room should have a 9-foot ceiling height. Open-shelf filing of X-ray films should be located in the corridor adjacent to the cysto rooms. Cysto rooms often have a 5-foot-high ceramic tile wainscot on all walls and may have a wall-mounted urinal. Furthermore, the room should have an exhaust fan.

It should be noted that some urologists, in deference to their budget, use a bucket for waste disposal instead of a floor drain and vinyl asbestos tile instead of ceramic tile or sheet vinyl on the floor. Likewise, many do not provide a private dressing or recovery area in the cystoscopy room.

There are no special requirements in this specialty in terms of interior design.

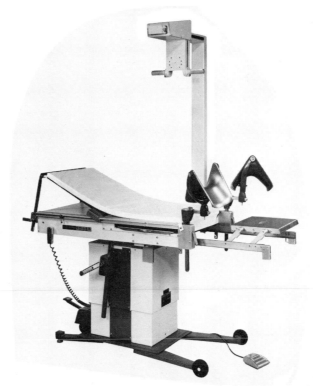

Fig. 4-72. Cystoscopic table. (Courtesy Ritter, Mfg. by Sybron Medical Products Div., Rochester, New York.)

Table 4–10. Analysis of Program. Urology

No. of Physicians:	1	2	3
Business Office	12 × 14 = 168	16 × 18 = 288	16 × 20 = 320
Waiting Room	12 × 16 = 192	12 × 18 = 216	14 × 20 = 280
Toilets	2 @ 5 × 6 = 60	3 @ 5 × 6 = 90	3 @ 5 × 6 = 90
Storage	6 × 8 = 48	6 × 8 = 48	8 × 8 = 64
Consultation Room	12 × 12 = 144	2 @ 12 × 12 = 288	3 @ 12 × 12 = 432
Exam Rooms	2 @ 8 × 12 = 192	4 @ 8 × 12 = 384	6 @ 8 × 12 = 576
Cysto/Exam (no X-ray)	—	12 × 11 = 132	2 @ 12 × 11 = 264
Cysto (with X-ray)[a]	12 × 18 = 216	12 × 18 = 216	12 × 18 = 216
Laboratory	10 × 10 = 100	10 × 10 = 100	10 × 16 = 160
Subtotal	1120 ft²	1762 ft²	2402 ft²
15% Circulation	168	264	360
Total	1288 ft²	2026 ft²	2762 ft²

[a] Includes darkroom, control, film filing and dressing cubicle.

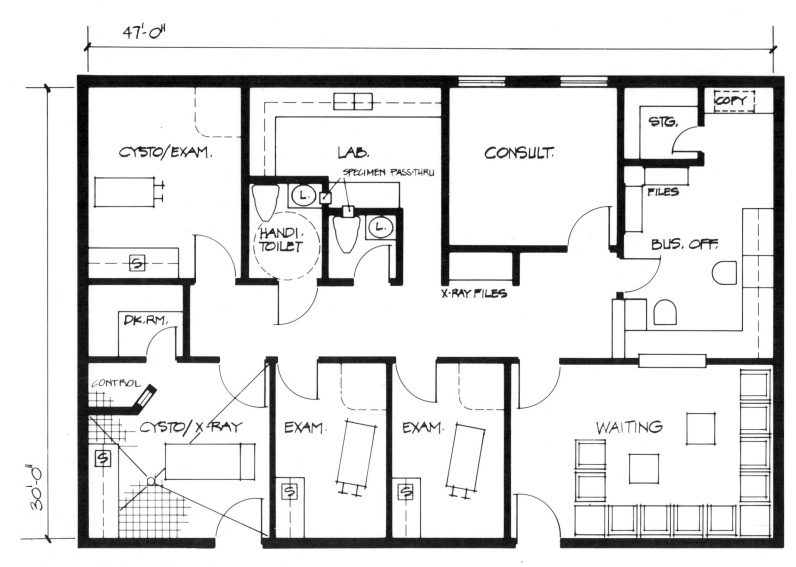

UROLOGY

1410 SQ FT.

Fig. 4-73. Suite plan for urology, 1410 square feet.

130

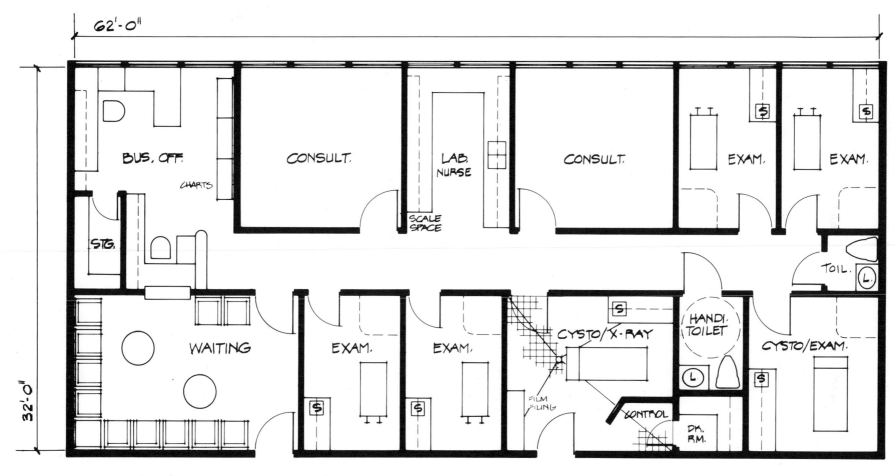

UROLOGY
1984 SQ. FT.

Fig. 4-74. Suite plan for urology, 1984 square feet.

ORTHOPEDIC SURGERY

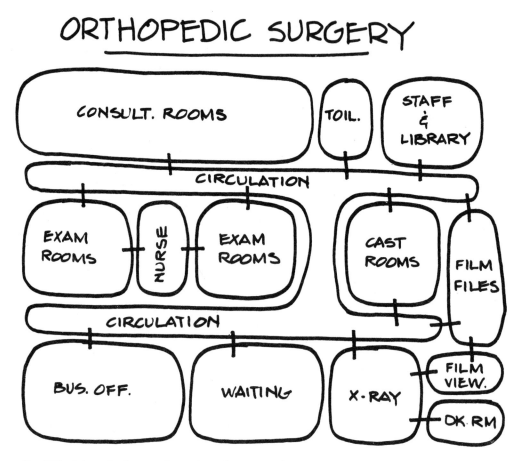

Fig. 4-75. Schematic diagram of an orthopedic surgery suite.

ORTHOPEDIC SURGERY

An orthopedic surgeon deals with diseases, fractures, or malformations of the bones, as well as arthritis, birth defects, industrial accidents, and sports injuries that affect the bones and joints. Some orthopedic surgeons specialize in hand surgery. With a tendency to group in large practices, it is not uncommon to find six or seven physicians working in the same office. Schedules may be arranged so that each doctor performs surgery two days a week and is in the office the balance. Therefore all the surgeons are seldom in the office at once.

A two-physician practice would typically have four exam rooms, one cast room, a small nurses' station, two consultation rooms, a large business office, a large waiting room, a radiology room and darkroom, a toilet room, and a large storage and film filing room. A larger practice might also have a physical therapy room and a staff lounge, additional cast rooms and exam rooms, and a sit-down film viewing area adjacent to the radiology room (Fig. 4-76).

Exam rooms may be as small as 8 × 10 feet (if a dressing area is not desired) since an orthopedist uses a 24 to 27-inch-wide by 72-inch-long table (usually custom built), which is frequently placed against the wall, and he or she usually examines the patient from one side only. Some orthopedists prefer to place the head of the table perpendicular to the wall so that they can walk around three sides of it (Fig. 4-77, Plate 10). The table will frequently have pull-out leaves for examination of limbs, and the lower portion of the table may be closed in for bulk storage. Sometimes there will be a row of drawers built into the table alongside the bulk storage portion of the cabinet. A hand surgeon needs only a desk with a

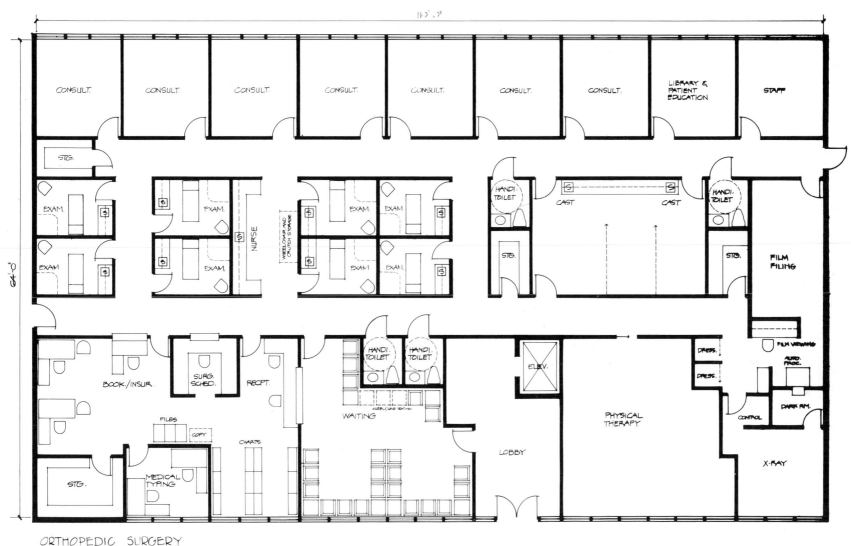

ORTHOPEDIC SURGERY
7040 SQ.FT.

Fig. 4-76. Suite plan for orthopedic surgery, 7040 square feet.

133

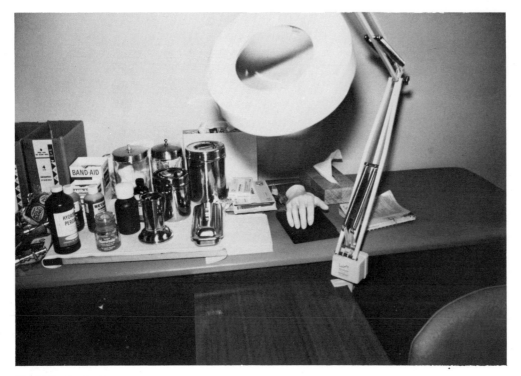

Fig. 4-78. Hand table.

pull-out dictation board (Fig. 4-78). The patient would be seated alongside the desk and place an arm or hand on the desk or pull-out dictation board. Of course, a treatment room or cast room (Fig. 4-79) would still be required for dressing wounds, removing stitches, and building casts. Each exam room and cast room must have a double-panel X-ray film illuminator (Fig. 4-82) recessed in the wall or surface mounted, at a stand-up height (see Appendix).

The cast room will have one full wall of cabinets designed precisely to accommodate the numerous splints, bandages, plaster, and other tools of the trade (Fig. 4-83). The design of a cast cabinet is extremely important to the efficiency of the room. The plaster comes in rolls 2, 3, 4, and 6 inches wide. Slots in the face of the cabinet will permit the rolls to feed through for use by the surgeon. Stockinette may be fed through other slots. Drawers will hold padding, open bins will hold elastic bandages, and one drawer will contain cast tools. A large hinged trash bin should be built into the cabinet if space permits. If possible this bin ought to be vented to the outside since the cast cutoffs have a foul odor. If this is not possible, at least the room should have an exhaust fan. The sink in the cast cabinet should have a single-lever faucet, a gooseneck spout (so that a bucket can be put under it), and a plaster trap. Each orthopedist seems to have a preferred arrangement of drawers, slots, and bins on the cast room cabinet, but all cast cabinets are composed, in one arrangement or another, of the above components (Fig. 4-84). One ought to bear in mind that the surfaces of the cast room must be washable since the room is prey to plaster dust when casts are sawed off and wet drippings when new casts are built. A sheet vinyl floor and vinyl wallcoverings are recommended.

The consultation room will usually be used as the doctor's private office and as a place to return phone calls and to review X-ray films. For this purpose, a two-panel or four-panel illuminated film viewer should be located to the side of or behind the physician at a sit-down height, usually mounted over the credenza (Figs. 4–85 and 4–86).

The cast room(s), radiology room, and film viewing area should be located in proximity to each other (Fig. 4–87). The reader is directed to Chapter 3 under *General Practice* for layout details on an X-ray room, control area, and darkroom. Open shelves (or lateral file cabinets) must be provided for film filing. The shelves should have vertical dividers every 24 inches since the films are heavy and unwieldy and tend to slump over if not packed tightly between divider supports. X-ray jackets (the paper storage envelope) are 14 1/2 × 17 1/2 inches, and the shelves should be shallow enough so that about 2 inches of the film jacket hangs over the edge of the shelf for ease of access.

The corridors of the suite should be 5 to 6 feet wide for easy passage of patients on crutches and in wheelchairs. The corridor is also used as a gait lane. Sometimes a small patient education room is included in the suite. Surgeons are finding it time-saving to purchase videotapes explaining certain frequently performed procedures to patients (inserting a pin in the hip, a plastic knee joint, etc.).

The toilet rooms in this suite must be designed to accommodate the handicapped (see Appendix). The waiting room must be large enough to accommodate people in wheelchairs without ambu-

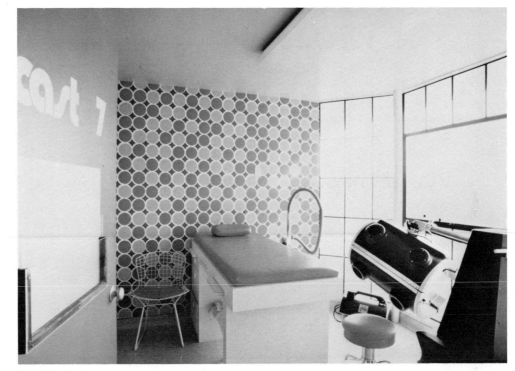

Fig. 4-79. Cast room.

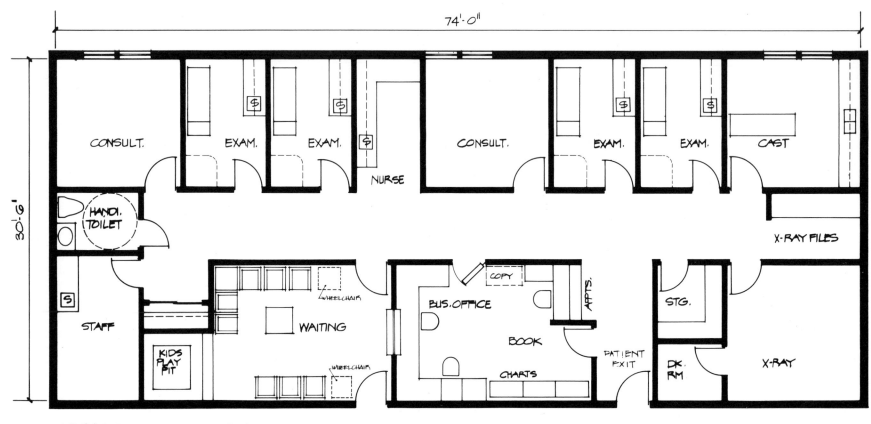

ORTHOPEDIC SURGERY
2257 SQ. FT.

Fig. 4-80. Suite plan for orthopedic surgery, 2257 square feet.

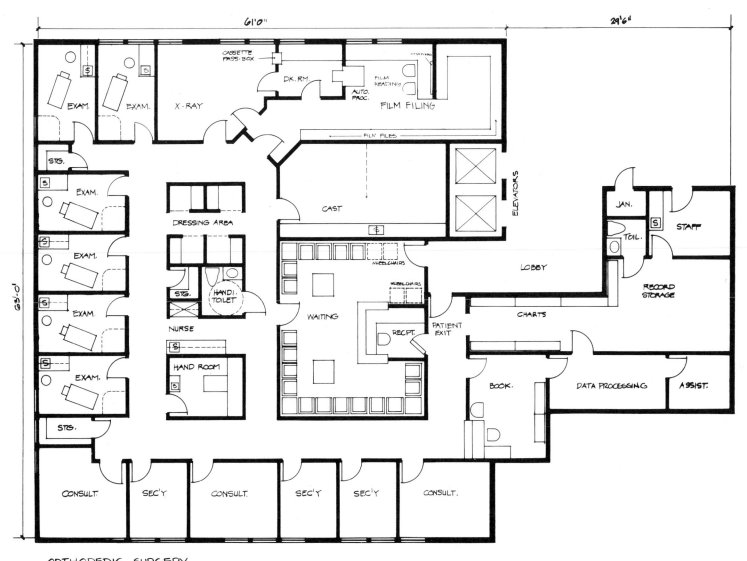

ORTHOPEDIC SURGERY
4464 SQ. FT.

Fig. 4-81. Suite plan for orthopedic surgery, 4175 square feet.

137

Fig. 4-83. Cast room.

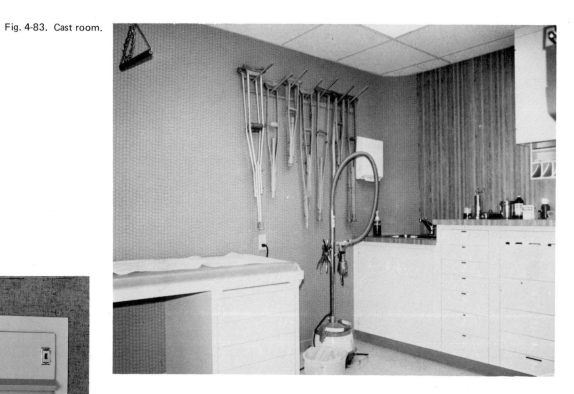

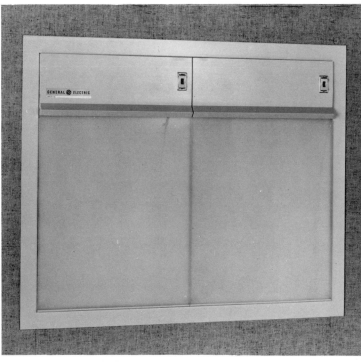

Fig. 4-82. Double-panel view box. (Courtesy General Electric Co., Medical Systems Div.)

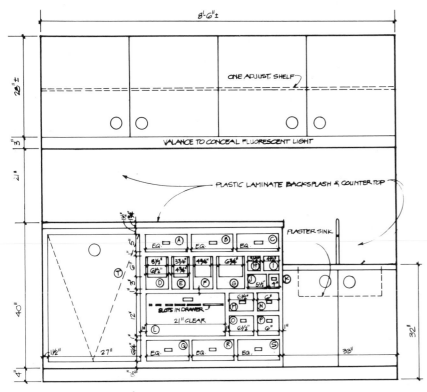

ONE ADJUST. SHELF

VALANCE TO CONCEAL FLUORESCENT LIGHT

PLASTIC LAMINATE BACKSPLASH & COUNTERTOP

PLASTER SINK

SLOTS IN DRAWER

21" CLEAR

EQ.

8'-6"±

28"±

3"

21"

40"

4"

11½"   27"

32"

33"

BASE CABINET IS 24" DEEP
UPPER CABINET IS 12" DEEP

CAST CABINET

Fig. 4-84. Cast cabinet diagram.

DOOR & DRAWER SCHEDULE	
Ⓐ Ⓑ Ⓒ Ⓡ Ⓢ	DRAWERS W/SIDE ROLLERS, ABC MUST HAVE CLEAR DEPTH OF 4" INSIDE
Ⓓ Ⓔ Ⓕ Ⓖ	NO SIDE ROLLERS - BOTTOM DWR. GLIDE ONLY. THESE DRAWERS ARE RARELY OPENED
Ⓗ Ⓘ Ⓙ	OPEN SHELVES FOR SPLINTS (CUBBY HOLES)
Ⓚ	DRAWER FOR 4" BIAS. DRAWER GLIDE ON BOTTOM
Ⓛ	STOCKINETTE DRAWER - SLOT OPENINGS MUST BE SANDED VERY SMOOTHLY. (NO SNAGS)
Ⓜ Ⓝ Ⓞ Ⓟ	DRAWERS FOR PADDING
Ⓣ	TILT-OUT TRASH BIN. (HOLDS LARGE PLASTIC TRASH CAN)

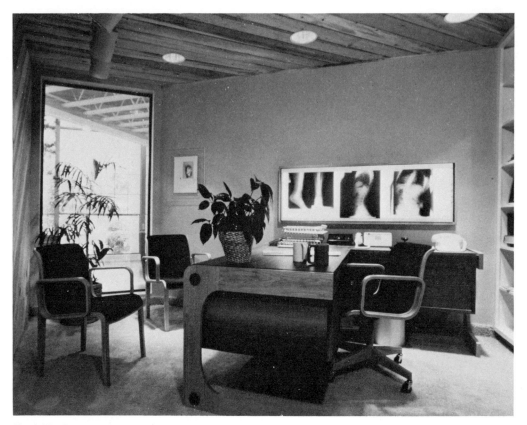

Fig. 4-85. Consultation room.

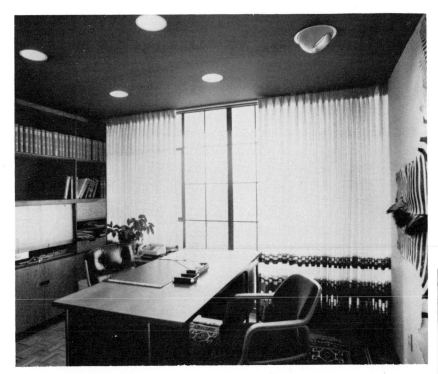

Fig. 4-86. Consultation room.

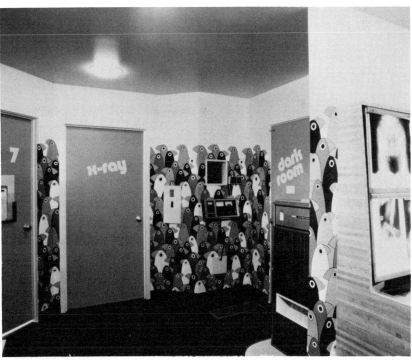

Fig. 4-87. X-ray/cast room area.

141

latory patients tripping over them. Chairs should be firm, with a high seat and with arms to aid an arthritic person, for example, to raise himself or herself out of the chair. The chair should be well balanced to avoid tipping when a patient leans on it for support (see Fig. 4–88, Plate 10).

The interior design of the suite must be pleasing to patients of all ages. Wall decor might include sports photos or perhaps educational exhibits dealing with birth defects, arthritis, or other orthopedic problems. All floors except the cast rooms and X-ray room can be carpeted with a tightly woven level loop commercial carpet glued

to the slab with no pad. Any other type of installation will be unsuitable for wheelchairs and people walking on crutches. A firm feeling underfoot is desirable here.

If the budget allows, the walls (at least the corridor walls) should be covered with commercial wallvinyl since wheelchairs and crutches abuse the walls. Doors should be 3 feet wide on all rooms where patients might be in wheelchairs, although the standard 2-foot 8-inch door often suffices. The door to the X-ray room must be 3 feet wide in order to move in the equipment, and the ceiling height of this room must be at least 9 feet.

Table 4–11. Analysis of Program.
Orthopedic Surgery

No. of Physicians:	2	4	6
Consultation Rooms	2 @ 12 × 12 = 288	4 @ 12 × 12 = 576	6 @ 12 × 12 = 864
Exam Rooms	4 @ 8 × 12 = 384	8 @ 8 × 12 = 768	8 @ 8 × 12 = 768[a]
Cast Rooms	12 × 12 = 144	2 @ 12 × 12 = 288	2 @ 12 × 12 = 288
Business Office	14 × 16 = 224	20 × 20 = 400	20 × 26 = 520
Office Manager	—	10 × 10 = 100	10 × 10 = 100
Toilets[b]	2 @ 5 × 6 = 60	2 @ 5 × 6 = 60	3 @ 5 × 6 = 90
Staff Lounge	8 × 10 = 80	10 × 12 = 120	14 × 16 = 224
Waiting Room	16 × 20 = 320	24 × 30 = 720	24 × 30 = 720
Physical Therapy	—	16 × 20 = 320	20 × 25 = 500
Nurse Station	(Located in corridor circulation area)		
Radiology	10 × 12 = 120	10 × 12 = 120	10 × 12 = 120
Darkroom	4 × 6 = 24	4 × 6 = 24	4 × 6 = 24
Storage and Film Filing	10 × 12 = 120	10 × 12 = 120	12 × 16 = 192
Film Viewing	4 × 6 = 24	4 × 6 = 24	4 × 6 = 24
Subtotal	1788 ft²	3640 ft²	4434 ft²
20% Circulation	358	728	886
Total	2146 ft²	4368 ft²	5320 ft²

[a] In a six-person practice, it is unlikely that more than three or four surgeons would be in the office at the same time.
[b] One toilet room should be equipped for the handicapped.

Chapter 5
Diagnostic Medicine

RADIOLOGY

We are all familiar with the general principles of radiology. A limb is exposed to X-rays that penetrate body tissues, exposing film mounted on a cassette that is positioned on the other side of the limb. Since body tissues absorb different amounts of radiation, bones, fat, gas, etc., make different exposures compared with the surrounding tissues, which allows the observation of internal body parts without pain and with small exposures to radiation. In addition to the examination of limbs, radiology procedures are used to diagnose the presence of gallstones and kidney stones, tuberculosis, arthritis, and bone tumors; to discover foreign bodies in soft tissue and enlarged or malfunctioning glands; to scan the brain, to reduce tumors (radiation oncology); to monitor a child in the womb (ultrasound); and to diagnose dozens of other diseases. (See Fig. 5–1.)

Making an X-ray film of a limb or the chest requires no special preparation, but filming organs such as the gallbladder or the gastrointestinal tract require that the patient fast before the procedure and then drink a special liquid or receive an injection that makes the organs visible to the radiologist. Since the designer must understand such procedures in order to plan an efficient suite, a brief outline of diagnostic radiology techniques follows.

Fluoroscopy

Fluoroscopy enables the radiologist to watch internal body structures at work. The patient swallows or receives an injection of a contrast medium—air, barium sulfate, or organic iodine compounds—which causes the soft tissue systems of the body to be outlined. X-rays passed through to body cast shadows on a fluorescent screen that is held by the radiologist. If the equipment includes an image intensifier and a cine camera, the screen images can be converted into a motion picture for future study or reference.

Contrast media injected into a blood vessel (angiography) travels with the blood supply to a specific organ and allows the radiologist to determine the health of that organ. For a study of the large intestine, a patient is given a barium enema. The radiologist makes sequential radiographs while the barium travels through the large intestine. After the patient eliminates, further films

RADIOLOGY

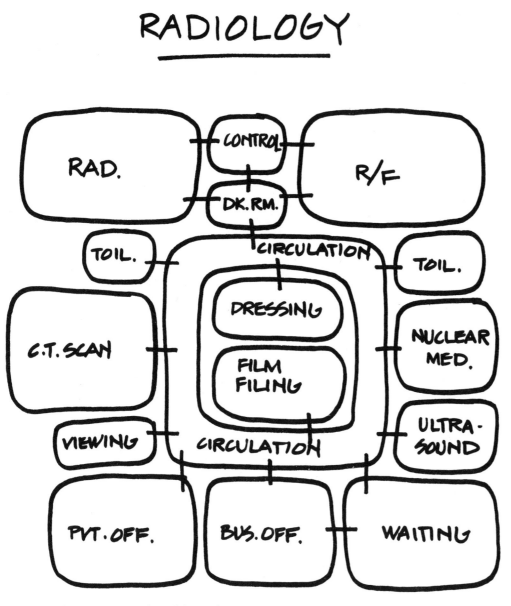

Fig. 5-1. Schematic diagram of a radiology suite.

are made. To study the digestive system, the radiologist performs gastrointestinal studies. A patient drinks barium and the radiologist makes films of it as it travels to the intestines.

Ultrasound

Ultrasound does not involve radiation. A high-frequency sound bounces off internal body structures much like sonar. Ultrasound is particularly useful in examining soft pelvic tissue masses, gallbladders, and fetuses in the womb—procedures where even low doses of radiation might be dangerous.

Nuclear Medicine

Nuclear medicine deals with the diagnosis and treatment of disease with radioactive isotopes—chemicals that are unstable and break down, giving off radioactivity. The isotope may be given to the patient orally or by injection. The substance is specific to a particular gland or organ (for example, iodine travels to the thyroid gland). The amount of the isotope absorbed by the gland permits the radiologist to determine the function of the organ and to trace its outline. Nuclear scans are useful for diagnosing brain tumors and malfunctioning of the kidneys, pancreas, and thyroid.

Computerized Tomography

Computerized Axial Tomography (CAT) is perhaps the most revolutionary diagnostic tool since the advent of radiography. Slices of tissue are scanned in a noninvasive procedure that is painless and risk-free. The patient lies on a table that slides through a rotating doughnutlike enclosure. X-rays scan narrow cross sections of the body—as many as 180 scans just one degree apart may be taken of an area. The numerous images are collected by a detector and reconstructed by a computer into a composite scan of the organ or tissue. The ability to see cross sections of internal body structures enables the radiologist to discover tumors embedded in soft tissue or organs which, until now, could not be seen by radiographic procedures. CAT scans have eliminated much exploratory surgery and offer the patient greater safety by reducing the need for more dangerous, often painful, tests.

Electron Radiography

This is a new technique not yet in wide usage. The patient lies on a table and X-rays are sent through the body into a gas chamber (in the table under the patient) instead of onto film. Gas particles are broken down and form an image on a plastic sheet.

Components of a Radiology Suite

1. Business Office
2. Waiting Room
3. Patient Dressing
4. Film Viewing and Consultation
5. Film Processing
6. Radiography Rooms

Business Office. The business office can be small since this is a referral practice and a patient's medical record remains with the referring physician. The radiologist stores only the X-ray films and a brief report on each patient.

Waiting Room. Allow 2.5 waiting room seats per

radiography room and provide a suitable space out of the traffic lane for a patient in a wheelchair. At times a patient may be brought in on a stretcher or a gurney. This should be taken into account when laying out the space. A 2 × 6-foot stretcher must be able to be wheeled from the waiting room (or a private staff entrance) through the corridor and into a radiography room without causing damage to walls and needlessly jostling the patient.

Patient Dressing. Allow two dressing rooms for each radiographic room. The rooms can be as small as 3 feet wide × 4 feet deep, but they should have a chair or built-in bench, a mirror, a shelf for disposable gowns, and one or two hooks for clothing (Fig. 5–2, Plate 11). Sometimes the rooms have a buzzer for summoning the staff. In a small clinic patients will leave their clothing in the dressing rooms, which are usually closed off only by a drapery and are not locked. In larger clinics sufficient dressing rooms are provided so that patients can lock their personal effects in the dressing rooms, or else lockers may be located outside of the dressing rooms where clothing and handbags may be stored, so as to not prevent others from using the dressing rooms. The dressing area should be carpeted since patients may be walking barefoot. It is advisable to make one dressing booth double width so that the bench is long enough to serve as a recovery cot in case a patient feels ill. This oversized dressing room also accommodates a patient in a wheelchair. (An alternative plan is to have a removable partition between two standard-size dressing booths and a folding bench that drops down to become the recovery cot.)

Film Viewing and Consultation. View box illum-

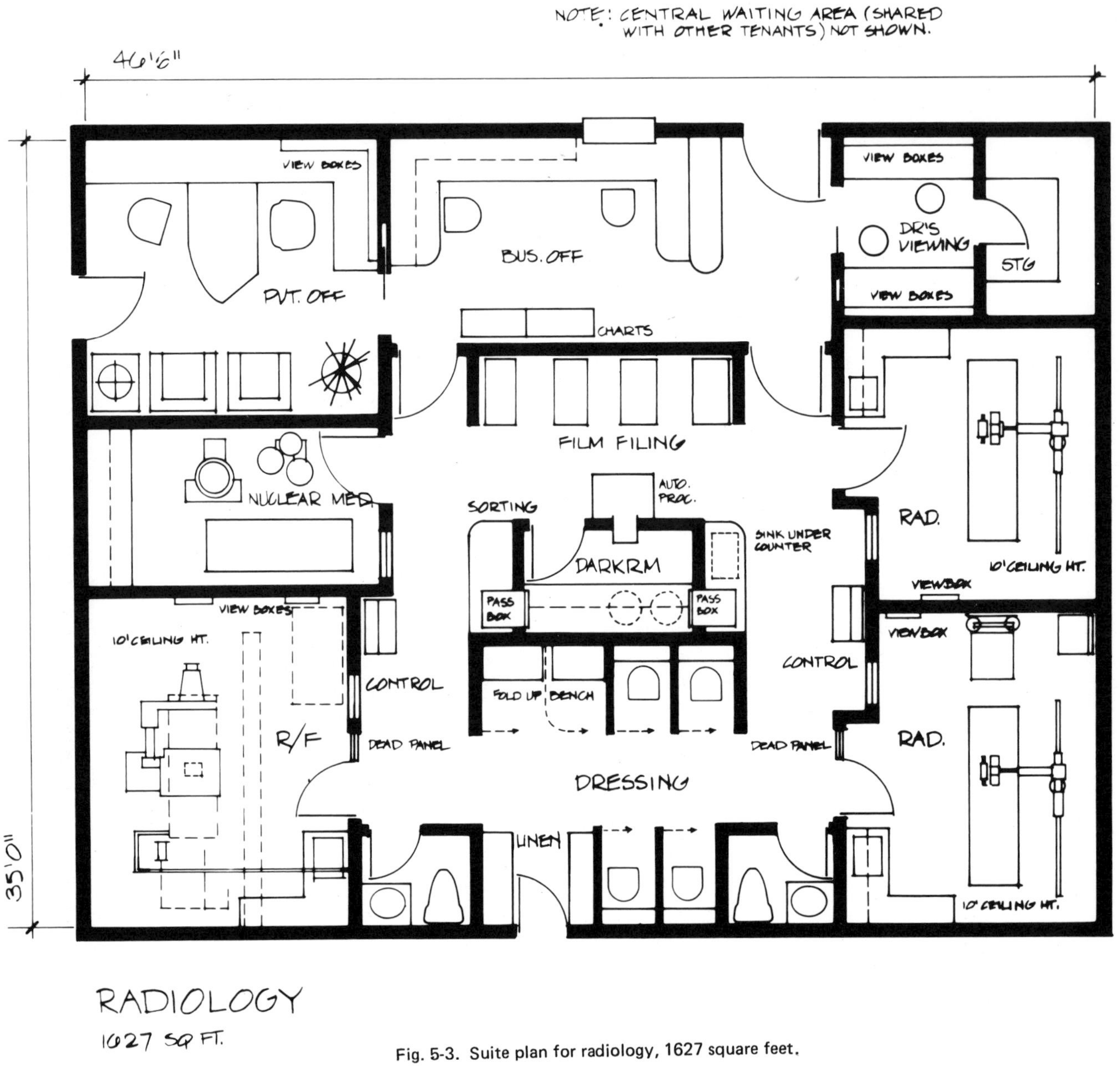

NOTE: CENTRAL WAITING AREA (SHARED WITH OTHER TENANTS) NOT SHOWN.

46'6"

35'0"

VIEW BOXES

PVT. OFF.

BUS. OFF.

VIEW BOXES

DR'S VIEWING

STG

VIEW BOXES

CHARTS

FILM FILING

NUCLEAR MED.

SORTING

AUTO. PROC.

SINK UNDER COUNTER

DARKRM

RAD.

10' CEILING HT.

VIEW BOXES

10' CEILING HT.

PASS BOX

PASS BOX

VIEWBOX

CONTROL

VIEWBOX

CONTROL

R/F

DEAD PANEL

FOLD UP BENCH

DEAD PANEL

RAD.

DRESSING

LINEN

10' CEILING HT.

RADIOLOGY

1627 SQ. FT.

Fig. 5-3. Suite plan for radiology, 1627 square feet.

146

inators will be required in several places. Usually a two-panel unit at stand-up height will suffice for the technician's use while checking films as they come out of the processor and for sorting them (Fig. 4–82). These view boxes should be located at the discharge side of the processor or darkroom. (See Appendix for mounting heights of view boxes.) Sometimes the film reading area is an alcove off the corridor near the consultation room (Fig. 5–3). Space for a minimum of eight illuminator panels should be provided at sit-down height. The illuminators should be mounted over a plastic laminate countertop (Fig. 5–4). Under the countertop would be compartments for sorting films.

In addition to this viewing area the radiologist will usually have 8 to 16 illuminator panels in the consultation room (four over four or perhaps eight over eight) mounted on the wall behind and to the side of the desk, with a sorting shelf underneath (Fig. 5–5). Each radiography room may have a one-panel or two-panel illuminator as well.

The consultation room is used as a private office. The radiologist does not consult with patients, but he or she does consult with referring physicians. This may take place in the consultation room or in the film reading alcove. A sophisticated radiology suite may provide closed circuit T.V. in the film reading/viewing room. This is an aid to referring physicians who may wish to observe a fluoroscopic procedure in progress. The film reading alcove or doctors' viewing room should be located near the radiologist's office for ease of consultation. It should also be positioned near the front of the suite so that the doctors do not have to intrude upon the functional flow of patients. Since the front of the suite is the administrative area, this also gives the conferring

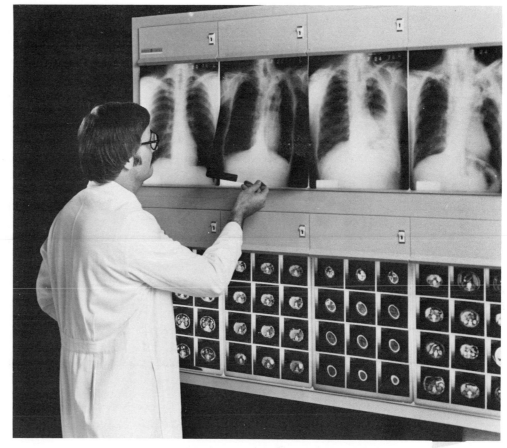

Fig. 5-4. Six over six view boxes. (Courtesy General Electric Co., Medical Systems Div.)

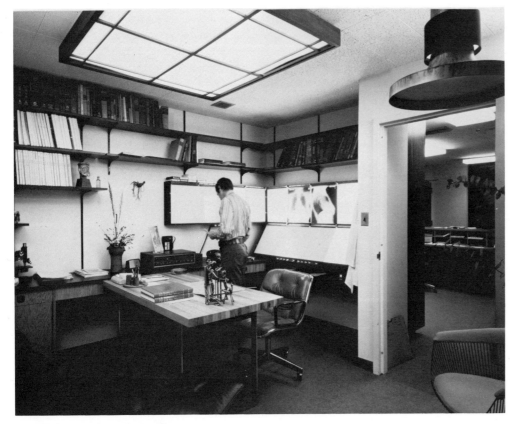

Fig. 5-5. Radiologist's private office.

physicians more privacy—there is less likelihood that diagnostic discussions will be overheard by patients.

Sufficient storage for X-ray films must be provided in lateral file cabinets. The films are placed in color-coded paper jackets and stored on open shelves for easy retrieval (Fig. 5-6).

Film Processing. Modern darkrooms contain automatic developers or "processors," but they may also contain manual tanks as an added precaution in case the processor fails. Some technicians feel it is not necessary to provide manual tanks with an automatic processor because, if the automatic processor breaks down and the technician starts to develop films manually, the exposures are so different from the automatic that it takes half a day to become accustomed to them. Thus it is better to shut down for a few hours until the serviceman arrives. Normally service is quite speedy on this type of equipment.

The size and design of the darkroom and processing area depends somewhat on the equipment, the number and arrangement of radiographic rooms around it, and the volume of film to be processed. In any case, there would be a "wet" side and a "dry" side. The wet side is where the developer and washing tanks are located. With manual processing, space must be allocated on the wet side for the developer and washing tanks, developer and fixer replenisher storage tanks, drying frames or an automatic film dryer, and bottles of chemicals. With an automatic processor, space must be allocated for replenisher tanks and a large sink for washing the rollers. Once a week the rollers have to be removed from the processor and cleaned. This sink may be located in the darkroom or outside of it, and near the side of the processor from which the rollers are removed. A sink 30 inches wide × 8 inches deep is adequate, and if provided with a hinged plastic laminate top, it may double as a work surface when not in use as a sink.

The automatic processor (Fig. 5–7) may be located inside the darkroom or, more commonly, outside the darkroom feeding through a light-sealed opening in the wall into the darkroom. The processor requires a 3 or 4-inch-diameter floor drain, a vent to the outside for the film dryer component, and a thermostatically controlled water supply. (Manual tanks also require a thermostatically controlled water supply.)

The dry side of the darkroom is where the film storage bin is located and where cassettes are loaded with film. One or more cassette pass boxes will be built into the wall for the transfer of unexposed and exposed film cassettes. Since these are very heavy lead-lined boxes, the wall in which they will be supported will require reinforcement. The pass box or boxes will be located in the wall of the darkroom closest to or contiguous with the radiography rooms (Fig. 5–8). If the darkroom is not contiguous with the radiography rooms (Fig. 5–3), the pass boxes would be located on a darkroom wall accessible to the radiography room corridor.

A darkroom should have two sources of light. A 100-watt incandescent fixture, either recessed or surface mounted to the ceiling, will serve for normal work, but a red safelight must be provided for work with exposed film. The safelight can be plugged into an outlet at 60 to 72 inches off the floor, and it can work by a pull chain or be wired to a wall switch. If the latter, the switch should be located away from the incandescent light switch so that the technician does not accidentally hit

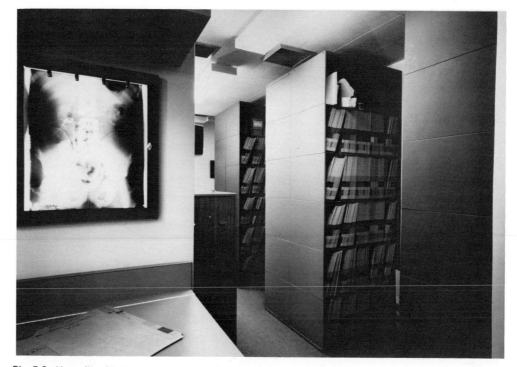

Fig. 5-6. X-ray film filing.

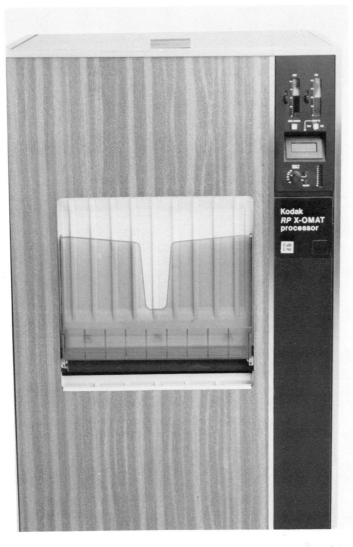

Fig. 5-7. X-OMAT automatic processor. (Courtesy Eastman Kodak Co.)

the wrong switch while working with exposed film. Any recessed light fixtures and the exhaust fan must have a light-sealed housing. Similarly, the darkroom door must have a light seal. Codes in some cities require a lightproof louver ventilation panel in the darkroom door.

Countertop work surfaces in a darkroom may be at a 36-inch or 42-inch height, depending on personal preference. A 6 to 10-inch deep shelf mounted at 12 to 14 inches above the countertop is convenient for storing bottles of chemicals. There is no need for "closed" storage in a darkroom. All shelves should be open shelves. It should be noted that the walls of darkrooms need not be dark. In fact, many technicians prefer white walls.

Acid-resistant waste piping should be used in a darkroom, and the waste lines should have vacuum breakers. It is imperative to have some system of warning to let people know when someone is in the darkroom. This can be accomplished with a red warning light over the door which is activated whenever developing is in process.

Radiography & Fluoroscopy. Not all radiography rooms are equipped for fluoroscopy. A diagnostic X-ray suite may have two radiography rooms and one radiography & fluoroscopy combination room or perhaps one radiography room and two R & F rooms. The R & F room should be at least 12 × 15 feet and must be close to a toilet. The toilet may have a door to the R & F room and another door to the corridor (Fig. 5–8). In a busy practice this presents problems, since a patient entering the toilet from the corridor may, by mistake, exit through the door to the R & F room while the machine is in use. Special hardware that locks the toilet door from the R & F room side solves

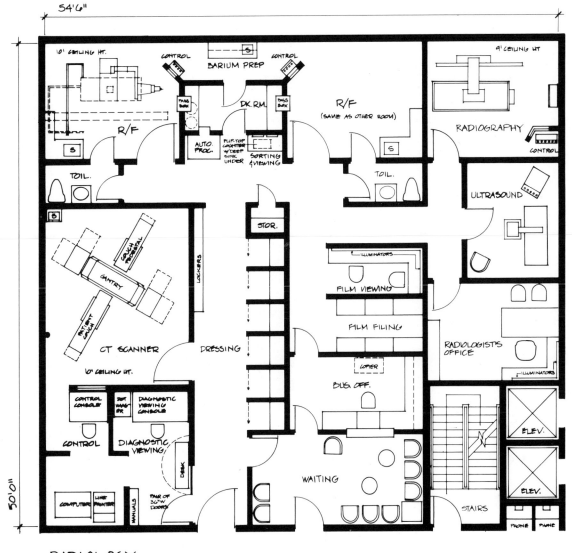

RADIOLOGY
2522 SQ. FT.

Fig. 5-8. Suite plan for radiology, 2522 square feet.

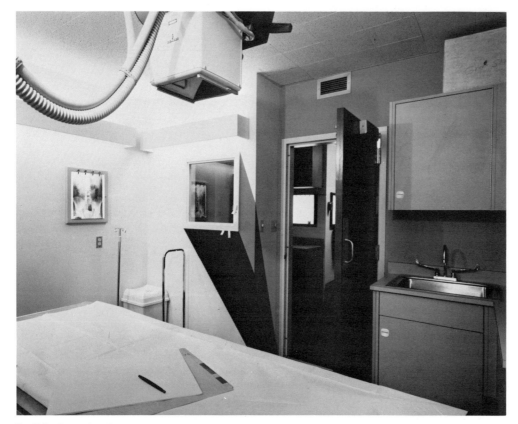

Fig. 5-9. General radiology room.

this problem provided the technician always remembers to lock to door, but it does not solve the problem of the toilet room being occupied when the patient in the R & F room has to discharge an enema. Thus, although one occasionally sees this sort of room layout in R & F suites, the author does not recommend it in a high-volume practice. Alternatives are a shared toilet room between two R & F rooms (this is satisfactory provided that two patients are not scheduled simultaneously for procedures that require access to the bathroom) or a separate toilet room for each R & F room.

In addition to a toilet room, an R & F room must have a barium prep area or "kitchen," which is a countertop with a double-compartment sink and plaster trap for preparation of barium or contrast media and an under-counter refrigerator. The R & F room should have at least a 9-foot ceiling height. All lighting should be controlled by dimmers (preferably a fluorescent light valance around the perimeter of the room as in Fig. 5–9), and the door of the room must be weatherstripped for light leaks. The walls and door must have lead shielding, the thickness and location of which will have been specified by a radiation physicist. The physicist will prepare a radiation study based upon the type of equipment in use, the volume of films produced daily, and the location of the room within the suite and within the medical office building. The physicist's recommendations must be strictly followed lest the architect or designer be held responsible should the room fail to meet the required standards. A lead-lined door is very heavy and will require a door closer. The door to a radiography room should be at least 3 feet wide with a 4-foot frame and a 1-foot dead panel (lead lined) that can be removed when equipment has to be brought into or removed from the room.

The size of a radiographic room will vary in accordance with the size of the X-ray machine and the ancillary equipment. A fluoroscopy room with an image intensifier, for example, must be larger than one without it. A radiography room without fluoroscopy should be a minimum of 11 × 13 feet, but 12 × 14 feet is better. If the room is to be used by a technician only (as is true with orthopedic and urology procedures, for example) the room can be smaller than if it is used by the radiologist, since he or she may be doing special procedures that require more than one person to be in the room and perhaps more portable equipment.

Manufacturers of X-ray equipment will supply spec sheets and suggested room layouts for their equipment. These spec sheets give the critical distances between various components and specify the required electrical and plumbing. There must be conduit connecting the control unit to the tube stand and the transformer. It should be noted that there are literally dozens of radiology accessory items that have to be accommodated in one way or another in the suite. These items are too numerous to detail or photograph; thus the reader would do well to obtain a radiology supply catalog that contains photos, dimensions, and electrical specifications on hundreds of items that may be used in a radiology practice. The book published by General Electric Co., Medical Systems Division is a particularly good reference.

Radiography rooms without fluoroscopy need not have sinks, but they still should have a built-in cabinet and shelves for storage of sandbags, foam supports, measuring devices used with the X-ray machinery, and disposable items needed

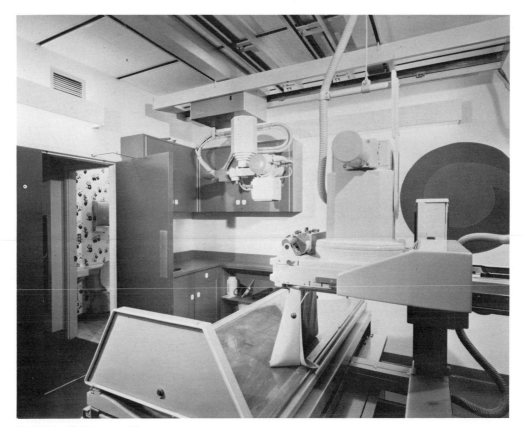

Fig. 5-10. Radiology and fluoroscopy room.

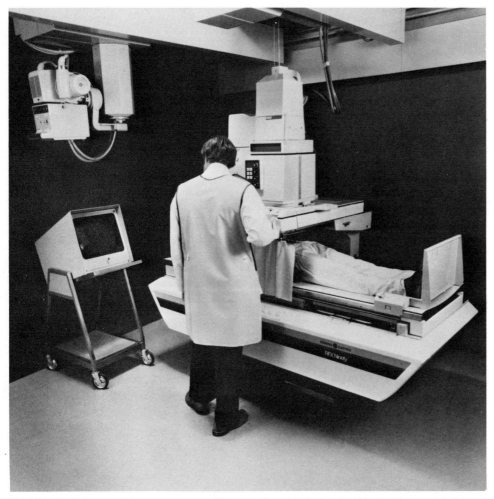

Fig. 5-11. Radiology and fluoroscopy room. (Courtesy General Electric Co., Medical Systems Div.)

154

for procedures. As an aside, some radiologists request emergency call buzzers in the procedure rooms and sometimes in the dressing rooms and toilet rooms. The annunciator panel would be located at the receptionist's desk.

Control Area. Note, when laying out radiographic rooms, that *the tables tilt so that the right side goes down and left up when one is standing on the working side.* The control area, then, should be on the right end so that the technician can see the patient at all times. Figure 5–8 shows a frequently utilized layout with two radiography rooms on either side of the darkroom. The problem with this, although it is convenient with respect to the darkroom, pass boxes, and barium prep, is that a right-handed and a left-handed room have been created. The R & F room on the right puts the technician behind the patient's head. The control area may be outside the radiography room (Fig. 5–3) behind a lead-shielded wall (the operator or technician looks through a lead-shielded window at the patient) or it may actually be in the radiography room (Fig. 5–8), provided the control partition and window are lead shielded. Prefabricated lead-lined control partitions and lead-shielded windows may be purchased from X-ray supply dealers and are illustrated in the aforementioned catalog.

If the control area is outside the room, the designer may wish to provide for a lead-lined speaking grille (or a microphone in the control room and loudspeakers in the R & F rooms) in the wall to enable the technician to communicate instructions to the patient. As a safety precaution, the control console may be wired to a red signal light outside of each radiography room to prevent entry when the machine is in use.

Dark Adaptation. A topic seldom considered by space planners is the problem of dark adaptation in a diagnostic radiology suite. Patients travel from the high illumination of the waiting room to the low illumination of the R & F rooms. And the technicians must retain their dark adaptation as they go back and forth from the darkroom to the R & F room and between fluoroscopic examinations in spite of the doors' being opened. A solution is to equip the corridors with a secondary lighting source of red bulbs to facilitate dark adaptation. If this is not within the scope of the project, the normal corridor lighting should at least be dimmer controlled. One does not want a high level of illumination in the corridors, dressing areas, R & F rooms, or adjacent toilet rooms. (See Figs. 5–10 and 5–11.)

It should be noted that radiography machinery, particularly R & F units, is visually intimidating. There are lots of cables and clutter at the ceiling and the equipment virtually dwarfs the individual. It seems to fill the whole room. The designer ought to make every attempt to balance the weight of the equipment with colorful wallgraphics which distract the patient and make the equipment less noticeable. In fact, the high-tech design of radiography machinery lends itself to a space-age type of decorative treatment. Mylar wallcovering (Fig. 5–12) lends an interesting effect, mirroring the equipment in a subdued way but one would not want to actually mirror a wall.

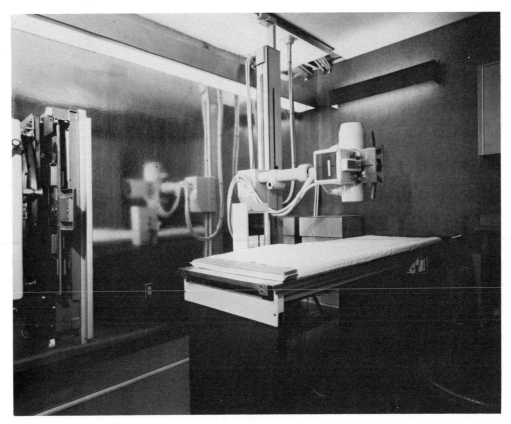

Fig. 5-12. General radiology and special procedures room.

155

Ultrasound

Since ultrasound does not utilize radiation, there is no need for lead shielding. The room need be only 10 × 12 feet in size with a 3-foot door. The patient lies on a standard gurney cart. The equipment consists of a portable console, approximately 24 × 36 × 48 inches high, which contains the computer and a mobile scanner arm unit (Fig. 5–13). The equipment usually has no special lighting or electrical requirements other than a clean line—a separate circuit. The room is darkened for the procedure.

Nuclear Medicine

This room needs to be approximately 10 × 14 feet and it need not be lead shielded. Only the isotopes need shielding, and these may be stored on the countertop with protection provided by a lead screen or lead bricks. Nuclear scan equipment varies significantly in size and number of components from manufacturer to manufacturer. Some units will fit in a room as narrow as 7 feet wide. The technician remains in the room with the patient. Since the procedure involves a measurement of the amount of the isotope that has been absorbed by the gland or organ under study (a detector measures the radiation), there is no danger of radiation to the technician. The room should have a 4 or 5-foot-long countertop with small sink and storage below. The patient lies on a gurney or stretcher cart. Special power requirements should be verified with the manufacturer of the equipment. An interesting treatment, *relevant art,* is illustrated in Fig. 5–14, Plate 11. A 4 × 5-inch thyroid scan has been blown up to 8 × 10 feet and applied to the wall like wallpaper. The patient probably thinks it is abstract art, but the physicians who pass by and glance in the window get a kick out of seeing a giant thyroid scan.

Computerized Axial Tomography

The CAT suite consists of a *scanner* or *procedure room,* an *equipment room,* a *control room,* and a *diagnostic viewing room.* Since this equipment is very complex it is necessary to follow the manufacturer's recommendations for layout. Manufacturers will supply an engineering data sheet with line drawings of each piece of equipment, dimensions, and power requirements. A floor plan will indicate the optimum room layouts and critical relationships between components.

The *procedure room* is where the scanner gantry is located. The patient is positioned on a table that slides back and forth under a rotating doughnut like enclosure (Fig. 5–15). The gantry is a large, highly sophisticated piece of machinery that nearly fills the room and takes weeks to install. The size of the procedure room will vary with different brands of equipment, but 15 × 20 or 18 × 20 is an average. In addition to the gantry, the room needs a built-in work surface with a sink and properly designed storage for the various accessories used in CAT procedures. Again, accessories vary with the manufacturer, but some of these items are: large water-filled Plexiglas calibration disks called "phantoms," which are used each morning to calibrate the scanner (these are awkward and delicate and apt to be stepped on or be knocked off a countertop if not properly stored), foam wedges and blocks, arm supports, head and shoulder restraints, upholstered cradle pads, and phantom holder assembly. The author has designed pull-out shelves lined with commercial (antistatic) carpet for storage of the calibration phantoms. Drawers should be partitioned for storage of alcohol preps, disposable syringes, injectibles, contrast media, tubes, tape, vomit pan, etc.

The ceiling of the room should be at least 9 feet high and the door should be 4 feet wide with a heavy-duty closer. The walls will have to be lead

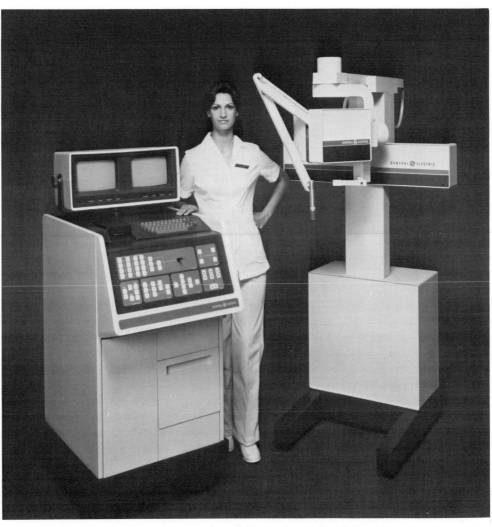

Fig. 5-13. Ultrasound equipment. (Courtesy General Electric Co., Medical Systems Div.)

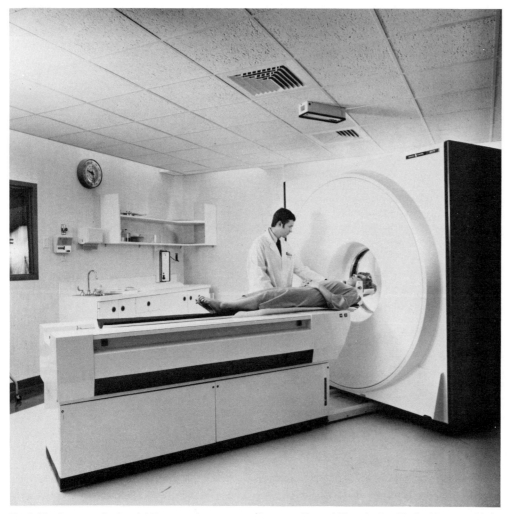

Fig. 5-15. Computerized Axial Tomography scanner. (Courtesy General Electric Co., Medical Systems Div.)

shielded according to the recommendations of the radiation physicist's study. The lighting in this room must be controlled by a dimmer. A valance of fluorescent lighting around the perimeter of the room will keep the glare out of the patient's eyes. The mass of equipment in this room is frightening to patients. A room with cheerful colors and a mural or artwork on the walls would do much to allay patients' fears.

The *equipment room* is where the computer is located. Some manufacturers recommend that this be a separate room which must be air conditioned and humidity controlled. Others locate the computer equipment in an alcove of the control room. Depending on the manufacturer, the equipment requires an area 6 × 8 to 8 × 10 feet. The room should be well illuminated since this is where a technician will have to work when the unit needs service. Some manufacturers recommend a raised computer floor for this room and for the control room so that the technician has ready access to the electrical cables for repairs.

The *control room* is where the operator or technician sits during the procedure. It must have a window facing the procedure room so that the patient is always in view. The control console and usually a writing surface (a small desk or countertop) are located in this room. The dimmer control for the procedure room lighting should be accessible from the control room. Although the size of this room depends upon the brand of equipment, 8 × 10 feet is usually adequate.

The *diagnostic viewing room* contains the viewing console from which the radiologist works. This unit is approximately 3 × 5 or 3 × 6 feet in size. Usually another piece of equipment will be located in the room as well. From this console the radiologist can recall scans from the computer's memory, and he or she can manipulate the image by changing contrast or by enlarging or reducing it in order to study the diseased organ more closely. After the scanner has scanned the patient's tissue, the multiple images are reconstructed by the computer and appear as a film printout on the diagnostic viewing console. It is here that the radiologist makes the diagnosis. Alongside the viewing console, or at right angles to it, should be a built-in work surface with multiple X-ray view boxes mounted above it and film sorting compartments below it. An area of 10 × 12 feet would be adequate for most diagnostic viewing rooms. Lighting should be variable—high for most uses but dim when maximum contrast with film illuminators is desired.

Storage for tapes and floppy disks should be planned in either the equipment room or the control room. A small bookcase for technical manuals may be located in the control room or the viewing room. There are many optional components marketed with the CAT scanner. Some suites have only the basic equipment and others have all the options as well, necessitating large rooms to accommodate it all.

Interior Design

Most diagnostic radiology suites are brutally clinical in appearance. Every effort should be made to make these suites cheerful and to distract the patients' attention from the massive equipment, the maze of cables, and the stainless steel surfaces which are cold to the touch. It takes great thought and imagination to render such spaces humane—to soften them through the use of color, lighting, carpet, wallcoverings, and artwork. The patients should be protected

Table 5-1. Analysis of Program. Radiology

No. of Physicians:	1		2-3	
Waiting Room	12 × 16 =	192	14 × 18 =	252
Business Office	12 × 12 =	144	12 × 16 =	192
Dressing Booths	5 @ 3 × 4 =	60	10 @ 3 × 4 =	120
Radiography Rooms	12 × 14 =	168	12 × 14 =	168
Radiography and Fluoroscopy Rooms	12 × 16 =	192	2 @ 12 × 16 =	384
Barium Prep Area	5 × 6 =	30	5 × 6 =	30
Ultrasound	10 × 12 =	120	10 × 12 =	120
Nuclear Medicine	10 × 14 =	140	10 × 14 =	140
CAT Scanner Suite[a]	—		18 × 40 =	720
Toilets	2 @ 5 × 6 =	60	2 @ 5 × 6 =	60
Darkroom and Processing	8 × 12 =	96	8 × 12 =	96
Film Filing	6 × 12 =	72	12 × 12 =	144
Private Office	12 × 12 =	144	3 @ 12 × 12 =	432
Viewing Area	6 × 8 =	48	6 × 8 =	48
Subtotal		1466 ft^2		2906 ft^2
15% Circulation		220		436
Total		1686 ft^2		3342 ft^2

[a] Includes procedure, equipment, control, and diagnostic viewing rooms.
Note: The above is an approximation since radiography rooms must also have control areas which may be inside or outside the room and many radiologists do not have a CAT scanner. Some may have both a private office and a viewing area, others only a private office which also serves then as the viewing area for conferring with physicians.

LABORATORY

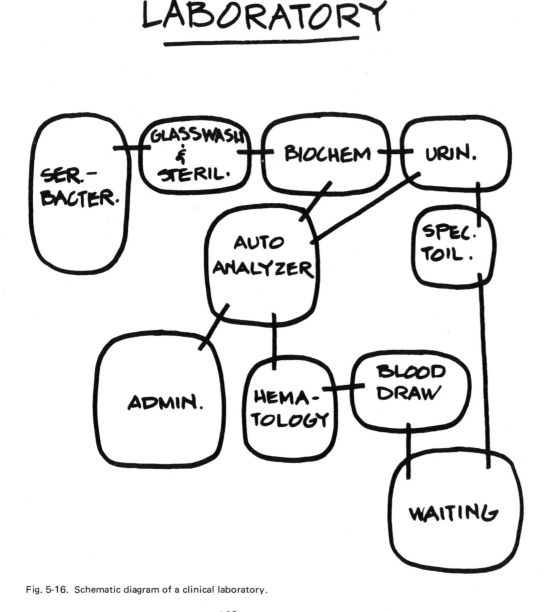

Fig. 5-16. Schematic diagram of a clinical laboratory.

and given as much privacy as the design will allow so that they do not have to wander half-naked in their paper gowns from the dressing rooms to the radiographic rooms. Such distances should be as short as possible. Walking barefoot on a cold tile floor increases the patient's anxiety, and such discomfort is really unnecessary when there are such inexpensive yet durable and easy-to-clean commercial carpets on the market today. It is particularly important to select a carpet that is permanently antistatic since this suite contains so much sensitive electronic equipment. equipment.

Note: For requirements of small X-ray rooms as found in orthopedic, urology, or general practice suites, the reader is referred to Chapter 3 under *General Practice.*

CLINICAL LABORATORY

Laboratory tests are a vital tool in diagnosing disease. A basic part of a thorough examination, these studies may be performed in a small room within the physician's office or in a sophisticated clinical laboratory within a medical office building. Or the lab may be located in an adjacent hospital. A physician may take a blood or urine specimen from a patient but send it out for processing. Others will do simple tests in the office, but send out the more complicated ones. It is unlikely, however, that a *large* clinical lab will be included in a medical office building if that building is adjacent to a hospital. The designer of a medical office building will most often encounter small clinical labs. Large labs, employing a pathologist, will normally be designed by a specialist who is experienced in the organization and efficient utilization of trained personnel and the physical requirements of large clinical

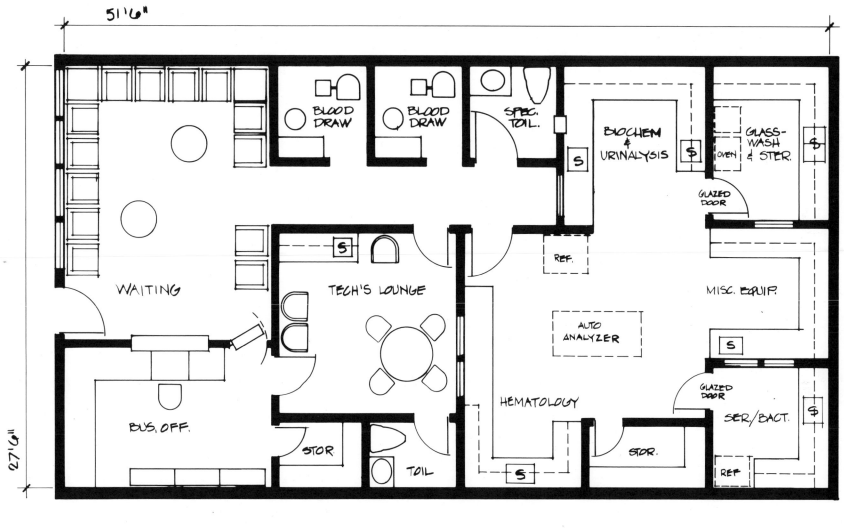

CLINICAL LABORATORY

1416 SQ. FT.

Fig. 5-17. Suite plan for clinical lab, 1416 square feet.

laboratories. This discussion, then, will be limited to introducing the reader to basic laboratory processes and space requirements—some of which will occur in a small laboratory facility. (See Fig. 5–16.)

Development of the Program

As with all medical suites, the success of a well-designed laboratory is dependent upon a thorough understanding of the program—a written description of all requirements that must be incorporated into the design. The following checklist* will serve as a guide.

1. Determine which services are to be provided.
2. Determine space requirements to accommodate equipment and personnel in the following areas:
   a. Administrative
   b. Technical
   c. Auxiliary (includes washing, sterilizing, storage, and locker facilities)
3. Divide the technical areas into functions or units such as: hematology, biochemistry, parasitology, bacteriology, histology, urinalysis, serology.
4. Determine where the procedures are to be performed:
   a. Those to be combined in the same work area
   b. Those to be done in completely separate work areas

5. Estimate the volume of work in each area or unit, allowing for future increases in workload.
6. Indicate the number of personnel requiring a work station in each unit.
7. Describe the major equipment in each unit.
   a. If possible, indicate the linear feet of bench space (countertop) required and how the space may be arranged.
   b. List the equipment that requires utility lines and indicate the location.
   c. List equipment, such as refrigerators, centrifuges, hoods, desks, that may be jointly used by technicians from different work stations.
8. Indicate the desirable functional arrangements. (For example, the bacteriology unit must be located at the extreme end of the lab, to reduce the contamination hazard, and the washing area should be next to the bacteriology unit; hematology must be next to the waiting room, adjoining the examination and specimen area.)
9. Indicate which work units may be expected to expand. (It may be possible to locate those areas at one end of the department to facilitate efficient, coordinated expansion.)
10. In the technical area, a standard module for the work areas is suggested.
11. List the utilities to be provided and any special requirements for instruments such as electronic counters. Separate electrical circuits for some electronic instruments are necessary in order to avoid fluctuating voltage, which affects the accuracy of these instruments.
12. List environmental requirements, such as light, ventilation, color, and isolation of

* This material reprinted (with minor modifications) by permission of *Architectural Record* from article "Planning the Laboratory for the General Hospital" (McGraw-Hill, Inc. Feb. 1961 © with all rights reserved.)

PLATE 1

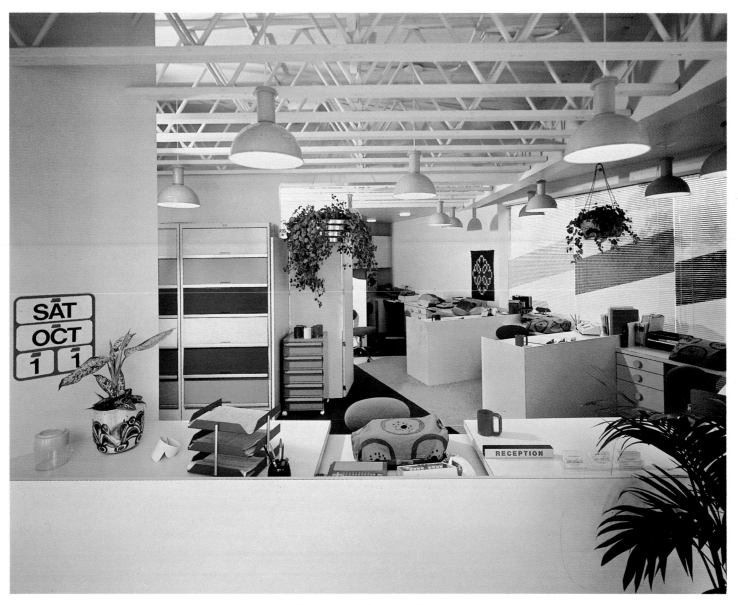

Fig. 3-3. Reception/business office.

PLATE 2

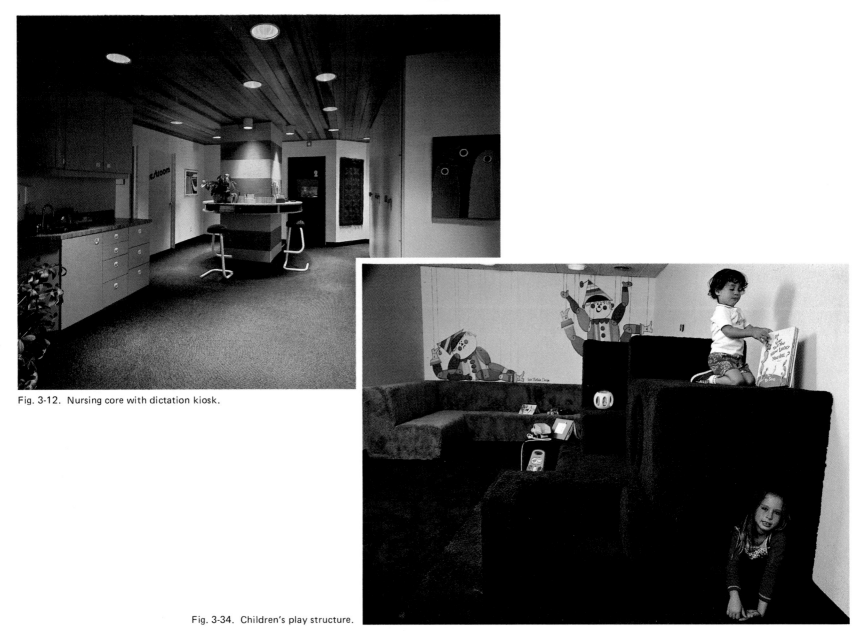

Fig. 3-12. Nursing core with dictation kiosk.

Fig. 3-34. Children's play structure.

PLATE 3

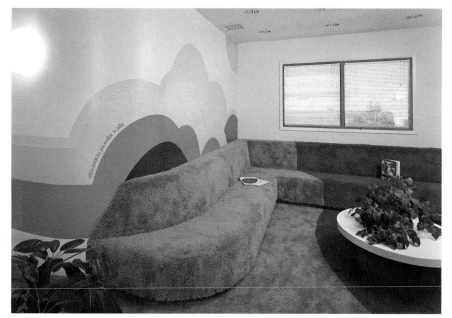

Fig. 3-37. Pediatric waiting room.

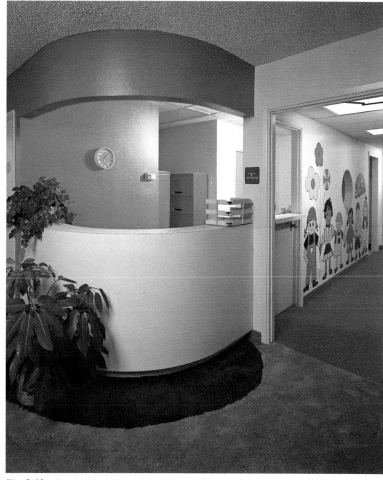

Fig. 3-40. Reception desk and corridor wallgraphic.

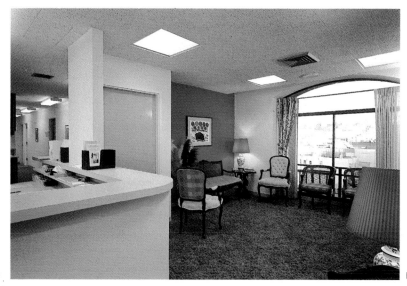

Fig. 4-2. Waiting room.

PLATE 4

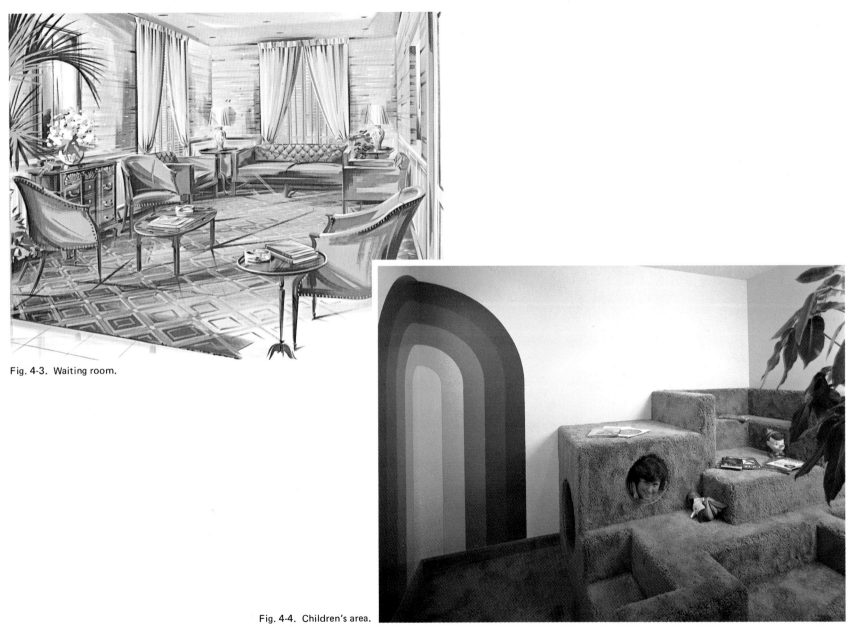

Fig. 4-3. Waiting room.

Fig. 4-4. Children's area.

PLATE 5

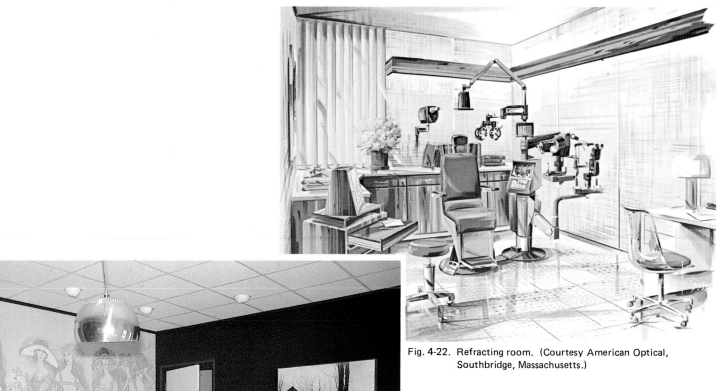

Fig. 4-22. Refracting room. (Courtesy American Optical, Southbridge, Massachusetts.)

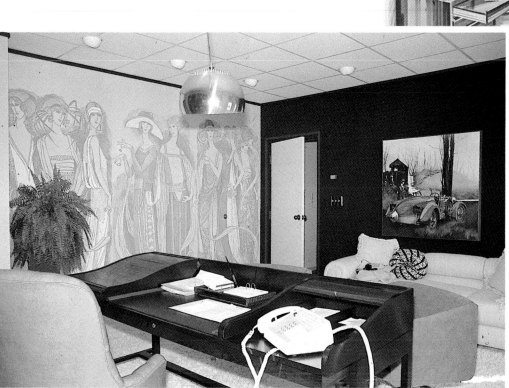

Fig. 4-9. Consultation room.

PLATE 6

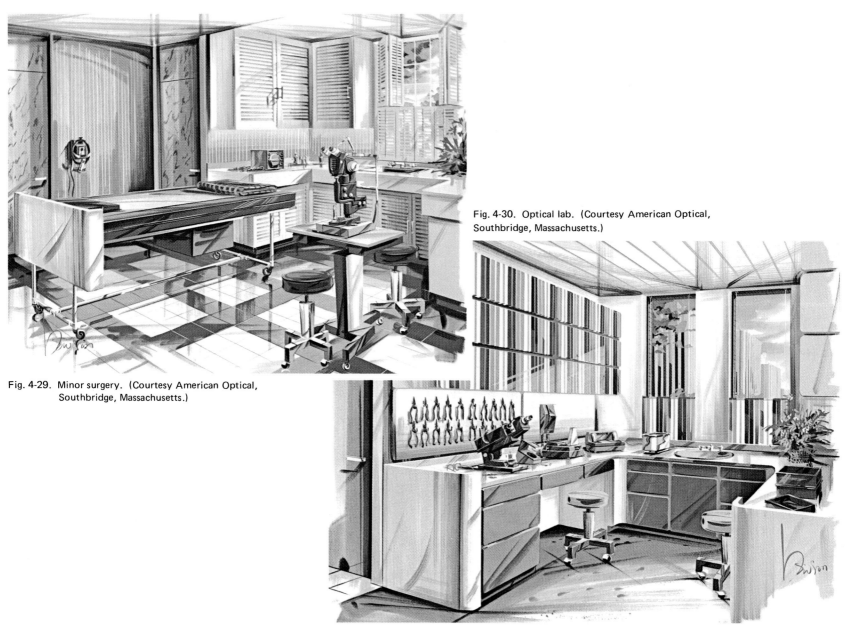

Fig. 4-30. Optical lab. (Courtesy American Optical, Southbridge, Massachusetts.)

Fig. 4-29. Minor surgery. (Courtesy American Optical, Southbridge, Massachusetts.)

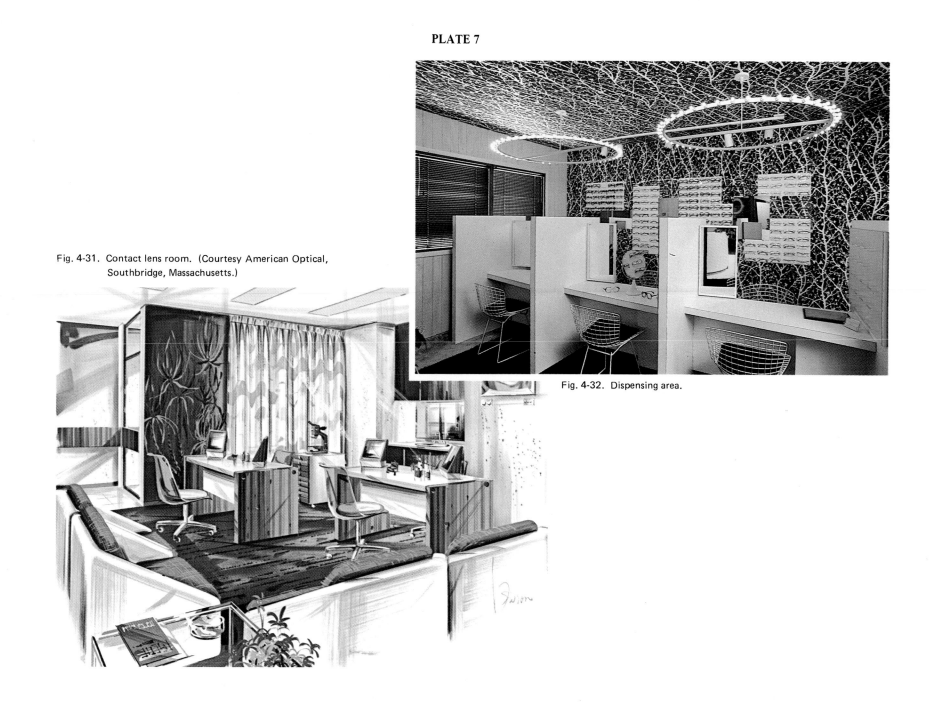

PLATE 7

Fig. 4-31. Contact lens room. (Courtesy American Optical, Southbridge, Massachusetts.)

Fig. 4-32. Dispensing area.

PLATE 8

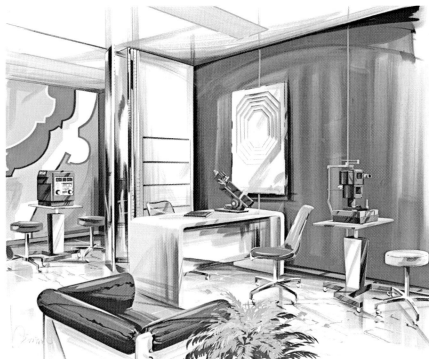

Fig. 4-33. Data collection room. (Courtesy American Optical, Southbridge, Massachusetts.)

Fig. 4-37. Waiting room. (Courtesy American Optical, Southbridge, Massachusetts.)

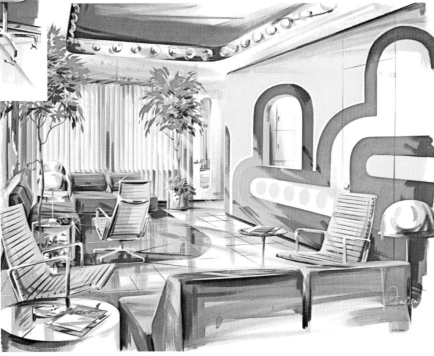

PLATE 9

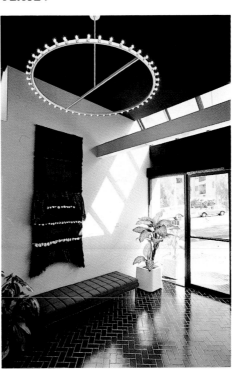

Fig. 4-49. Entry foyer.

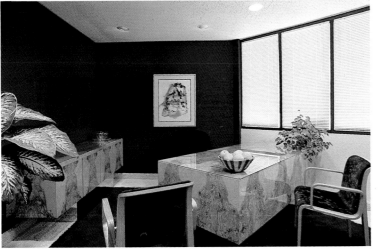

Fig. 4-48. Consultation room.

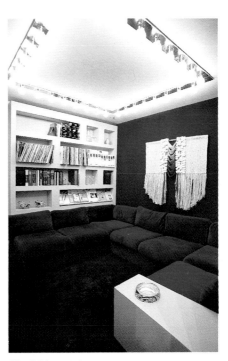

Fig. 4-51. Waiting room.

PLATE 10

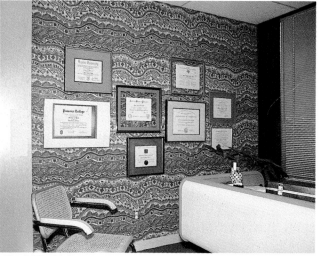

Fig. 4-62. Diplomas.

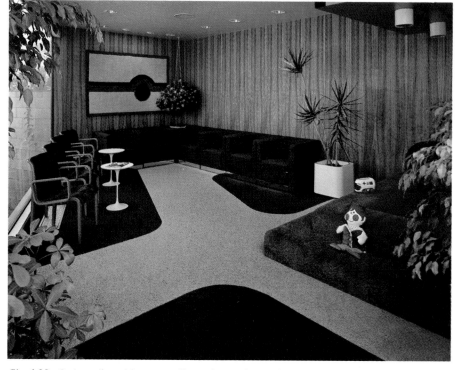

Fig. 4-88. Orthopedic waiting room allows plenty of space in center of room for people on crutches.

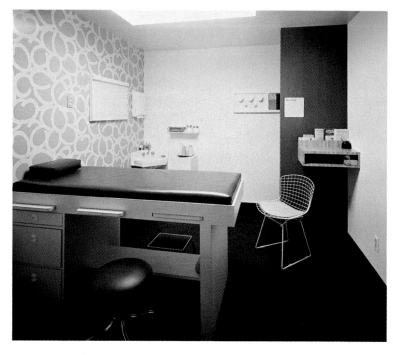

Fig. 4-77. Orthopedic exam room.

PLATE 11

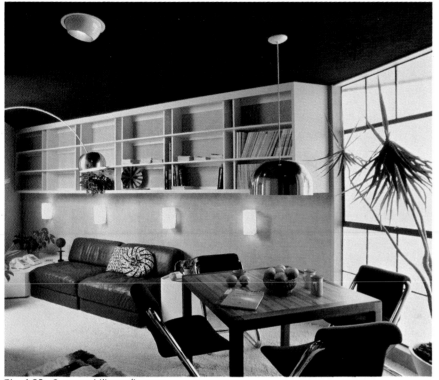

Fig. 4-89. Surgeons' library/lounge.

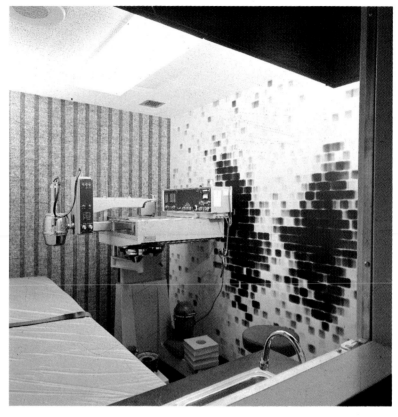

Fig. 5-14. Thyroid scan wallgraphic.

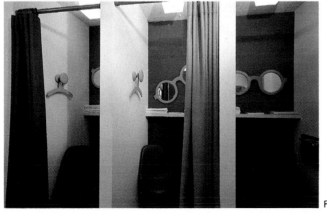

Fig. 5-2. Radiology dressing rooms.

PLATE 12

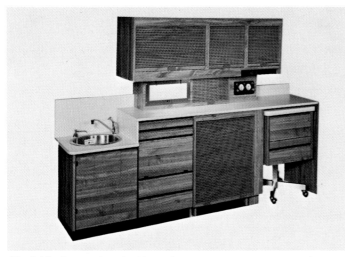

Fig. 8-10. Custom dental cabinet. (Courtesy Hamilton Industries.)

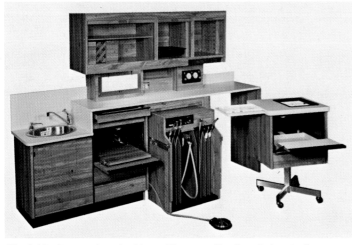

Fig. 8-11. Custom dental cabinet. (Courtesy Hamilton Industries.)

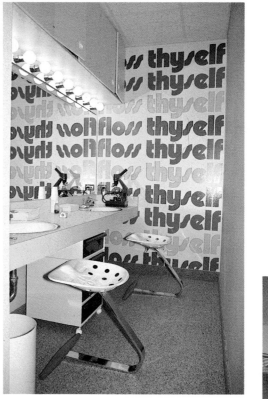

Fig. 8-27. Patient education graphic.

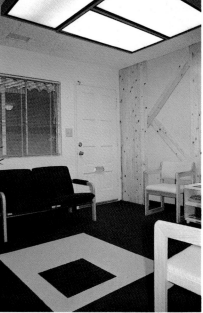

Fig. 8-31. Dentist's waiting room.

PLATE 13

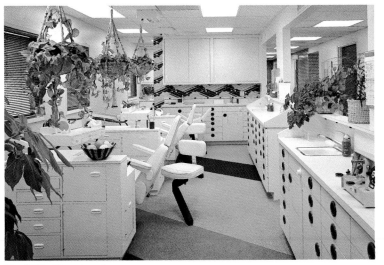

Fig. 8-52. Operatory bay.

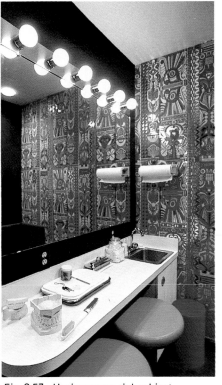

Fig. 8-57. Hygiene room sink cabinet.

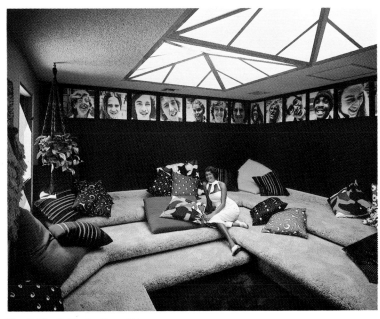

Fig. 8-55. Orthodontic waiting room.

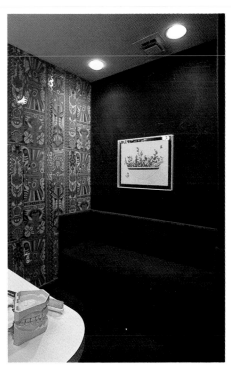

Fig. 8-58. Hygiene room carpeted bench.

PLATE 14

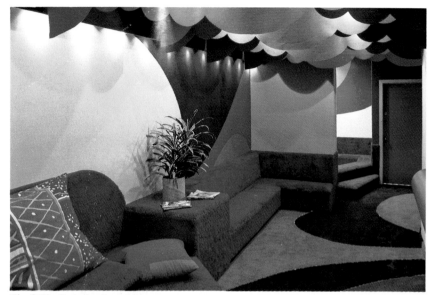

Fig. 8-59. Pedodontic waiting room.

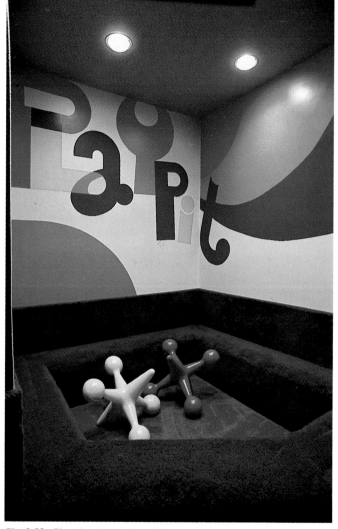

Fig. 8-60. Playpit pedodontic waiting room.

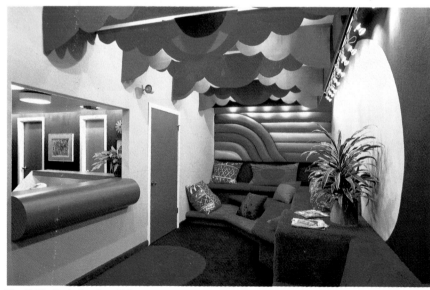

Fig. 8-61. Pedodontic waiting room.

PLATE 15

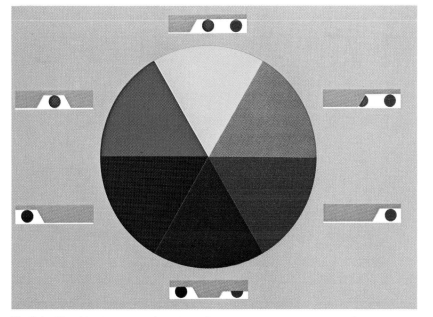

Fig. 9-1. The old color wheel. (Reprinted from *The Theory and Practice of Color,* by Frans Gerritsen, by permission of Van Nostrand Reinhold, publishers, New York, 1974, p. 172.)

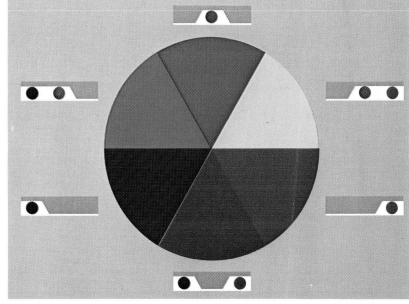

Fig. 9-2. The new color wheel. (Reprinted from *The Theory and Practice of Color,* by Frans Gerritsen, by permission of Van Nostrand Reinhold, publishers, New York, 1974, p. 173.)

PLATE 16

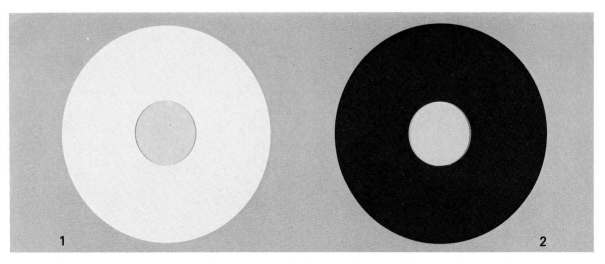

Fig. 9-3. Simultaneous contrast. (Reprinted from *The Theory and Practice of Color,* by Frans Gerritsen, by permission of Van Nostrand Reinhold, publishers, New York, 1974, p. 128.)

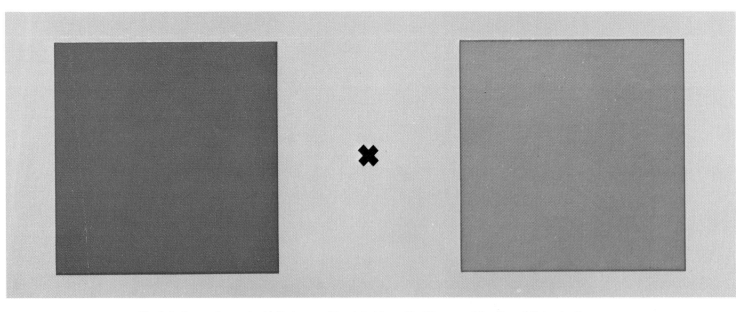

Fig. 9-4. Successive contrast/afterimage. (Reprinted from *The Theory and Practice of Color,* by Frans Gerritsen, by permission of Van Nostrand Reinhold, publishers, New York, 1974, p. 146.)

equipment that may be noisy or may produce heat when used.

Technical Modules

Hematology. This is the study of the chemical components of blood. Thus it should be located close to the venipuncture (blood draw) booths. One-half of the module should be set aside for procedures such as sedimentation rates, hemoglobin tests, staining, and washing of pipettes. Another portion of the work surface (at 30-inch height) should have knee spaces for sit-down work at the microscope. The microhematocrit centrifuge, due to its noise and vibration when in use, should be placed in an area outside the hematology module where it is less likely to disturb someone. A refrigerator and desk should be located outside the module at a location convenient to the urinalysis and chemistry modules so that these items can be shared by all three.

Biochemistry. A variety of chemical procedures are performed here. Most work is done at a 36-inch-high countertop, but a lowered knee-space area should be provided for titrations and other seated procedures. The countertop should have reagent shelves (for chemicals used during the procedures), a utility sink in each chemistry work area, and drawers and cabinets below the countertop.

An instrument table (36 inches high) should be located away from the prep and test area for the colorimeter, flame photometer, spectrophotometer, and carbon dioxide gas apparatus. By locating these instruments away from the busy work area, others can share them and there is less likelihood of accidental chemical spillage. Near the instrument table the analytical balance

should be located on a vibration-free stand or support. The centrifuge, refrigerator, and desk are shared with the hematology unit. The work area will require a fume hood for removal of vapors and gases and outlets for compressed air, vacuum, and gas. Optional equipment are an automated blood gas analyzer and electrophoresis apparatus. It should be noted that much of this work can be done by automated machines in less space than would be required for the equipment needed to do the procedures manually, but some small labs can not afford to buy such sophisticated machinery.

Urinalysis. This unit is located in the same module as the biochemistry unit. One half of the urinalysis work counter is used for microscopic examinations and the other half for chemical procedures. The work surface should be 30 inches high and should have a sink. Urinalysis would share the hematology centrifuge.

Histology. This is the study of tissues. Thin slices of diseased specimens are examined by microscope. During surgery (or autopsy), for example, sections of tumors would be sent to the lab for a pathologist's report on possible malignancy or other cellular deformities. Small labs in a medical office building would usually not have a histology unit and would not have a pathologist. Normally this work would be performed in a hospital's clinical lab. Thus the requirements in equipment and work space will not be discussed here.

Serology-Bacteriology. Serology is the study of blood serum and bacteriology is the study of bacteria and their effect on the body. These units are usually combined. Culture media for use in bacteriology are prepared in the bacteriology work area and sent to the sterilization area to be sterilized. Since most work is done in a seated position, the countertop should be 30 inches high with a knee space for each technician, and it should have shelves for reagents. A sink with garbage disposal should be provided in the serology area and a sink for staining slides should be provided in the bacteriology area. A fume hood should be provided to prevent the spread of infection (and noxious odors) during preparation of specimens of tuberculosis, fungus, viruses, or stool cultures. *Parasitology*, the study of parasites (normally performed on feces), is often included in the bacteriology module. A centrifuge, refrigerator, and incubator should also be located in the unit. If at all possible, the bacteriology unit should be separated from the other units by full-height partitions and a door to reduce contamination of air and the chance of infection transmitted to other lab personnel.

Automatic Analyzer. Many laboratories, even small ones, now have automatic microprocessor biochemical analyzers which reduce the number of technicians required and eliminate a good deal of the equipment necessary for manual analysis. The automatic analyzers vary considerably in their size and in their capacity. They save an incredible amount of time. One may feed a blood or urine specimen into the machine, and in approximately one minute, the machine will complete 10 to 20 tests simultaneously and produce a printout with the results. The large machines can process upwards of 150 samples per hour and do a thorough analysis—error free—of each, thus fractionalizing the time required by lab personnel to

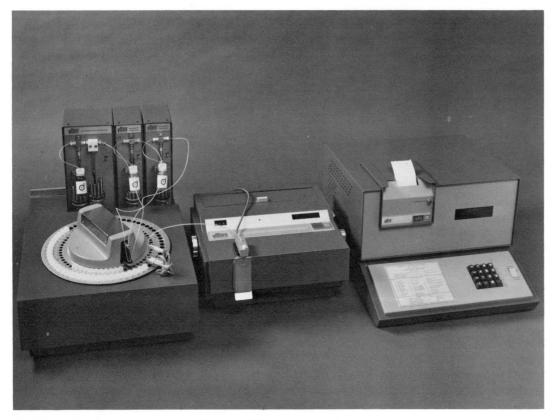

Fig. 5-18. Tabletop automatic analyzer. (Courtesy Gilford Instrument.)

perform these tests individually and manually. Some of the analyzers fit on a countertop (Fig. 5-18) and others may occupy a 4 × 6-foot or larger floor space (Figs. 5-19, 5-20, 5-21, and 5-22).

Administrative Area

The administrative area consists of a waiting room, a business office/reception room, and sometimes a private office for the pathologist or director of the lab. These areas should be separated from the technical areas so that nonlab personnel need not enter the lab work areas.

Specimen Toilet

The specimen toilet for collection of urine specimens should have a small pass-through door that opens into the technical area so that urine samples can be picked up by the urinalysis technician.

Blood Draw

Blood draw (venipuncture) can be performed either in a small booth or cubicle (equipped with a straight chair and a 24 × 36-inch table) or in a prefabricated special blood draw chair with tablet arm which may be located in an open room without any enclosure or behind a screen. The screen is intended to protect those waiting from the view of blood being drawn. Often persons watching become faint.

Other Procedures

Basal metabolism rate (BMR) studies no longer require special equipment. They are now done by

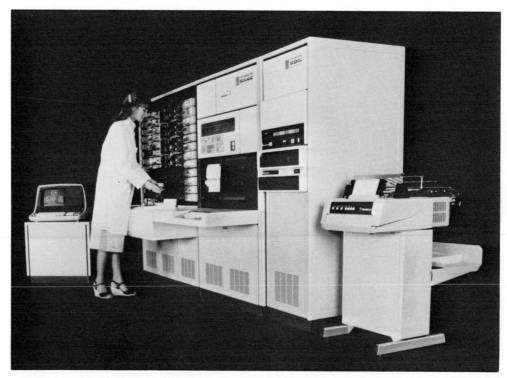

Fig. 5-19. Automatic clinical analyzer, SMAC/SDM. (Courtesy Technicon Instruments Corp.)

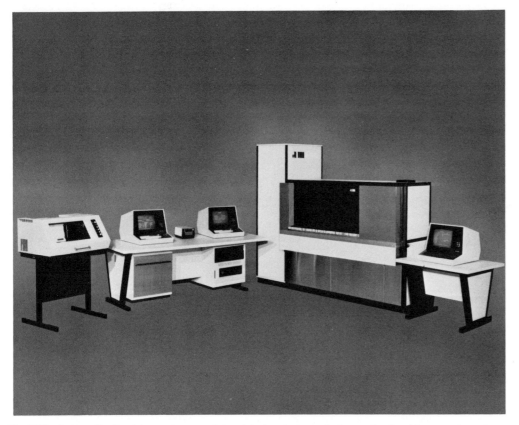

Fig. 5-20. Automatic chemistry analyzer: printer, data terminals, control console, chemistry console, and secondary terminal. (Courtesy American Monitor Corp.)

a radioimmunoassay and all that is necessary is a blood sample.

EKG studies are sometimes performed in a clinical lab. The reader is referred to Chapter 3 under *Internal Medicine* for a discussion of EKG and pulmonary function lab equipment and procedures.

Dressing Area For Employees

A large lab may provide lockers and a dressing area where technicians may change clothes. A staff toilet room may also be included.

Auxiliary Services

The *glass-washing* and *sterilization* unit should be located close to the serology-bacteriology and biochemisty units, since they utilize these services more frequently than the other modules. This unit should contain a water still, a pressure sterilizer, sterilizing oven, and pipette washer. Storage of glassware, chemicals, reagents, and paper supplies would be provided in cabinets. A hood over the sterilizers and water still would exhaust the heat generated by the equipment.

It should be mentioned that the glass-wash and sterilization area would be different if all lab procedures were done manually than if they were done by computerized biochemical analyzers. The standard procedures and equipment have been made obsolete by the microprocessor instrumentation. Thus it is important to study the capabilities of any computerized analyzers the lab may have and then plan the other areas around them. The manufacturers of the autoanalyzers may also make recommendations as to the requirements for their units and any support facilities that may be needed.

Utilities

A clinical laboratory requires gas, vacuum, and compressed air in addition to water and waste systems. Because of the importance of these systems (and the need for continuity of service) the piping should be easily accessible (but not exposed) and should have an ample number of valves, traps, and cleanouts to facilitate repairs. Each individual piping system should be color coded and should be of a noncorrosive material. The waste from the pipes should be discharged to a dilution pit or should be carried to a point in the system where the discharged material will be diluted by the waste from other areas. Laboratory sinks should be of a noncorrosive material. The countertop work surfaces should be of a chemical-resistant plastic laminate or special ceramic lab tops.

Air Conditioning and Ventilation

The need for a well-planned, functional air-conditioning and ventilation system is critical in a laboratory. Chemical fumes, vapors, gases, heat from equipment, plus the impracticality of open windows create a health hazard to those in adjacent medical suites as well as to the laboratory staff who suffer repeated exposure. It is not adequate simply to exhaust these vapors out of the roof of the building without considering the dispersion to nearby persons and buildings. The ventilation requirements for each work unit must be carefully studied so that airflow patterns can be regulated by proper location of supply and exhaust grilles. A competent mechanical engineer should be consulted to prepare this study. The serology-bacteriology unit should be slightly pressurized (by supplying more air to it than is ex-

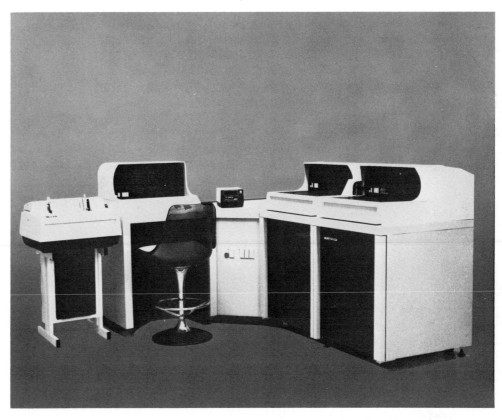

Fig. 5-21. KDA micro chemistry analyzer. (Courtesy American Monitor Corp.)

167

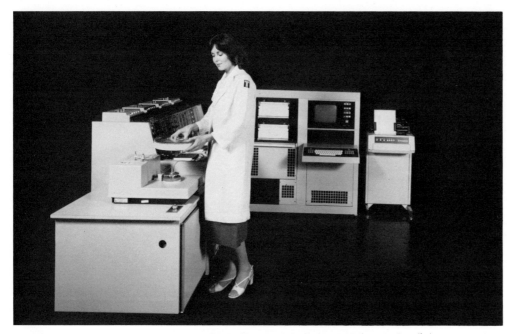

Fig. 5-22. Automatic chemistry analyzer, SMAII. (Courtesy Technicon Instruments Corp.)

each work surface countertop should have a continuous plug-mold strip and a separate circuit every 8 to 10 feet. Because certain pieces of equipment may draw as much as 15 amperes initially when warming up, a careful inventory must be made of the power requirements of each major piece of equipment. Automated analyzers are sensitive to voltage fluctuations and may require a constant voltage regulator as well as a separate circuit. The work areas require shadow-free light, so if the unit contains upper cabinets, a fluorescent "shelf" light will be mounted to the bottom of the upper cabinets. Otherwise the light would be supplied totally by ceiling-mounted fluorescent luminaires in sufficient quantity to assure a level of at least 100 footcandles for close work and 50 footcandles for general illumination.

The Small Laboratory

The small laboratory, which may be part of a group practice suite or perhaps will serve a small medical office building, would perform the more common and simple laboratory tests, while specimens requiring complex bacteriological or chemical procedures would probably be sent to a large outside laboratory. Diseased tissue specimens would most likely be sent to a pathologist at a nearby hospital. Thus the small lab (650 to 750 square feet) would have separate areas for hematology, biochemistry, urinalysis, and bacteriology, allowing approximately 6 lineal feet of countertop for each plus two blood draw cubicles, a specimen toilet, a small reception/waiting area, a storage room, and a glass-wash/sterilization area. Many of the computerized biochemical analyzers are designed for the needs of the small laboratory (Fig. 5–18).

hausted from it) to reduce the possibility of infiltration of aerosols which might contaminate the specimens being processed. Exhaust air from the fume hoods should be conducted through noncorrosive ducts to the roof of the building and not be recirculated. A slightly negative air pressure relative to the other areas of the medical building should be maintained in the laboratory in order to prevent odors and contaminants from spreading.

Power Requirements

A laboratory demands maximum flexibility; thus

168

Chapter 6
Group Practice

There is an ever-increasing trend toward group practice. Although some physicians do not feel psychologically geared to practice in a big organization and some fear a loss of individual authority in medical matters, the fact is that group practice increases a physician's productivity and lowers the cost of health care.

A shortage of doctors is a major impediment to quality health care in the United States. One solution is to make each doctor more productive by eliminating the waste and inefficiencies inherent in solo practice. A solo practitioner may be working a 60-hour or 70-hour week, but about a quarter of his or her time is spent on management of the office—bookkeeping, scheduling, ordering supplies, etc. A large group practice can afford to hire sufficient personnel to perform these nonmedical tasks thereby enabling the physicians to concentrate solely on medical matters.

Another advantage of group practice is the convenience of having a fully staffed radiology department and clinical lab right in the physician's own office. Equipment that might be too costly or underutilized in the small medical office can easily be justified in a large group practice. Other benefits of a group practice are greater freedom with regard to leisure time. The partners can cover for each other with no lack of continuity in care for the patient. And the physicians in a multispecialty group provide each other with immediate access to specialists in other fields. This pooling of resources provides patients more efficient and complete professional services than each physician could individually.

Of course economics plays a prime role in motivating physicians to practice together. Eight physicians in *private* practice would require *eight* business offices, *eight* waiting rooms, *six to eight* X-ray rooms, *six to eight* minor surgery rooms—a great duplication of space and personnel. Together, as a group, the eight could do with two minor surgeries, two X-ray rooms, one large waiting room, and one centralized business office. More efficient use of space and personnel equals more take-home profit for the physicians and perhaps even lower costs for the patient. In addition, certain lab tests or X-rays that might be sent out could be done within a properly equipped suite, netting the extra fees for the group practice to reduce office overhead.

There are four types of group practice. The

169

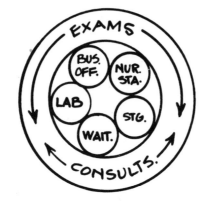

CENTRALIZED PLAN
SINGLE SPECIALTY GROUP

Fig. 6-1. Schematic diagram of a centralized plan for a
single-specialty group.

single-specialty group is comprised of physicians (rarely more than eight) who are all of the same medical specialty. This type of group permits a physician a great deal of freedom since patients usually will accept treatment from any member of the group. This allows for better utilization of all the doctors' time.

The *mixed-specialty group* might typically be a large clinic offering internal medicine, OB-GYN, urology, pediatrics, family practice, ENT, or any combination of medical specialties. A group such as this could offer many of the outpatient services provided by a hospital: clinical lab studies, diagnostic radiology, physical therapy, respiratory therapy, renal dialysis, and multiphasic medical screening. A mixed specialty group might be comprised of 20 to several hundred physicians as in an HMO.

The *internal medicine group* might be a group of internists each with a different subspecialty: pulmonary medicine, cardiovascular disease, hematology, oncology, gastroenterology, or endocrinology. A large enough group could support its own clinical lab, radiology department, cardiovascular rehabilitation lab, and pulmonary function lab.

The *general practice group* enables general physicians to expand beyond their individual resources in purchasing equipment and staffing an office. Large general practice groups are often found in small towns and sometimes they have one or more specialists on staff in an effort to offer the community a wider range of services.

Health Maintenance Organizations

Any of these groups may be organized as a health maintenance organization, although HMOs tend to be multispecialty groups offering services to its group of subscribers on a prepaid fee basis, or they may charge a fee at the time the service is rendered as do the majority of physicians. It should be remembered that HMOs stress health maintenance (it is less costly to keep people healthy than to treat them when they are sick), so any clinic set up as an HMO should be designed to accommodate many more patients than a mixed-specialty group of the same number of physicians. Many more paramedic aides will be employed in an HMO to do health screening and other procedures aimed at preventive medicine. An HMO will usually have a large physical therapy department, an inhalation therapy department, a cardiopulmonary lab, an allergy department—all of which may process a large volume of patients daily who do not have to see a doctor.

The bookkeeping system is somewhat simplified in an HMO since subscribers prepay a monthly fee that entitles them to office visits for a routine flat fee of $1.00 to $2.00 plus a minimal charge for lab tests and X-rays. Subscribers are issued an embossed identification card that is presented to the receptionist upon checking in and checking out of the clinic. This saves time in heading up a form for each patient visit, and the identification plate has the patient's billing code and other pertinent information on it. Thus, although an HMO may have more subscribers than a similar sized mixed-specialty that charges a fee for service, the billing procedures are often less complicated (there are no insurance claims to file) and are assisted by data processing and computer systems.

Health maintenance organizations are regulated by the state and are subject to close scrutiny by various health planning regulatory agencies. This accounts for the low number of HMOs and also for the fact that they are usually very large multispecialty groups that have met strict requirements with regard to their medical services, their utilization of personnel, and their schedule of fees.

SINGLE-SPECIALTY GROUP

This suite would be composed of the same elements as a standard medical office for a solo practitioner except on a larger scale. (The reader is referred to Chapter 3 under *General Practice*). The functions of administration, patient care, and support services remain the same. It is the relationship of the rooms that becomes critical as the suite becomes larger. It is no longer possible for all rooms to be close to each other as they are in

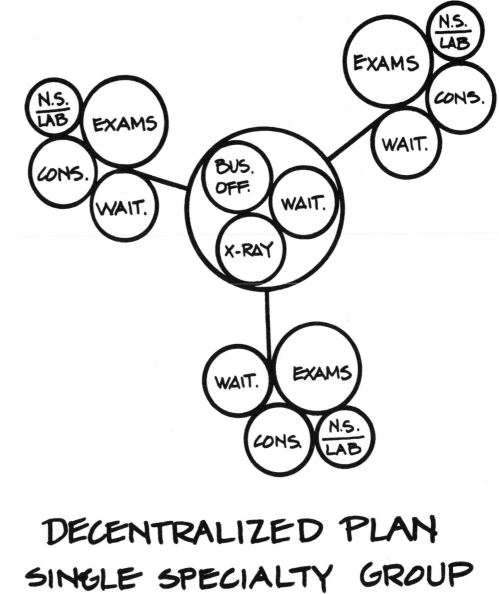

DECENTRALIZED PLAN SINGLE SPECIALTY GROUP

Fig. 6-2. Schematic diagram of a decentralized plan for a single-specialty group.

171

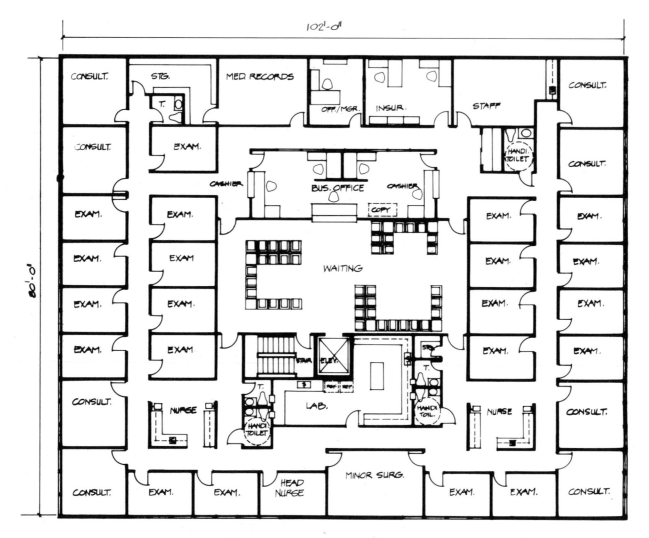

SINGLE SPECIALTY GROUP - OB/GYN
CENTRALIZED PLAN
8160 SQ. FT.

Fig. 6-3. Suite plan for single-specialty group, OB-GYN, centralized plan, 8160 square feet.

a small suite. The administrative and support services may be *centralized* or *decentralized*—that is the major decision to be made at the outset. With a centralized plan (also known as an "island" plan), the business office, nurse station, lab, and supply room would be grouped together, forming the core of the suite, with the patient areas (exam and treatment rooms, consultation and waiting rooms) grouped around the perimeter of the core (Fig. 6–3).

With a decentralized plan, the administrative and support services would be divided into units each serving a certain number of exam and treatment rooms. The exam and treatment rooms would be grouped into pods (three to six exam rooms to a pod) with an adjacent nurse station/lab and one or two consultation rooms (Fig. 6-4). It would be impractical to have more than one business office, medical records area, or insurance office, so these services would have to be located so that a patient exiting from any pod of exam rooms would follow a path leading him or her past the cashier's desk and appointment desk and back into the central waiting room. Sometimes in a large suite, proper circulation must be reinforced by well-placed, easy-to-read signage plaques or wallgraphics (Figs. 6–3a and 6–3b).

MIXED-SPECIALTY GROUP

This type of clinic offers the greatest challenge to a designer. The space to be planned may be vast, and each specialty must be carefully analyzed for its relationship to the other specialties (see Figs. 6–5 and 6–6). Large multispecialty clinics tend to grow and change a good deal. Physicians leave and others join the group. Departments are sometimes shuffled around to realign them according to new priorities. The facility should be designed

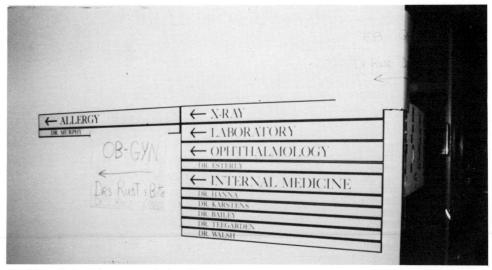

Fig. 6-3a. Clinic signage system "before."

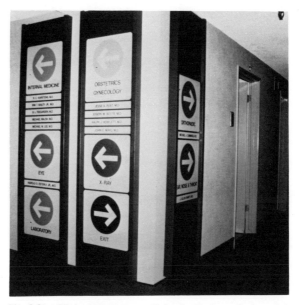

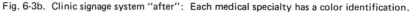

Fig. 6-3b. Clinic signage system "after": Each medical specialty has a color identification.

173

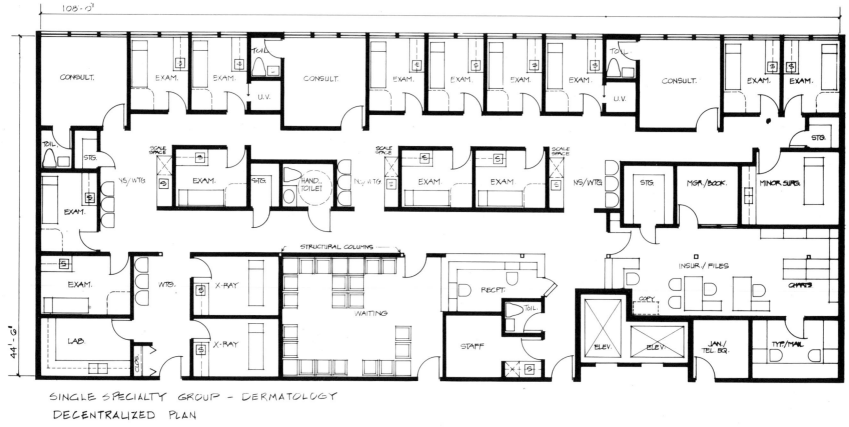

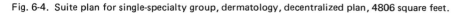

SINGLE SPECIALTY GROUP - DERMATOLOGY
DECENTRALIZED PLAN
4806 SQ.FT.

Fig. 6-4. Suite plan for single-specialty group, dermatology, decentralized plan, 4806 square feet.

174

for expansion with anticipation of which departments may outgrow their present limits. Radiology, for example, tends to expand. New equipment is introduced, and due to the scale of the machinery, a single piece may require its own room. Thus it is a good idea to locate the radiology department on the perimeter of the suite adjacent to the area allocated for expansion. Radiography rooms are very costly to build due to the special electrical, plumbing, and lead-shielding requirements; therefore it would not be economically feasible to abandon the existing radiology rooms, tearing them down to remodel for less specialized use such as additional examination rooms or an expanded waiting room. By locating the radiology department contiguous to the area of proposed future expansion, the existing radiology rooms need not be altered, but new rooms could be added.

Medical records is another area that often has to be expanded. Since this would typically be located in the core of the suite it is hard to enlarge it. It is better to initially project the realistic number of charts and growth for a seven-year period (physicians must keep medical records for seven years) and make the room large enough to begin with (Figs. 3–6, 3–7).

If the building is designed for and owned by the doctors, the architect can take liberties with the design and make the structure of the building really conform to the spatial requirements of the group's practice. A large clinic may be laid out with the administrative and support services in the core with each specialty department radiating out from it like spokes of a wheel. Each "spoke" would have its own nurse station and waiting room, but the clinical lab, medical records, insurance, business office, etc., would be in the

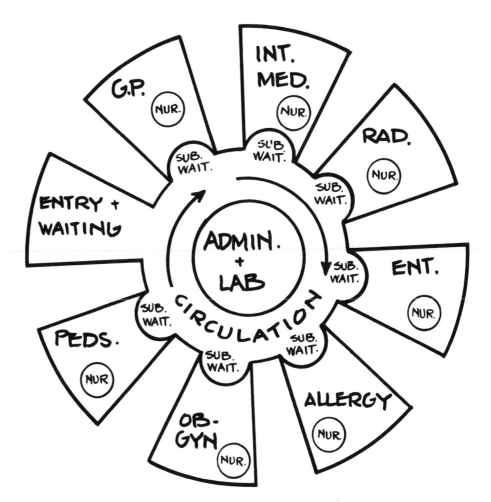

SATELLITE PLAN
MULTI-SPECIALTY GROUP

Fig. 6-5. Schematic diagram of a satellite plan for a multi-specialty group.

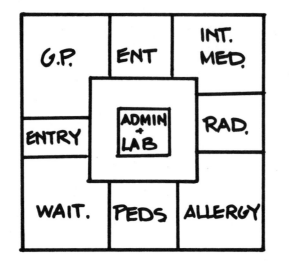

MULTI-SPECIALTY GROUP

Fig. 6-6. Schematic diagram for a multi-specialty group, showing the relationship of specialties for optimum function: keeping the highest volume toward the front, pediatrics close to allergy, radiology close to internal medicine, lab and business office central to all.

core area (Fig. 6-7). This is also known as the *satellite* plan. If the square footage of each specialty department is not great, one large waiting room may be designed near the reception and business office. Patients would be called from there to the various departments. But in the majority of cases, each specialty department would function independently with its own waiting room, reception desk, nurse station, and other support facilities. There may be a central reception desk and waiting room at the entrance of the clinic where an aide may head up a form which the patient carries to the subreception desk located at the specialty department. Upon checking out, the patient may book a future appointment either at the subreception desk or at the central reception desk depending upon how the flow of paperwork is set up. Payment for services would usually be made at the central reception desk or cashier's counter, if one exists, rather than at the specialty department.

Most large medical offices are using computer bookkeeping systems. The equipment varies somewhat depending on the manufacturer and the individual's requirements, so the designer must carefully review the sizes of the computer components, the electrical requirements, and the communication linkage between departments. The computer terminals at each subreception desk can give each department access to a patient's ledger or to the appointment schedule without having to phone or walk over to the central business office (Fig. 6-8).

INTERNAL MEDICINE GROUP

This is a single-specialty group, but due to the many internal medicine subspecialties, more

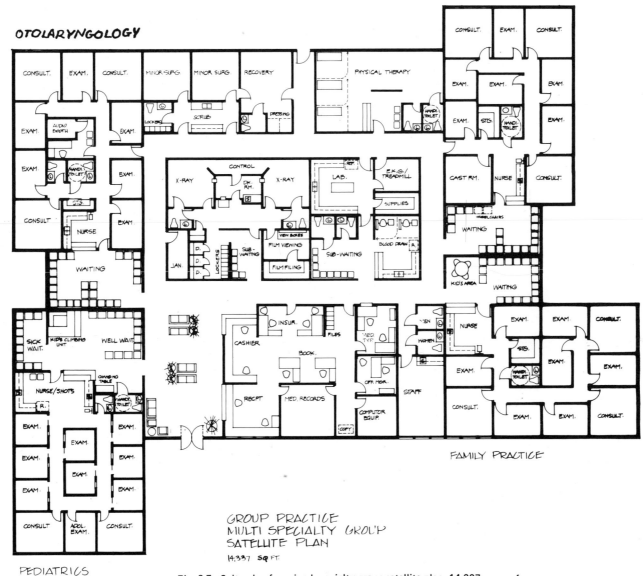

ORTHOPEDICS

OTOLARYNGOLOGY

PEDIATRICS

GROUP PRACTICE
MULTI SPECIALTY GROUP
SATELLITE PLAN
14,337 SQ FT.

FAMILY PRACTICE

Fig. 6-7. Suite plan for mixed-specialty group satellite plan, 14,337 square feet.

177

specialized rooms and a larger clinical lab and radiology suite are required than with most single-specialty groups. An internist specializing in cardiology or in pulmonary disease would need an EKG room and a cardiopulmonary lab. An internist specializing in gastrointestinal disease will require a proctology room, and if he or she wishes to do the G.I. series of X-rays in the office, will require a fluoroscopy room with adjoining toilet room and barium prep area. Endocrinologists order many lab studies some of which require patients to report to the lab in the morning and remain nearby for four to six hours with blood being drawn every hour. Thus the lab must be of sufficient size to accommodate a high volume of work and should have a comfortable lounge for waiting patients.

The suite for a group practice of internists would typically have five exam rooms for each two doctors (two for each plus a third shared between them), a consultation room for each physician adjacent to his or her pod of exam rooms, a toilet, and a nurse station. The proctology rooms, EKG rooms, cardiopulmonary lab, clinical lab, and radiology suite would be located in the core area central to all exam rooms. The business office, insurance office, cashier's desk, and waiting room would be located at the entrance of the suite so that each patient upon entering and upon leaving must pass by the reception and the cashier's desks (Fig. 6–9).

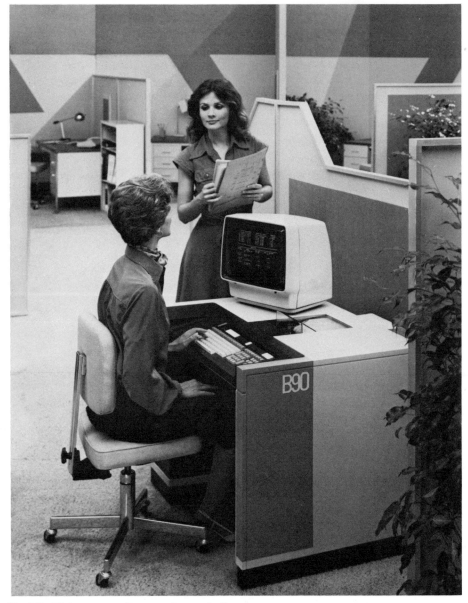

Fig. 6-8. Minicomputer. (Courtesy Burroughs Corp.)

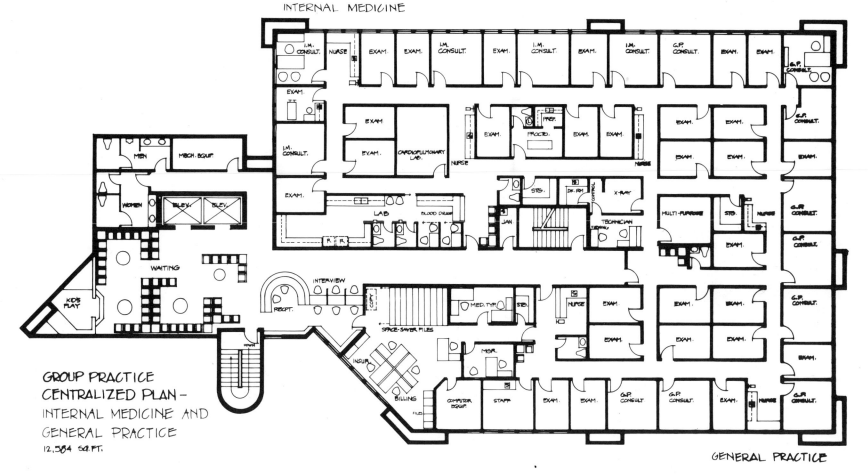

INTERNAL MEDICINE

GROUP PRACTICE
CENTRALIZED PLAN –
INTERNAL MEDICINE AND
GENERAL PRACTICE
12,584 SQ. FT.

GENERAL PRACTICE

Fig. 6-9. Suite plan for group practice, centralized plan, 12,584 square feet.

Table 6-1. Analysis of Program. Group Practice—Single Specialty

	Internal Medicine 8 Physicians		General Practice 8 Physicians	
Waiting Room(s)		$35 \times 35 = 1225$		$35 \times 40 = 1400$
Exam Rooms	20 @	$8 \times 12 = 1920$	24 @	$8 \times 12 = 2304$
Consultation Rooms	8 @	$12 \times 14 = 1344$	8 @	$12 \times 12 = 1152$
Nurse Stations		$12 \times 14 = 168$		$12 \times 14 = 168$
Toilets	4 @	$5 \times 6 = 120$	4 @	$5 \times 6 = 120$
Storage		$12 \times 12 = 144$		$12 \times 12 = 144$
Staff Lounge		$12 \times 16 = 192$		$12 \times 16 = 192$
Laboratory[a]		$24 \times 32 = 768$		$24 \times 32 = 768$
Minor Surgery		—	2 @	$12 \times 12 = 288$
Cast Room		—		$12 \times 14 = 168$
EKG Room[b]	2 @	$12 \times 10 = 240$		$12 \times 14 = 168$
Radiology[c]		$12 \times 26 = 312$		$12 \times 26 = 312$
Procto Room[d]		$12 \times 15 = 180$		—
Business Office[e]		$24 \times 24 = 576$		$24 \times 24 = 576$
Office Manager		$12 \times 10 = 120$		$12 \times 10 = 120$
Pulmonary Function Lab (optional)		$16 \times 20 = 320$		—
Medical Records		$12 \times 16 = 192$		$12 \times 16 = 192$
Insurance		$14 \times 16 = 224$		$14 \times 16 = 224$
Subtotal		8045 ft²		8296 ft²
15% Circulation		1207		1244
Total		9252 ft²		9540 ft²

[a] Includes lab waiting, blood draw, recovery, toilet.
[b] Includes mounting area.
[c] Includes darkroom, control, film filing, film viewing, dressing area. (Radiography room not equipped for fluoroscopy.)
[d] Includes prep area and toilet.
[e] Includes reception, bookkeeper's office, transcription, computer equipment.

Table 6-2. Analysis of Program. Group Practice—Single Specialty

	OB-GYN 8 Physicians		Orthopedics 8 Physicians	
Waiting Room(s)		$35 \times 40 = 1400$		$40 \times 40 = 1600$
Exam Rooms	21 @	$8 \times 12 = 2016$	12 @	$8 \times 12 = 1152$
Consultation Rooms	8 @	$12 \times 12 = 1152$	8 @	$12 \times 11 = 1056$
Nurse Stations	2 @	$8 \times 10 = 160$	2 @	$6 \times 8 = 96$
Toilets	6 @	$5 \times 6 = 180$	4 @	$5 \times 6 = 120$
Storage		$12 \times 12 = 144$		$12 \times 12 = 144$
Staff Lounge		$12 \times 16 = 192$		$12 \times 12 = 144$
Lab		$12 \times 16 = 192$		—
Minor Surgery		$14 \times 16 = 224$	4 @	$12 \times 12 = 576$
Cast Rooms		—		$12 \times 28 = 336$
Radiology		—		
Business Office		$16 \times 30 = 480$		$16 \times 30 = 480$
Office Manager		$10 \times 12 = 120$		$10 \times 12 = 120$
Insurance		$14 \times 16 = 224$		$14 \times 16 = 224$
Medical Records		$12 \times 16 = 192$		$12 \times 16 = 192$
Head Nurse's Office		$10 \times 10 = 100$		—
Physical Therapy		—		$25 \times 45 = 1125$
Subtotal		6776 ft²		7589 ft²
15% Circulation		1017		1139
Total		7793 ft²		8728 ft²

A large group practice will have a business manager or an administrator who will require a small private office preferably with window walls (starting at 48 inches off the floor) facing the business office, reception area, and internal corridors of the suite so that he or she can keep an eye on operations at all times.

Patients may at times report to the lab without having to see a physician, so the lab should be located at the front of the suite enabling a patient to enter and leave without mingling with the patients waiting for visits with a physician. In fact the lab might have an entrance from the street (or public corridor of the medical building) directly into the lab. The reader is referred to Chapter 5 for space planning requirements of a clinical lab.

The waiting room must accommodate one hour's patients per doctor. Thus if each doctor can see an average of four patients per hour and each has 2.5 examining rooms, an eight-physician group would need seating for approximately 44 persons in the waiting room or elsewhere within the suite when all doctors are seeing patients simultaneously. A formula for estimating the required number of seats is:

$$2P \times D - E = S$$

where

P = Average number of patients per hour per doctor

D = Number of doctors

E = Number of exam rooms

S = Seating

The formula assumes that each patient arrives with one other person, a friend or relative.

Allowing that some patients will arrive unaccompanied by a friend or relative and some will be directed to the lab, X-ray, procto room, or EKG

Table 6-3. Analysis of Program.
Group Practice—Mixed Specialty—9 Physicians

This program assumes the following: 2 internists, 3 general practitioners, 3 pediatricians, and 1 otolaryngologist; a central business office and lab will serve all; in addition to the central supply, several small storage rooms would be scattered throughout the facility.

Waiting Rooms	40 × 45 =	1800 ft²
Pedo Exam Rooms	2 @ 8 × 12 & 8 @ 8 × 8 =	704
Pedo Nurse Station	10 × 12 =	120
Pedo Consultation Rooms	3 @ 10 × 12 =	360
ENT Exams	2 @ 8 × 12 =	192
Audio Room	10 × 12 =	120
ENT Minor Surgery	12 × 12 =	144
ENT Consultation Room	12 × 12 =	144
ENT Nurse Station	8 × 8 =	64
I.M. Exam Rooms	5 @ 8 × 12 =	480
I.M. Consultation Rooms	2 @ 12 × 12 =	288
I.M. Nurse Station	8 × 10 =	80
Procto Room[a]	12 × 15 =	180
EKG/Cardiopulmonary Lab	16 × 18 =	288
G.P. Exam Rooms	9 @ 8 × 12 =	864
G.P. Consultation Rooms	3 @ 12 × 12 =	432
G.P. Nurse Station	8 × 10 =	80
Cast Room	12 × 12 =	144
Minor Surgery	12 × 12 =	144
Staff Lounge	14 × 16 =	224
Central Supply	12 × 16 =	192
Medical Records	12 × 16 =	192
Office Manager	12 × 10 =	120
Lab[b]	24 × 32 =	768
Radiology[c]	12 × 26 =	312
Toilets	7 @ 5 × 6 =	210
Business Office:		
Reception	10 × 12 =	120
Bookkeeper	14 × 16 =	224
Insurance	14 × 16 =	224
Transcription	10 × 12 =	120
Computer Equip./Clerical	12 × 12 =	144
Subtotal		9,478 ft²
15% Circulation		1,422
Total		10,900 ft²

[a] Includes prep area and toilet.
[b] Includes lab, lab waiting, blood draw, recovery, toilet, storage.
[c] Includes darkroom, control, film filing, viewing area, dressing area.

room, the 44 required seats might be reduced to 35 at the absoute minimum. Figuring 18 square feet per person, a waiting room that will accommodate 44 persons will have to be approximately 792 square feet in size.

GENERAL PRACTICE GROUP

The suite for a general practice group would be an expansion of a suite for a solo G.P. (refer to Chapter 3). It would also include cast rooms, an X-ray facility, a lab, a private office for a business manager, and maybe a small allergy suite. Often a group of G.P.s will include a general surgeon. The formula discussed above for estimating the number of seats in the waiting room applies here except that a G.P. can see up to six patients an hour and each G.P. should have the use of three exam rooms.

Chapter 7
Paramedical Suites

PHYSICAL THERAPY

There are seven basic methods of physical therapy:

1. Hydrotherapy
2. Diathermy
3. Heat or Cold
4. Massage
5. Ultraviolet Therapy
6. Exercise
7. Ultrasound

Hydrotherapy

Hydrotherapy involves immersion of a limb or, at times even the entire body, in water. The tank may be a portable whirlpool or a full-body Hubbard tank (Fig. 7–1). The latter is more apt to be found in a hospital physical medicine department. The large body tanks are usually installed with permanent water and waste connections. Smaller body tanks (Fig. 7–2) also require permanent connection. Since large amounts of hot water release a lot of steam, the walls of these rooms with large tanks should have at least a 5-foot-high ceramic tile wainscot with commercial vinyl wallcovering above. The floor should also be ceramic tile. It is possible to use sheet vinyl on the floor, but it is not nearly as hygienic or serviceable as ceramic tile.

Most physical therapy suites will have a couple of small portable tanks (Fig. 7–3), suitable for an arm or a leg, in addition to built-in whirlpools. Floor sinks must be provided for the portable tanks, which have to be drained and filled for each patient. A hose connection to a nearby tap may suffice for filling the tank. The whirlpool rooms or enclosures are usually 5 × 8 feet in size and are closed off on the open side by a cubicle drape. The walls of these enclosures should have a 2 or 3-foot-high wainscot of ceramic tile on all walls, and the wall above the tile must have a waterproof enamel finish or commercial vinyl wallcovering. The floors of these enclosures should be ceramic tile.

Diathermy

Diathermy equipment varies somewhat in size, so the designer must verify the specific equipment to be used. A mobile unit that can be wheeled

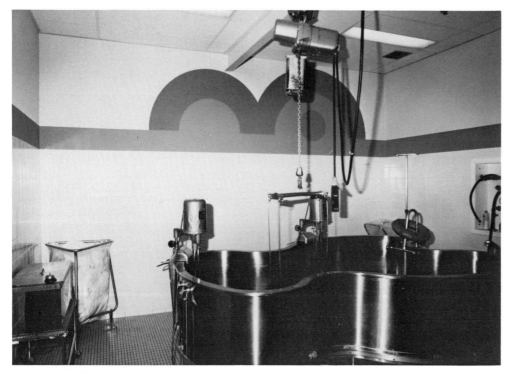

Fig. 7-1. Full-body immersion hydrotherapy tank.

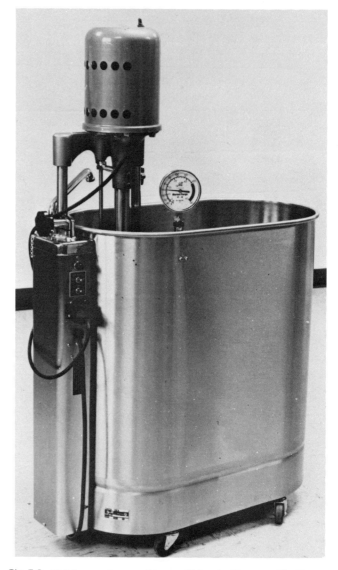

Fig. 7-2. Mobile arm, foot, and knee whirlpool. (Courtesy Ille Div. Market Forge, Everett, Massachusetts.)

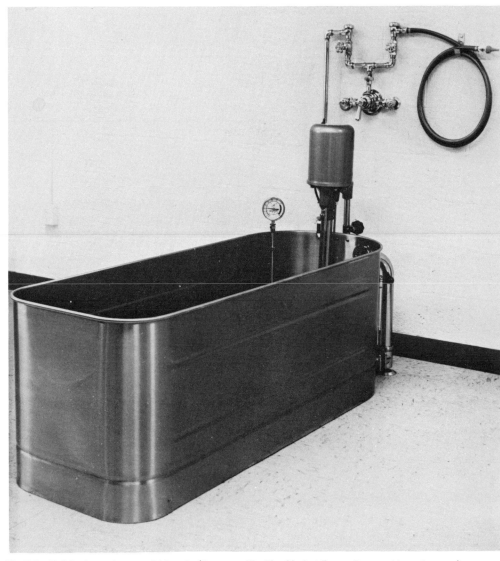

Fig. 7-3. Full-body stationary whirlpool. (Courtesy Ille Div. Market Forge, Everett, Massachusetts.)

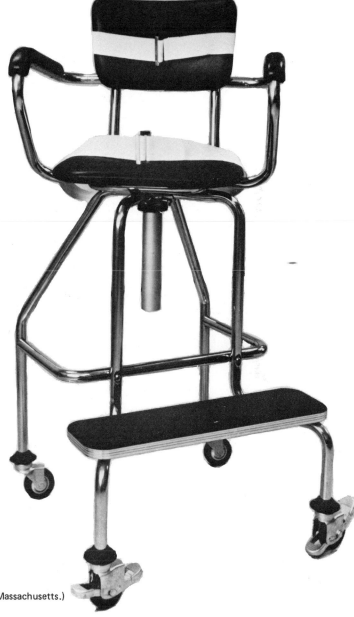

Fig. 7-4. Mobile adjustable high chair. (Courtesy Ille Div. Market Forge, Everett, Massachusetts.)

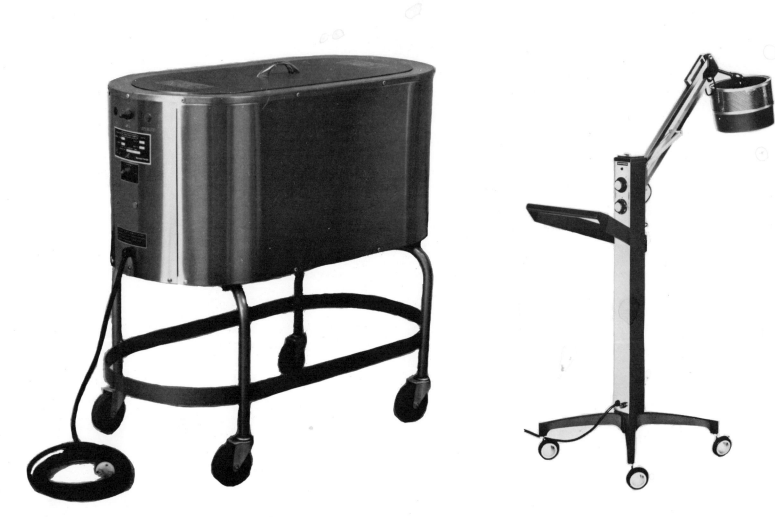

Fig. 7-5. Mobile arm, hand, and foot paraffin bath. (Courtesy Ille Div. Market Forge, Everett, Massachusetts.)

Fig. 7-6. Short-wave diathermy. (Courtesy Mettler Electronics Corp., Anaheim, Califronia.)

from room to room is commonly used (Fig. 7–6). Diathermy may be either microwave or short-wave, the latter being the most common. Thus high-frequency electromagnetic radiation or radio frequency current is directed at the affected part of the body to produce heat. This type of therapy is used with great caution due to the fact that it is easy to burn people and cannot be used on persons with pacemakers. Occasionally the rooms where this equipment is to be used must be shielded to contain the radio frequency or microwave radiation. Local codes must be consulted in this regard.

Heat or Cold

Heat is produced by a variety of methods from a simple electric heating pad to hot steam packs, or by soaking the affected part of the body in hot water or by infrared lamps. Cold is normally produced by cold packs or ice which are applied to the affected part of the body. Most of this equipment has no special requirements other than a suitable amount of storage space and convenient grounded electrical outlets. The hot-pack and cold-pack machines may be either stationary or mobile, the latter permitting more flexibility. They vary in size from 16 × 21 inches to 20 × 32 inches with an average height of 33 inches (Fig. 7–7).

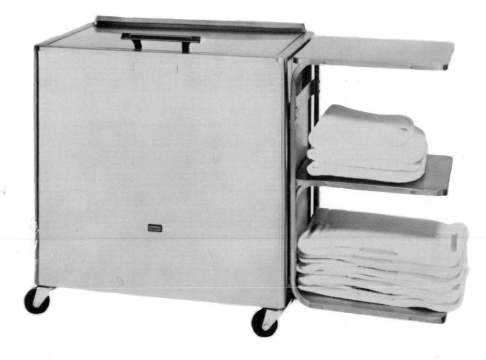

Fig. 7-7. Mobile hot-pack unit. (Courtesy Chattanooga Corp., Chattanooga, Tennessee.)

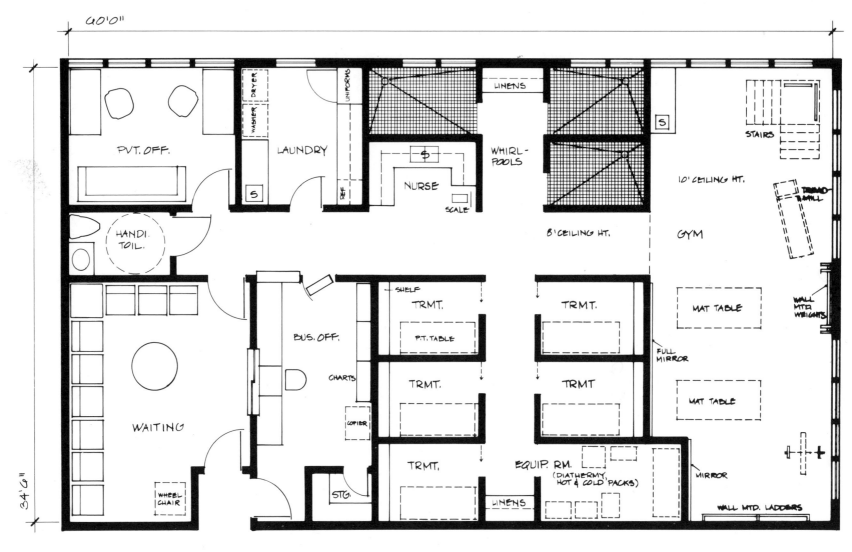

PHYSICAL THERAPY

2070 SQ. FT.

Fig. 7-8. Suite plan for physical therapy, 2070 square feet.

188

Massage

Massage is the oldest form of physical therapy. It is performed in private "cubicles," which may be constructed of standard partitions on three sides with a ceiling-mounted cubicle drape on the fourth side (Fig. 7-8), or the treatment cubicles may be contained in one large room, each one separated from the others only by ceiling-mounted cubicle drapes. In either case, the treatment modules need to be approximately 6 feet wide by 8 feet long. A physical therapy treatment table (Fig. 7-9) is 27 to 30 inches wide and 78 inches long. It would be placed along one wall. The room may also have a chair, a wall mirror, hooks for a patient's clothing, and a shelf for creams and ointments that may be used during the massage. A colorful accent wall in these rooms is a pleasant addition, and the cubicle drape fabric should be one of the many attractive stripes or plaids currently available in that product line. Various types of portable equipment such as a muscle stimulator or ultrasound unit may be wheeled into the cubicles as needed (Fig. 7-10).

Ultraviolet Therapy

Ultraviolet therapy is used to combat infection (kill bacteria) and to stimulate growth. A small hand-held light may be used or a hot quartz lamp on a mobile stand may be wheeled from room to room as needed. No special accommodations are required for ultraviolet therapy.

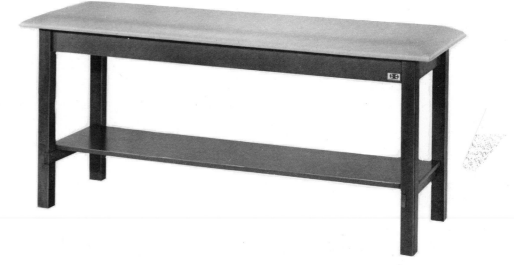

Fig. 7-9. Physical therapy treatment table. (Courtesy Hausmann Industries, Inc., Northvale, New Jersey.)

Exercise

A good deal of physical therapy involves the use of gym equipment. A large exercise room should be provided for therapeutic equipment some of which is wall mounted and some of which stands on the floor. Although windows and a nice view make exercising very pleasant, a good deal of wall space will be required for positioning wall-mounted equipment such as stall bars, weights, and pulleys.

The room may also have gait bars (Fig. 7-11), exercise bicycles (Fig. 7-12), barbells, an ambulation staircase (Fig. 7-13), a shoulder wheel (Fig. 7-14), as well as other gym equipment. The wall-mounted equipment must be located before construction begins, since the walls will require plywood reinforcement to support the additional weight. The room should have a 9-foot ceiling height and large mirrors which may be positioned so that people can see themselves using the equipment. Stylized wallgraphics of people exercising add vitality to the lackluster gym equipment (Figs. 7-15 and 7-16). Carpet is a nice addition to the gym functionally—it softens the blow if weights are dropped—and visually—it softens the geometry of the equipment.

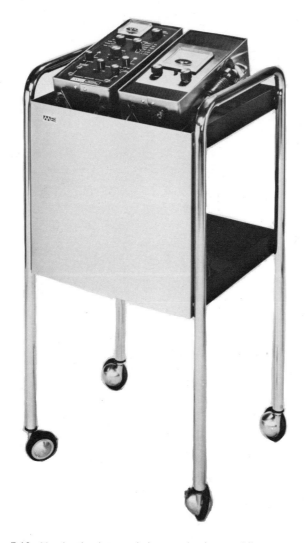

Fig. 7-10. Muscle stimulator and ultrasound unit on mobile cart. (Courtesy Mettler Electronics Corp., Anaheim, California.)

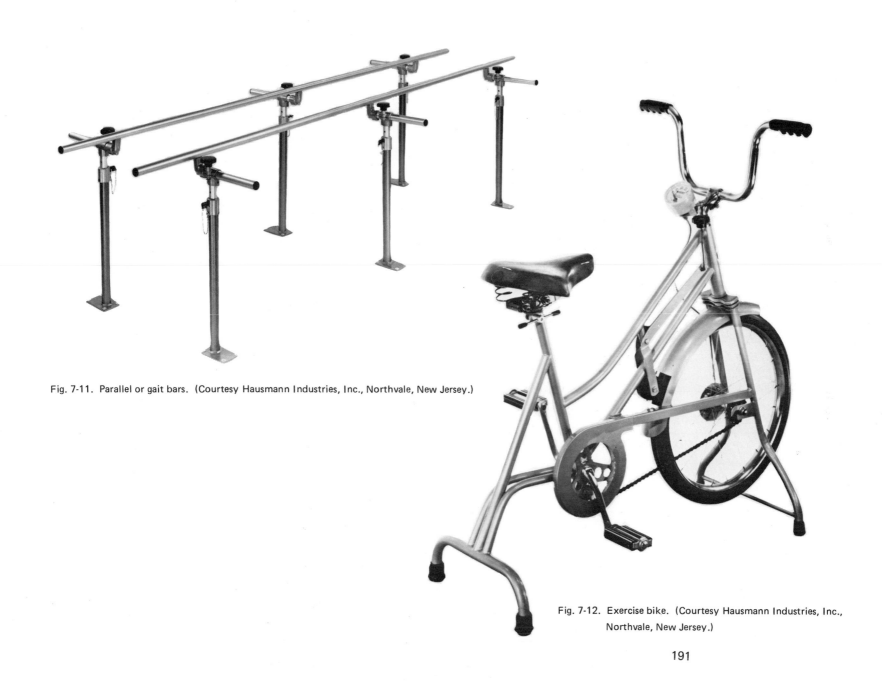

Fig. 7-11. Parallel or gait bars. (Courtesy Hausmann Industries, Inc., Northvale, New Jersey.)

Fig. 7-12. Exercise bike. (Courtesy Hausmann Industries, Inc., Northvale, New Jersey.)

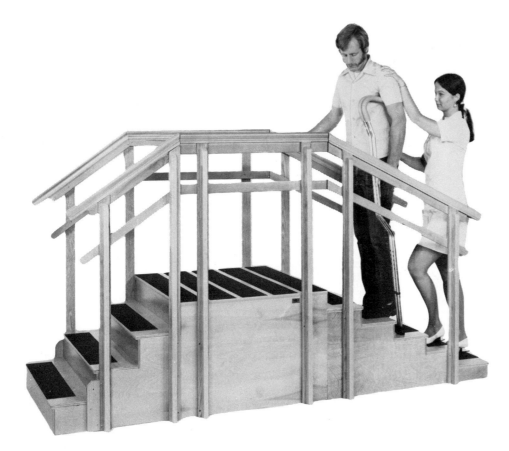

Fig: 7-13. Ambulation staircase. (Courtesy Hausmann Industries, Inc., Northvale, New Jersey.)

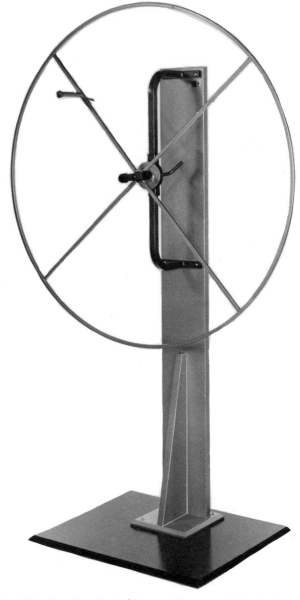

Fig. 7-14. Shoulder wheel. (Courtesy Hausmann Industries, Inc., Northvale, New Jersey.)

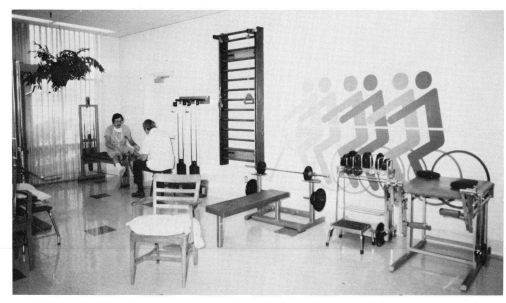

Fig. 7-15. Physical therapy gym.

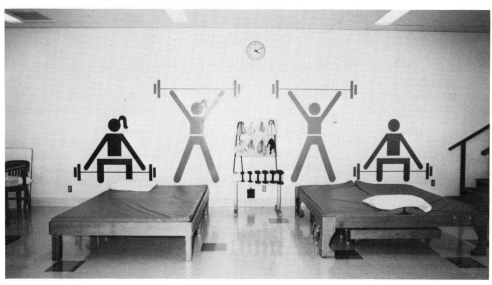

Fig. 7-16. Physical therapy gym.

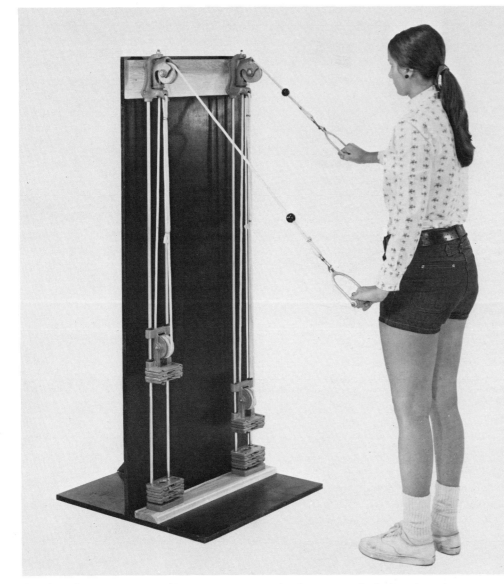

Fig. 7-17. Chest pulley weights. (Courtesy Hausmann Industries, Inc., Northvale, New Jersey.)

Ultrasound

Ultrasound involves an acoustic high-frequency vibration that is used to produce an analgesic effect on the nerves of the involved tissues. The ultrasound unit is small (Fig. 7-10) and can be wheeled on a mobile cart to a room as needed. It requires no special accommodation.

Other Areas

A physical therapy suite will also contain a small business office, a waiting room that will accommodate a wheelchair and people on crutches, a toilet that will serve the handicapped, a small private office, a nurse station, a laundry room with washer and dryer, and convenient storage of clean and dirty linen. All electrical outlets should be grounded, and local codes may require ground fault interrupters on baths and whirlpools. The massage area and any areas where water will be used should have sheet vinyl flooring or ceramic tile.

Table 7-1. Analysis of Program. Physical Therapy

Gym		15 × 27 =	405
Whirlpool Rooms	3 @	5 × 8 =	120
Nurse Station		6 × 9 =	54
Treatment Rooms	5 @	6 × 8 =	240
Waiting Room		14 × 16 =	224
Business Office		10 × 16 =	160
Toilet		6 × 8 =	48
Laundry		11 × 12 =	132
Private Office		11 × 12 =	132
Storage		6 × 8 =	48
	Subtotal		1563 ft²
15% Circulation			235
	Total		1798 ft²

PHARMACY

This discussion will be limited to pharmacies located in medical office buildings. Since the pharmacy's primary (and in some cases, total) source of business is the tenants in the building, it is wise not to plan the pharmacy's space until the tenants and their respective specialties are known. If the medical office building is isolated and not adjacent to neighborhood foot traffic, the pharmacy's referrals will come exclusively from the medical office building. If the pharmacy was in business in the neighborhood before moving into the new medical building, chances are a certain amount of "outside" business will follow the pharmacist to the new location due to loyalty or to prior business arrangements.

Thus it is necessary to analyze the source and number of prescriptions, both new and refills. Once the tenant population is known, the volume of prescriptions can be analyzed. A general practitioner or internist will see 25 to 35 patients per day and perhaps two-thirds of those patients will be given a prescription. Certain specialties tend to generate more prescriptions than others. When the estimated total of prescriptions to be derived from the tenant population has been determined, one must speculate on the percentage of those "scripts" that will end up at the building's pharmacy. If the physicians in the building "like" the pharmacist, if the pharmacist provides a comfortable place for patients to wait while a prescription is being filled, and if the pharmacy is located so that patients have to pass it upon exiting the building, approximately 70% of the building's "scripts" will be filled at the building's pharmacy. If the pharmacy is part of a group practice, approximately 80% of the group's prescriptions will filled at its own pharmacy. If the pharmacy hap-

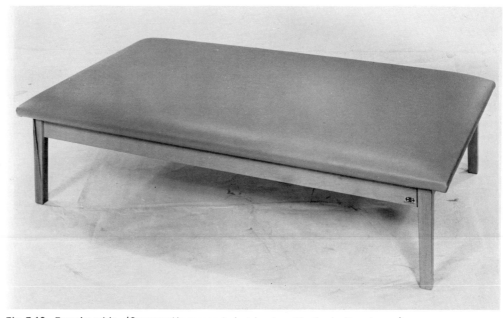

Fig. 7-18. Exercise table. (Courtesy Hausmann Industries, Inc., Northvale, New Jersey.)

pens to be located in a medical complex, but it is in a separate building and the patient has to walk outdoors to reach it, less that 40% of the complex-generated prescriptions will reach it. Some patients will remain loyal to a local pharmacy near their home or use one that will deliver.

After the volume of prescriptions is determined, the display space must be defined. If the pharmacy will sell prosthetic devices (crutches, braces, artificial limbs, colostomy supplies, etc.) a fitting room and a large storage room should be provided. Undoubtedly a certain amount of display space will be required even in a professional pharmacy for toothpaste, special soaps, first aid items, personal hygiene supplies, nonprescription drugs, and perhaps a limited line of cosmetics.

195

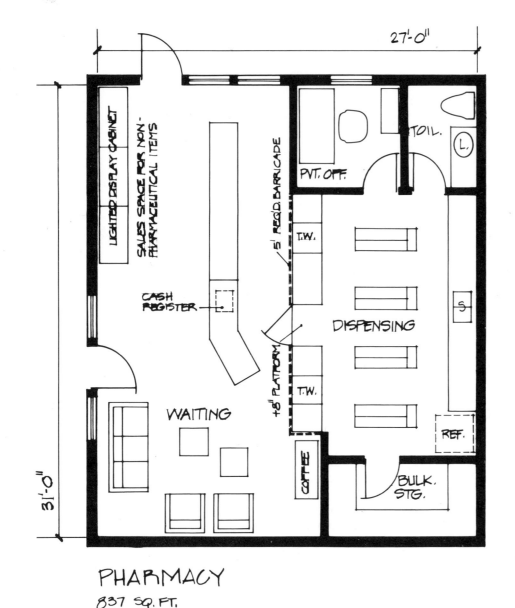

PHARMACY
837 SQ. FT.

Fig. 7-19. Pharmacy 837 square feet.

One pharmacist can usually fill 50 prescriptions in a day, which includes compounding, packaging, and dispensing. If he or she can prepackage certain frequently used medications, the scripts per day can be boosted to 70 per person. That is, certain physicians who are major sources of scripts may routinely prescribe certain medications in standard dosages. If the pharmacist knows this, he or she can, in slack periods, prepackage these items and store them on a shelf. When a patient requests them, only a label need be typed and the script is complete.

Each pharmacist requires 4 to 5 feet of countertop work surface for compounding and another 2 to 3 feet of countertop for typing and labeling. Each work station needs a phone. A full-size refrigerator and a built-in cabinet with a double sink should also be provided. Adjustable open shelving 8 to 10 inches deep is all that is required for storage of pharmaceuticals. Twelve lineal feet (6 feet high) of shelving is a minimum, with an additional 4 lineal feet per pharmacist. The dispensing area will have a raised platform floor (8 inches above floor of display and sales area), a required 5-foot-high security wall separating the dispensing and sales area, a required bathroom, and a bulk storage room. Sometimes a small private office is included. The bathroom is a code requirement based upon the reasoning that the pharmacist should never have to leave the store unattended while he or she leaves to use a public restroom. A professional pharmacy will occupy anywhere from 500 to 1000 square feet of space (Fig. 7-19).

Chapter 8
The Practice of Dentistry

The layout of dental facilities is far less standardized than the layout of medical facilities. Dentistry permits a wide range of options in preferred method of practice. In a dental suite the equipment largely determines the size and layout of the operating rooms. And therein lies the difficulty. The variety of equipment options is staggering, ranging from outdated units that have been modified to meet the fancy of a particular practitioner, to highly automated, sleekly contoured machinery. Dentistry allows for highly personalized practice methods, and the variables in equipment, location of utilities, and cabinetry reflect this diversity. This chapter, then, will acquaint the designer with the equipment and general requirements for the practice of dentistry, but each dentist-client must be interviewed thoroughly to determine his or her individual practice habits and preferences.

The broadest category of dentists is *general dentists.* Thus the basic elements of a dental suite will be discussed under *General Dentistry.* The modifications required for the primary dental specialties—orthodontics, pedodontics, and oral surgery—will be discussed thereafter.

GENERAL DENTISTRY

Office Circulation Patterns

The traffic flow within a dental office is from waiting room to X-ray (either a special room for this purpose or located in a standard operatory) to operatory. The patient should be able to enter the operatory and sit down on the right side of the chair (for a right-handed dentist) without walking around the chair or through the assistant's work area (Fig. 8-1). At the end of the procedure the patient walks to the reception area, repairs makeup or combs hair at the vanity or in the toilet room, books a future appointment if required, and pays for services.

The dentist's circulation is from private office to operatory and between operatories. He or she should be able to enter the operatory without having to walk around the chair or through the assistant's work area, wash hands, and be seated on the patient's right (if he or she is right-handed), as in Fig. 8-1. The assistant's path is from the sterilizing area to the operatories, darkroom, and lab. The assistant (also called the auxiliary), in

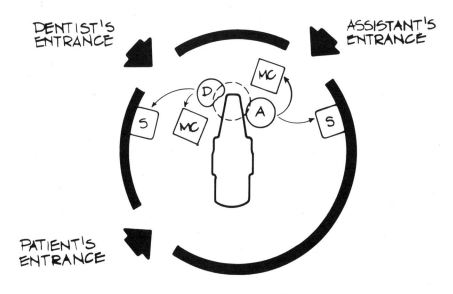

LEGEND

D = DENTIST
A = ASSISTANT
MC = MOBILE CABINET
S = SINK
FC = FIXED CABINET

DENTIST'S ENTRANCE

ASSISTANT'S ENTRANCE

PATIENT'S ENTRANCE

OPTIMUM TRAFFIC FLOW PATTERN FOR OPERATORY. DOTTED LINE INDICATES INSTRUMENT TRANSFER ZONE.

Fig. 8-1. Optimum traffic flow pattern.

most cases, will have to walk the greater distance in order to reach her work area since it is more important to maximize production that the dentists have the shortest route (Fig. 8–2, Plans A, C, D, and Fig. 8–3, Plan F). The office should be laid out to save as many steps as possible. Since the dentist and assistant are working in such confined areas, it is critical that these spaces be well planned and efficient. As with a medical office, a dental office should have a private entrance/exit for the staff and dentists so that they do not have to pass through the waiting room.

The Dental Assistant

The dental assistant or auxiliary performs many duties. Among them are cleanup of operatories, seating of patients in dental chair, preparing tray setups, taking X-rays, sterilizing instruments, loading anesthetic syringes, pouring impressions, mixing amalgams, charting and numbering teeth, handling suction, air, and water syringe, and assisting the dentist in dozens of restorative and surgical procedures.

Design Operatories for Flexibility

A right-handed dentist will work to the patient's right and a left-handed dentist to the patient's left. Traditionally, operatories were designed either for a right-handed dentist *or* a left-handed one. Today, flexibility is the key. New equipment is designed to accommodate change. In a practice composed of right-handed and left-handed dentists, an *ambidextrous* operatory can be designed (Fig. 8–4) in which the utilities are brought up under the toe of the chair and are mounted near the chair on a swing-away bracket that is designed to swing to either the left or the right of the chair. The X-ray head should be mounted over the fixed cabinet behind the patient, and the mobile cabinet used by the assistant may be used on either side of the chair. The mobile cabinet would slide into an opening in the fixed cabinet when not in use, and the hoses for water, compressed air, and suction would come from the wall behind the fixed cabinet or from a swing-away bracket on the chair, negating the need for a mobile cabinet.

Size of Operatories

Operatories may be as small as 8 × 10 feet or as large as 10 × 12 feet, 100 square feet is the average size. Figure 8–5 shows the minimum distances between the dental chair, cabinetry, and perimeter of the room. Dentists used to prefer small operatories when they worked alone so that while seated (or standing) they could reach everything they needed without walking. Now that most dentists use an assistant and the trend is toward longer appointments (it is more efficient to do a lot of work at one sitting), many dentists feel more comfortable working in a large operatory. If the dentist uses large mobile cabinets, a more spacious operatory is desirable so that the cabinets can easily be moved to any position in the room.

Number of Operatories

There is no rule governing the number of operatories per dentist since the dentist's temperament and practice methods have a lot to do with it. A dentist who works slowly or who does a lot of restorative work with long appoint-

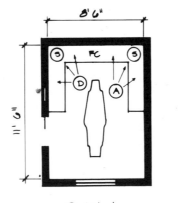

PLAN A

"U" DESIGN OPERATORY
DENTIST AND ASSISTANT WORK
OFF OF FIXED CABINETS.

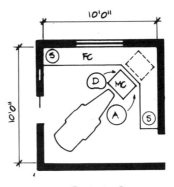

PLAN B

DIAGONAL CHAIR PLACEMENT
WITH SINGLE MOBILE CABINET
BEHIND PATIENT'S HEAD. DENTIST
AND ASSISTANT WORK OFF OF
MOBILE CABINET.

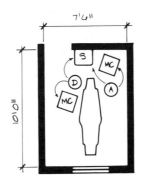

PLAN C

ASSISTANT AND DENTIST
WORK OFF OF SPLIT MOBILE
CABINETS. NO FIXED CABINETRY
IN ROOM.

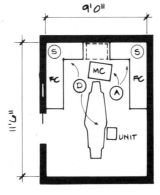

PLAN D

MODIFIED "U" ARRANGEMENT
WITH OPENING IN FIXED CABINETS
FOR STORAGE OF MOBILE CABINET.
ASSISTANT WORKS OFF OF MOBILE
CABINET BEHIND PATIENT AND
DENTIST WORKS OFF OF A DENTAL
UNIT WITH INSTRUMENTATION DELIVERED
OVER THE PATIENT'S CHEST.

Fig. 8-2. Plans A, B, C, D.

199

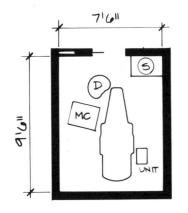

PLAN E

AN OPERATORY FOR A DENTIST
WHO WORKS WITHOUT AN ASSISTANT.

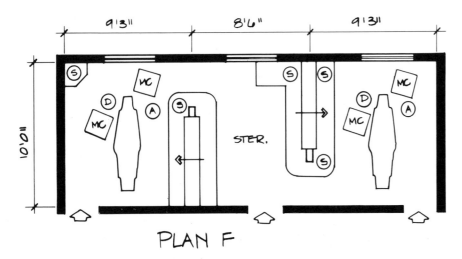

PLAN F

DENTIST AND ASSISTANT WORK OFF MOBILE CABINETS.
BOTH OPERATORIES HAVE PASS-THROUGH FEATURE WITH
STERILIZATION AREA WHICH PERMITS CLEAN TRAY SET-UPS
TO BE PLACED IN OPERATORY (AND DIRTY ONES REMOVED)
WITHOUT ENTERING THE ROOM.

Fig. 8-3. Plans E, F.

ments can be comfortable with two operatories. A dentists with many short appointments will need four operatories in order not to lose time during the change of patients and the preparation or cleanup of operatories. A rule of thumb is three operatories per dentist in a general practice.

Design of the Dental Operatory

This is the most important room in a dental office. Although analagous to the physician's examination room, it is far more critical to a dentist's practice than the medical exam room is to a physician's practice since the physician has ancillary rooms for diagnosis, testing, and treatment, but the dentist has only the operatory. In terms of economics, the physician has the opportunity to enhance his or her income from laboratory tests, X-ray films, and the use of medical aides to give injections, administer EKGs and EEGs, or to do physical therapy. But the dentist has only the operatory plus the laboratory and X-ray work from which to derive income. For this reason many time and motion studies focusing on operatory efficiency have been published in dental journals. And, in recent years, certain major changes have evolved as a result of these studies. Patients now recline in a contour chair with the dentist working from a seated position at the side of the patient. If right-handed, the dentist will be seated to the right of the patient and will work in an area that could be designated at from 9:00 to 12:00, imagining the face of a clock surrounding the patient. Most dentists use an assistant, which is called *four handed dentistry*. Some dentists use two assistants. Figure 8–1 illustrates the optimum traffic flow pattern for an operatory. However, the exigencies of the fixed structure of the space, the location of windows and other "given" features, have an impact on the layout of the space, and compromises sometimes must be made.

Instrumentation. There are four categories of instrumentation.

Handpiece Delivery System. This is composed of rotary tools with drill bits that are used to cut and shape teeth.

Evacuation System. Blood, debris, and water are removed from the mouth usually by suction (a vacuum system). This is normally performed by the dental assistant.

Hand-held Instruments. These tools include probes, scalers, forceps, etc.

Three-way Syringe. Often used by both the dentist and the assistant for spraying water, compressed air, or a combination thereof. In a well-equipped operatory, the assistant will have her own three-way syringe for drying or moistening preparations as well as for washing debris from the patient's mouth.

Methods of Delivery. The instrumentation can be delivered to the oral cavity of the patient by three methods.

Mobile Delivery System. The utilities (water, air, suction, electricity) can be delivered via mobile carts in *split* fashion (the dentist's cart has the handpieces and syringe, while the assistant's cart has a syringe and suction), or via a *single* cart from which the dentist's as well as the assistant's instruments are delivered. The single cart

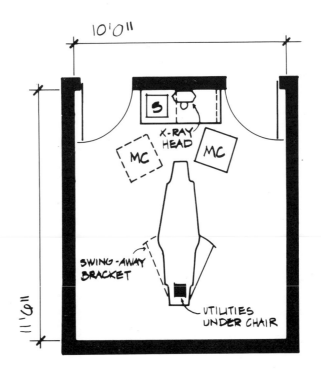

AMBIDEXTROUS OPERATORY

THIS ARRANGEMENT SERVES A PRACTICE COMPOSED OF RIGHT-AND-LEFT-HANDED DENTISTS. THE X-RAY HEAD IS MOUNTED BEHIND THE PATIENT. UTILITIES ARE UNDER THE TOE OF THE CHAIR AND THE ASSISTANT'S MOBILE CART CAN MOVE TO EITHER SIDE.

Fig. 8-4. Ambidextrous operatory.

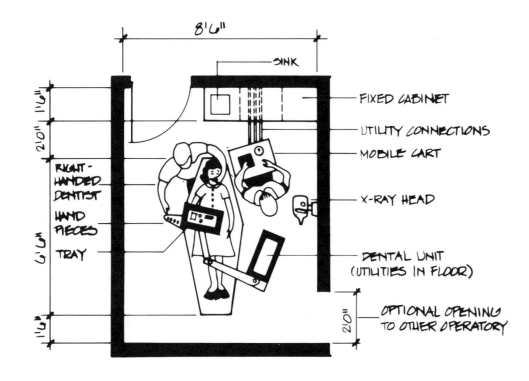

OPTIMAL SIZE OF OPERATORY

Fig. 8-5. Optimal size of operatory.

is usually located to the rear of the patient (Fig. 8-2, Plan B), while the split cart (for a right-handed dentist) would be located just below the patient's right shoulder and the split cart for the assistant would be located to the left of the patient's head (Fig. 8-1 and Fig. 8-2, Plan C). (See also Figs. 8-7, 8-8, 8-9, and Figs. 8-10, 8-11, Plate 12).

Rear Delivery System. Both the dentist's and the assistant's instrumentation are delivered from behind the patient's head from a fixed cabinet (Fig. 8-2, Plan A) with the systems built in. Delivery of instrumentation from a mobile cabinet behind the patient is discussed above.

Over-the-Patient Delivery System. Instruments and utilities are delivered from an area near the patient's left or right elbow or over the patient's chest. These kinds of delivery systems are usually attached to the chair so that even as the chair is adjusted up or down, the relationship of instrument location with respect to the oral cavity is constant (Fig. 8-3, Plans D and E).

There are combinations of the above delivery systems as well as other variables that must be considered. Two such items are the use of the cuspidor versus the more efficient central suction, and the number and placement of sinks in the operatory. Cuspidors (spittoons) can be purchased with central suction operation or with gravity drain (Fig. 8-17.) However, most modern dental offices use central suction with no cuspidor. The suction hoses at each operatory work off of a vacuum pump located in an equipment room near the operatories. The vacuum piping is PVC Schedule 40. Since the vacuum pump and air compressor are noisy, it is desirable to enclose them in a small sound-insulated mechanical equipment room.

As for sinks, an operatory must have at least one since the dentist and assistant must wash their hands upon entering the room. (Some dentists may prefer a foot lever or wrist action faucets.) Operatories may have an additional sink for the assistant in order to save steps and keep the assistant out of the dentist's path (Plans A, B, D, and F of Figs. 8–2 and 8–3). Regardless of number, operatory sinks may be quite small. Stainless steel bar sinks function well. (See Figs. 8–18 and 8–19.)

Another variable, and one that inspires controversy, is the number and placement of doors (or whether to have doors) in the operatory. A solid-core hinged door helps to block the sound of high-speed drills but makes it more difficult for the dentist and assistant to rotate quickly between operatories. Thus many operatories have sliding doors which remain open most of the time but can be closed for visual privacy (they offer little sound attenuation) when necessary. However, many dentists prefer openings without doors (Fig. 8–20) as well as openings between operatories so that they and the assistants can quickly move back and forth between the rooms. The author favors this option not just for efficiency but also because the patient feels less apprehensive when not closed up in a small room.

The method of instrumentation delivery and the number of sinks must be determined early in the space planning since the locations of air, vacuum, waste, water, and electric depend on it.

Gas. Gas is used to heat certain impression materials. As an option a dentist may want gas lines run into the operatories for a Bunsen burner. It is safer to locate the gas line in the wall behind the operatory cabinet (rather than near the dental chair) to avoid hot materials dripping on the pa-

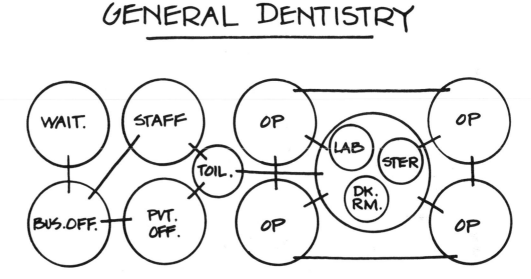

GENERAL DENTISTRY

Fig. 8-6. Schematic diagram of a general dentistry suite.

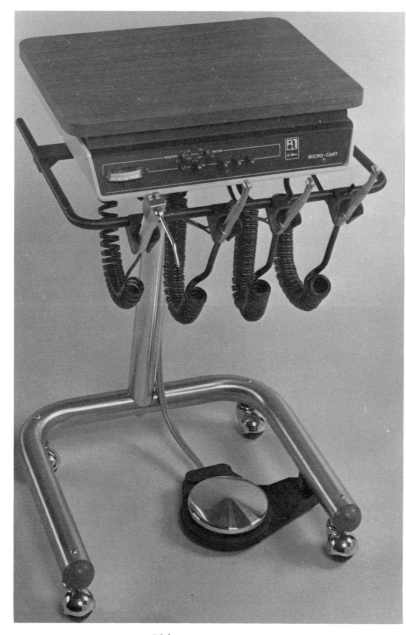

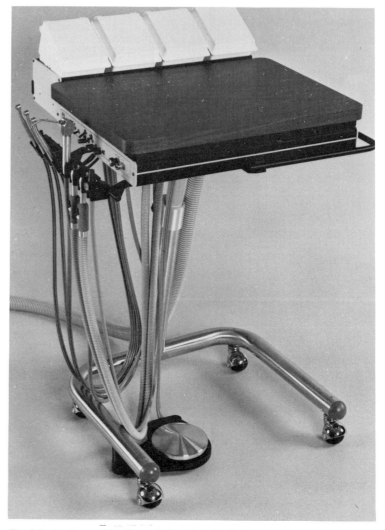

Fig. 8-8. Dual cart: Usually used directly behind chair or on assistant's side. (Courtesy Adec, Newberg, Oregon.)

Fig. 8-7. Dentist's cart. (Courtesy Adec, Newberg, Oregon.)

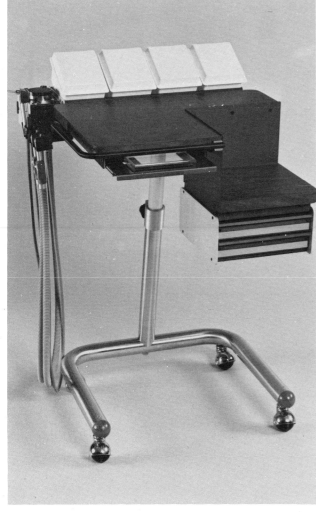

Fig. 8-9. Assistant's cart. (Courtesy Adec, Newberg, Oregon.)

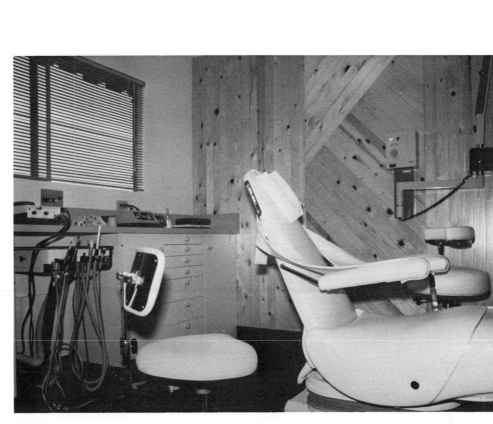

Fig. 8-12. Dental operatory.

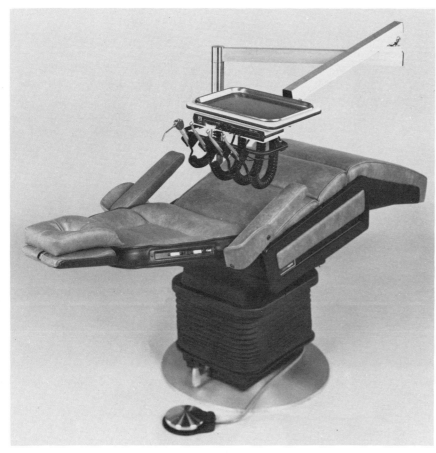

Fig. 8-13. Over-the-chair unit for dentist only. (Courtesy Adec, Newberg, Oregon.)

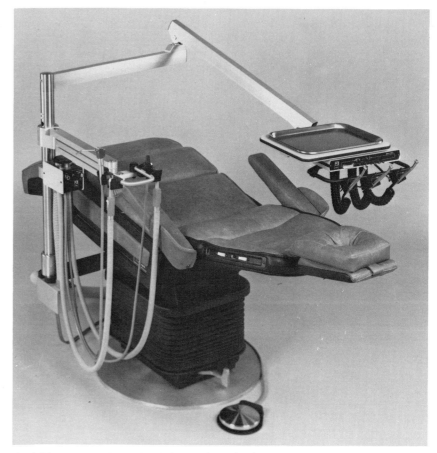

Fig. 8-14. Dual over-the-chair unit for dentist and assistant.
(Courtesy Adec, Newberg, Oregon.)

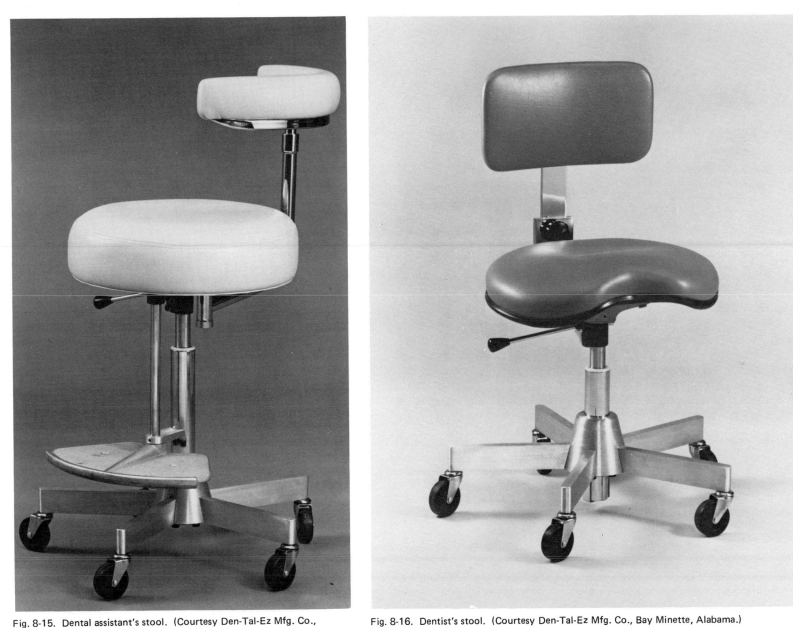

Fig. 8-15. Dental assistant's stool. (Courtesy Den-Tal-Ez Mfg. Co., Bay Minette, Alabama.)

Fig. 8-16. Dentist's stool. (Courtesy Den-Tal-Ez Mfg. Co., Bay Minette, Alabama.)

207

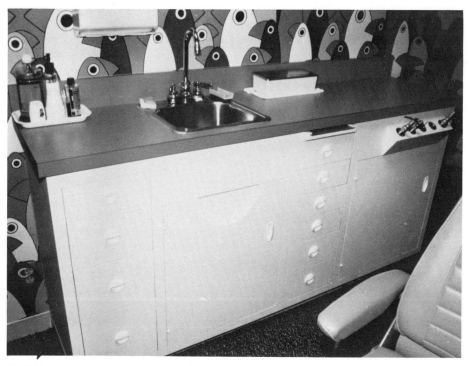

Fig. 8-18. Dental cabinet with trash slot and pull-out board for daily appointment schedule.

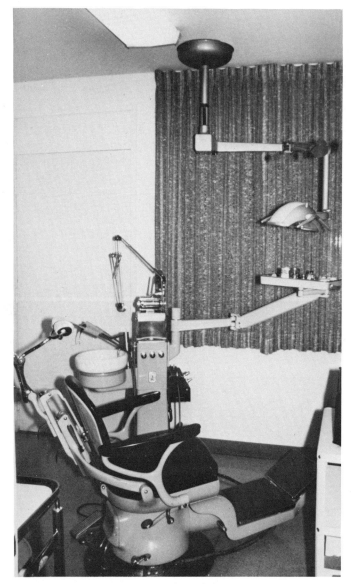

Fig. 8-17. Outdated dental chair with cuspidor.

tient. New equipment generally does not have a built-in Bunsen burner. Most dentists use a portable alcohol torch instead of gas because running a gas line into a building is very expensive. Medical office buildings often have a gas line in the building and the individual tenants must pay only for the piping to their suite.

Tray Setups

Instruments are sterilized and then set up in advance on trays for various procedures. These trays (size varies from 4 × 8 to 13 × 17 inches) may be stored in a central location (Fig. 8–21) or may be stored in each operatory for that day's work. Operatories that are contiguous with the sterilizing area (Fig. 8–3, Plan F) can have upper cabinets that open from both sides, permitting trays of sterile instruments to be placed in an operatory without someone actually entering the room (Fig. 8–22). "Dirty" instrument trays can be removed from the operatory by the same procedure. The upper cabinet would have a "clean" side and "dirty" side. During procedures, the instrument tray is placed where it is accessible to both the dentist and the assistant. This may be on a mobile cabinet, on a fixed cabinet, on a Mayo stand over the patient's chest, or on a shelf that is attached to the dental chair.

Design Considerations

In addition to the functional requirements, the operatory should meet certain psychological needs of the patient. A window is always desirable to give patients a psychological escape route and a pleasant view. In lieu of a window, a landscape mural or other wallcovering might be

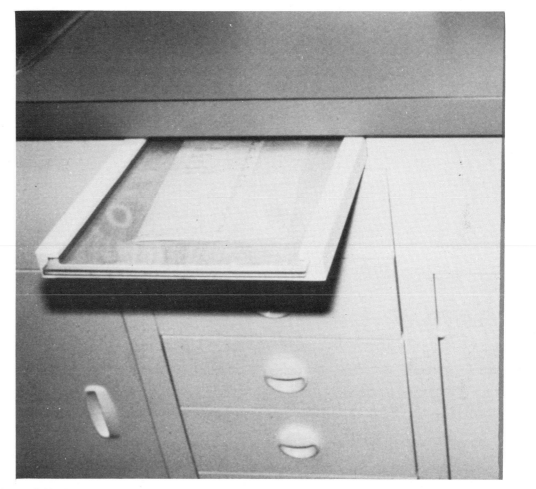

Fig. 8-19. Pull-out board for keeping daily lists of patients.

209

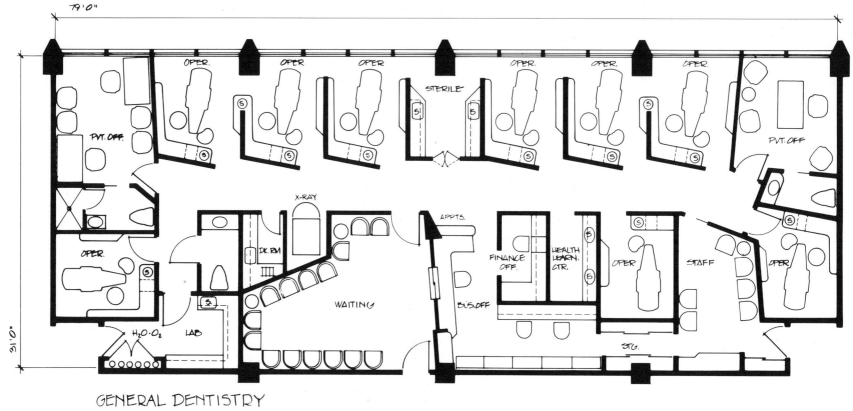

79'0"

31'0"

OPER. · OPER · OPER · STERILE · OPER. · OPER. · OPER · PVT. OFF.

PVT. OFF.

OPER.

X-RAY

DK. RM.

APPTS.

FINANCE OFF. · HEALTH LEARN. CTR.

OPER · STAFF · OPER

BUS. OFF.

WAITING

H₂O·O₂ · LAB

STG.

GENERAL DENTISTRY

2400 SQ. FT

Fig. 8-20. Suite plan for general dentistry, 2400 square feet.

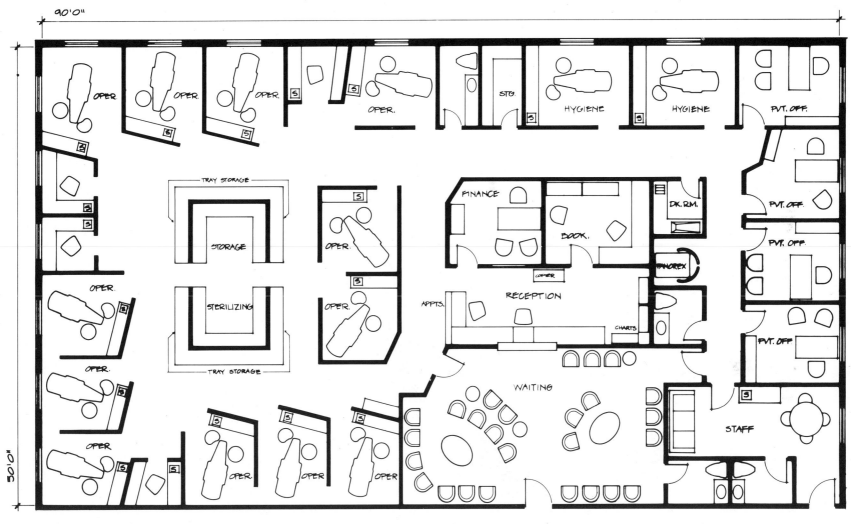

GENERAL DENTISTRY - GROUP PRACTICE
4500 SQ. FT.

Fig. 8-21. Suite plan for group practice, 4500 square feet.

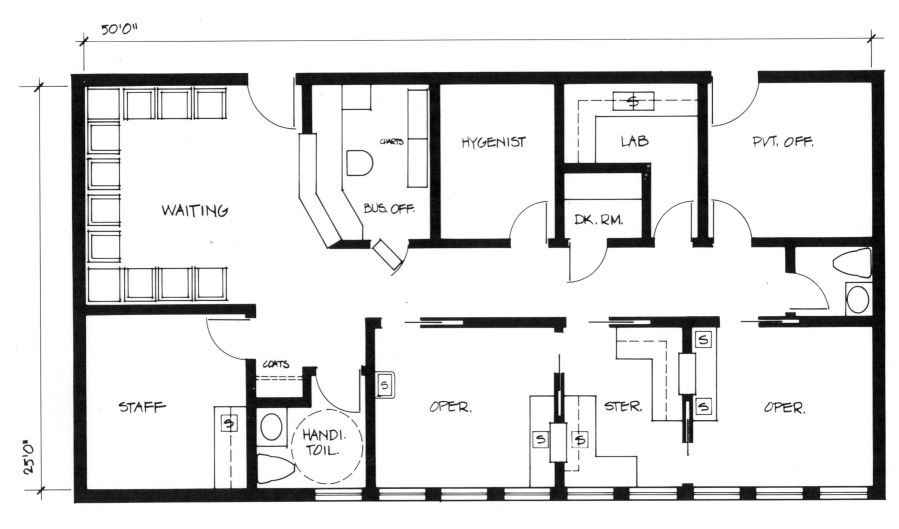

50'0"

25'0"

WAITING

CHARTS

BUS. OFF.

HYGENIST

LAB

$

DK. RM.

PVT. OFF.

STAFF

COATS

$

$

HANDI. TOIL.

OPER.

$

$

STER.

$

$

OPER.

GENERAL DENTISTRY

1250 SQ. FT.

Fig. 8-22. Suite plan, 1250 square feet.

installed. A mobile suspended from the ceiling so that the patient can see it while reclined in the chair is a distracting diversion. The dental chair and fixed and mobile cabinetry should be selected in attractive colors that coordinate with the room's interior design. The author prefers to use light, neutral colors for the cabinetry and dental units in order to make them blend into the background and be less obtrusive.

Other amenities in the operatory are a hook for a handbag, a tissue box accessible to the patient, and a waste receptacle. Operatories can successfully be carpeted with a low-pile commercial carpet glued directly to the floor. The carpet should be in place and all decorating complete before the dental equipment is installed. Carpet in dental operatories should have a synthetic backing (not jute) so that it does not rot in the event of a plumbing break. (Dental operatories are prone to plumbing disasters.) Live plants add a nice touch to an operatory and subliminally indicate that if the plants are thriving, so will the patient.

Sterilization

Sterilization can be performed in the lab if it is close to the operatories, or it can be done in an alcove in the corridor (Fig. 8–23) with cabinets, a sink, and space for an autoclave and an ultrasonic cleaner. If the clean tray setups are stored here, a larger area will be needed and the upper cabinet would be fitted with slots into which the trays slide. There are three methods of sterilization each with advantages and disadvantages:

Dry Heat—Long cycle at high temperature. Good because it does not rust or dull sharp instruments, but the oven gives off lots of heat and it is a slow process. Used by endodontists who use tools made of carbide steel.

Steam—Fast, but dulls instruments; however, there are products available that protect the instruments from rusting and dulling. Steam autoclave combines live steam and pressure.

Chemical—Alcohol-based chemical vapor sterilizes.

Most dentists use either steam or chemical sterilization. A few dentists use both, and some use steam plus dry heat. The sterilizing sequence is: Dirty instruments are scrubbed in a sink, then cleaned in an ultrasonic cleaner, wrapped or bagged, sterilized by one of the methods above, then placed in storage trays or cabinets. It should be noted that many sterilizers require a separate circuit. (See Figs. 8–24 and 8–25.)

Laboratory

The size of the laboratory will vary greatly depending upon whether the dentist sends out most of the lab work or whether he or she employs lab technicians. If two workbenches are arranged so that they face each other, a dental engine, lathe, and other tools can be shared. If the work load demands it, two separate work stations should be set up so that one person does not interfere with the other. Upper cabinets should be positioned so that they are accessible to seated technicians

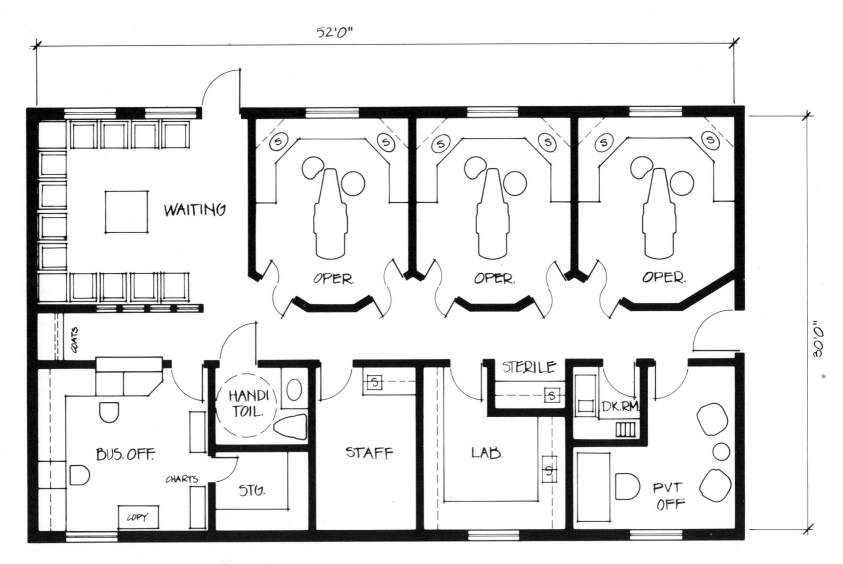

52'0"

30'0"

WAITING

S S S S S S

OPER. OPER. OPER.

COATS

HANDI TOIL.

BUS. OFF.

CHARTS

STG.

COPY

STAFF

LAB.

STERILE

S

S

S

DK.RM.

PVT OFF

GENERAL DENTISTRY

1560 SQ. FT.

Fig. 8-23. Suite plan, 1560 square feet.

214

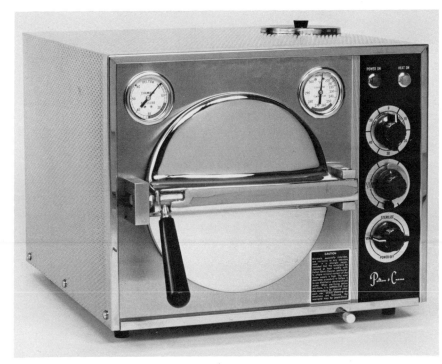

Fig. 8-24. Steam autoclave. (Courtesy Pelton & Crane, Charlotte, North Carolina.)

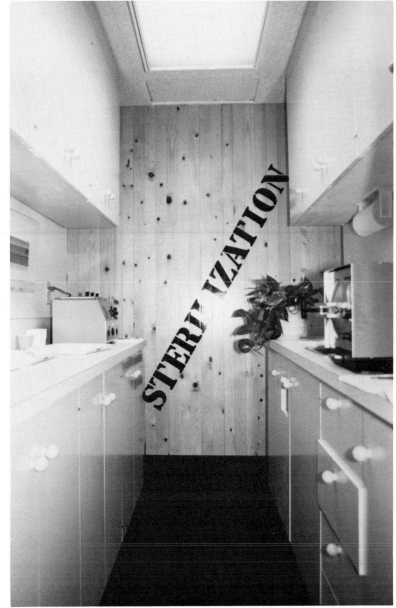

Fig. 8-25. Sterilization/lab.

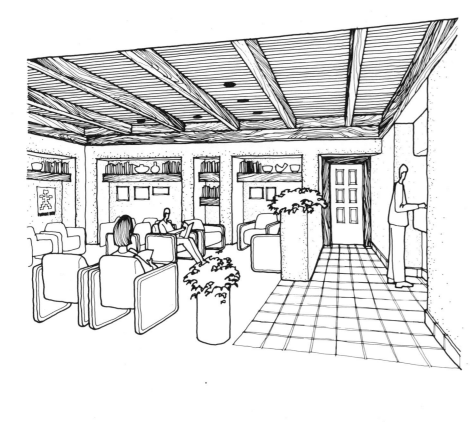

WAITING

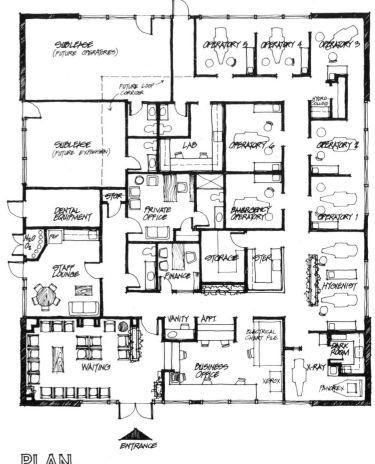

PLAN

Fig. 8-26. Suite plan for general dentistry. (Courtesy Michael T. Hadley, AIA: Quadrasource.)

without too much stretching. The sink should be positioned in a central location. The air compressor and vacuum may be located in the lab to supply the lab and the operatories, unless it is located in a mechanical equipment room. The lab requires gas, compressed air, water, waste (acid-resistant drainage lines and sink with plaster trap), a plaster bin, and many electrical outlets (continuous plug strips should be mounted above the countertops). It is important to design the electrical service large enough to accommodate the high usage requirements of various pieces of equipment. The lab may be located near the operatories to meet demands of immediate impression pouring, but if a considerable number of noisy procedures are performed it is wise to keep the laboratory a distance from the operatories. Since labs tend to be messy, it is advisable to supply a door so that patients cannot see into the room.

Vanity Area

A mirror and shelf or vanity cabinet should be located near the reception area if space permits. Thus a patient can comb hair or repair makeup while the receptionist is scheduling a future appointment (Fig. 8-26).

Audiovisual Room

Many dentists have small patient education rooms that consist of a built-in countertop at a 29-inch height, stools or chairs, and several electrical outlets for plugging in an audiovisual training machine—either photographic or video. Patients may watch or listen to presentations on how to floss teeth or reduce dental caries, or on how a complicated dental procedure is performed. This saves the dentist and staff from repeating this information. Sometimes this room does not have A.V. equipment but is used as a patient education-hygiene room, in which case it is equipped with two or three sinks (built into the countertop) and a wall-to-wall mirror so that a dental assistant can explain and demonstrate dental flossing and proper brushing techniques. This should be a cheerful area with an attractive vanity counter and wallpaper or perhaps a supergraphic design reinforcing good dental hygiene (Figs. 8-27, Plate 12 and 8-28).

Hygiene Operatory

The hygienist performs many duties. She takes X-rays, processes and mounts the film, performs dental prophylaxis, instructs patients on proper

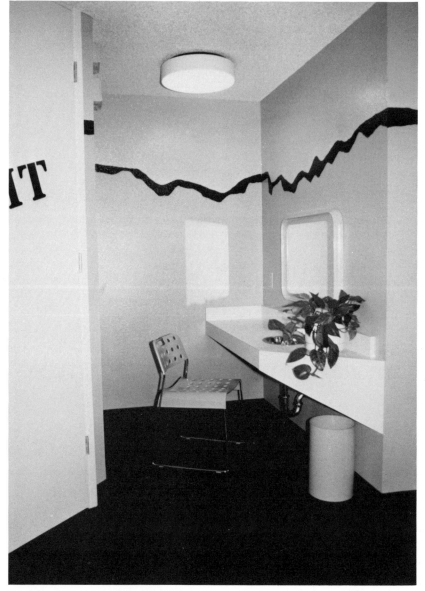

Fig. 8-28. Patient education alcove.

brushing and flossing techniques, discusses nutrition in regard to prevention of dental caries, and maintains the patient recall system.

Many dentists set aside one operatory for the use of the hygienist, while others schedule a hygienist perhaps two or three afternoons a week and use one of their standard operatories. Thus this room may have the normal dental equipment or it may have specialized equipment. The room should not (as is sometimes seen) have funky antique dental chairs because, although interesting in terms of interior design, it puts the hygienist at a functional handicap. A modern dental hygienist should have modern, full instrumentation equipment.

Since one wishes to positively reinforce good dental hygiene, this room should be attractively decorated and be uplifting so that a good impression lingers after the patients departs.

Analgesia and Anesthesia

The use of analgesia (medications that decrease sensitivity to pain but that do not put the patient to sleep) is very common in dental practice today. Local anesthetics, such as Novocain or Xylocaine, make dentistry painless and require no special accommodation in the room or suite. However, analgesia, usually a mixture of nitrous oxide (N_2O) and oxygen (O_2), requires special handling. These gases may simply be portable tanks that are wheeled into the operatory as needed or tanks that are located in a small storage room either inside or outside of the suite. *Building and fire codes are very strict regarding where and how medical gases are to be stored.* Specifically, they may not be stored in a location in which flame or electrical sparks are produced such as a dental laboratory. In addition, tanks should be stored in a place that is easily accessible for servicing. Medical gases that are stored in this fashion are piped through degreased, sealed copper tubing (using only silver solder) to a flow meter in each operatory or surgery. If the tanks are stored outside of the suite, a zone shutoff valve assembly and alarm system must be located within the suite to monitor the supply. Nitrous tanks and valve are always placed to the left of the oxygen tank and valve as one faces them. This convention permits a fire fighter to enter a smokey room and locate the more combustible oxygen tanks quickly.

The use of anesthesia (medications that put patients to sleep) is confined mainly to oral surgeons. They normally use Sodium Pentothal administered to the patient via the arm.

Special Plumbing and Electrical Requirements

There exist many variables in the proper location of plumbing and electric to service the dental unit, the chair, the mobile carts, and the X-ray equipment. It would be virtually impossible for the designer or architect to keep current with each manufacturer's specific requirements. Thus it is mandatory to work closely with a qualified, reputable dental equipment dealer. Such dealers offer planning services either free with an equipment order from the dentist, or for a small fee. It is wise to work with the dealer in laying out the equipment in the room. There are many critical dimensions and complex plumbing and electrical requirements specific to each manufacturer. Normally equipment dealers will also service the equipment, which is another reason that it should be laid out according to their specifications.

Most dental equipment has its own water supply and shutoff valve, but in addition, it is advisable that each operatory have its own water and air shutoff valves so that repair work can be done in one operatory without closing down the entire office. The ideal location for these shutoff valves, and one that is easily accessible, is in the cabinet under the sink in each room.

Business Office

The business office of a dental suite is generally smaller than that of a similar-size medical office since the procedures are often fewer and do not require the volumes of paperwork associated with numerous lab tests and batteries of X-ray films. Dental records are not as bulky as medical charts and the X-ray films are considerably smaller. Nevertheless, as dentists begin to add computer billing equipment to their offices and as they begin to offer health maintenance organization prepaid plans to subscribers, and since there are now numerous dental insurance plans in operation, the dental business office will have to expand. High-volume practices such as pedodontics and orthodontics process a lot of patients, and the business office must reflect this volume of transactions. The reader is referred to Chapter 3 under *Business Office* for a more complete discussion of this topic.

Waiting Room

The reader is referred to Chapter 3 under *Waiting Room* for a general discussion of waiting rooms. Dentists tend to have smaller waiting rooms than medical offices of the same square footage since the patient volume is lower. A family practice

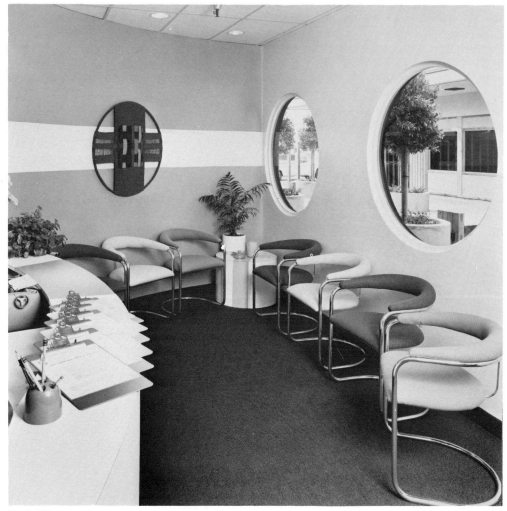

Fig. 8-29. Waiting room.

physician may see upwards of six patients per hour, while a general practice dentist may see only two or three, depending upon the complexity of the procedure and whether the appointment is primarily for examination and diagnosis or for restorative work. In cold-weather climates where persons wear coats and galoshes and use umbrellas, a coat closet or coat rack should be located where it can be supervised by the business office staff. A patient should be able to enter the waiting room, proceed to the reception window to check in, then select a magazine and be seated without tripping on furniture or patients' feet. The waiting room should have carpet and sound-absorbing wallcoverings since it would make waiting patients anxious to hear the sound of the drill in a nearby operatory. Many patients are terrified of a visit to the dentist. Every opportunity should be seized to reduce this anxiety. Relaxing colors, textured wallcoverings, a luxurious carpet, pleasant music, comfortable furniture, and interesting artwork should be employed to this end. Both the dentist and the patient are influenced by the physical climate of the office and the attitudes and personality of the staff. A patient's past experiences with dentists and the dentist's feeling of success or failure are the basis for the tension system in which the patient finds himself or herself. A dentist with a positive attitude, who schedules his or her day effectively and who employs well-trained auxiliary help who are sensitive to both the dentist's and the patients' needs can effectively break the tension system.

As a rule of thumb, two seats in the waiting room should be provided for every operatory and hygiene room. High-volume practices such as orthodontics and pedodontics, which are characterized by many short appointments, should have three to four seats per dental chair, if space permits (see Fig. 8–31, Plate 12).

Private Office

Dentists tend to have very small private offices, sometimes as small as 8 × 9 feet. Patients rarely enter a dentist's private office, so it is used primarily to read mail, return phone calls, or relax between procedures. Sometimes, in order to save space, dentists will share a private office (Fig. 8–36).

X-ray

Some dentists equip all operatories for X-ray; others confine the X-ray to one operatory or to a special room that is equipped with a panoramic X-ray as well as an intraoral one (Fig. 8–37). In some practices, the operatories are set up for intraoral X-rays but a small room (approximately 5 × 8 feet) or a niche in the corridor is set aside for the panoramic X-ray unit (Figs. 8–37, 8–38, 8–39), one in which the patient sits in a special chair, or stands, and the X-ray head revolves around the patient, making a film of the complete mouth rather than just the limited area of the bitewing X-ray. Certain dentists will also have a cephalometric X-ray unit, which takes a film of the whole

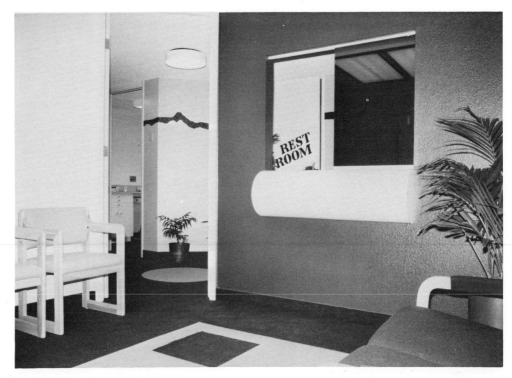

Fig. 8-30. Reception window.

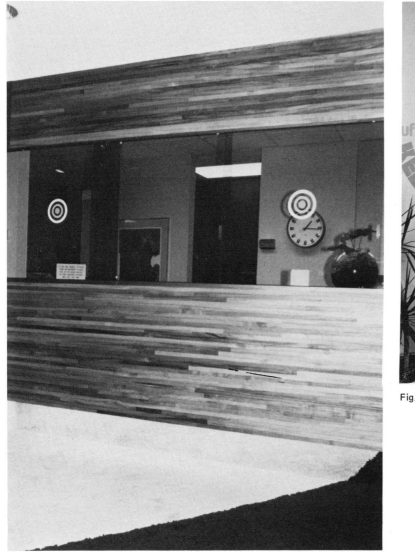

Fig. 8-32. Reception window: Note teak butcher block and recessed light under base.

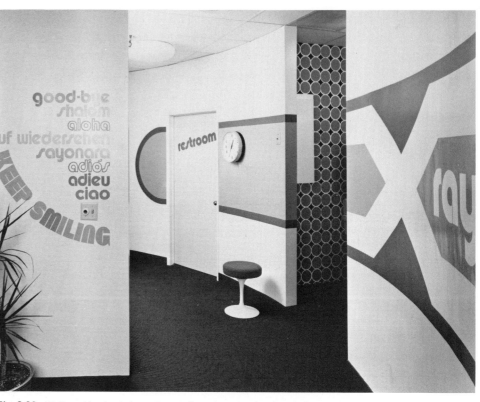

Fig. 8-33. Wallgraphics lend themselves well to the curved walls of plan in Fig. 8-37.

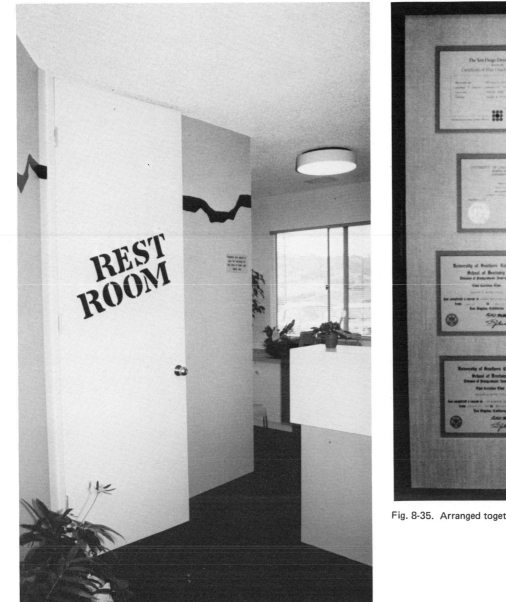

Fig. 8-34. Appointment desk.

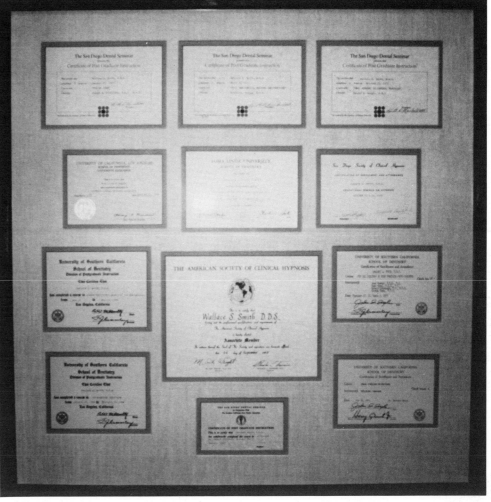

Fig. 8-35. Arranged together, these diplomas make an impressive piece of wall decor.

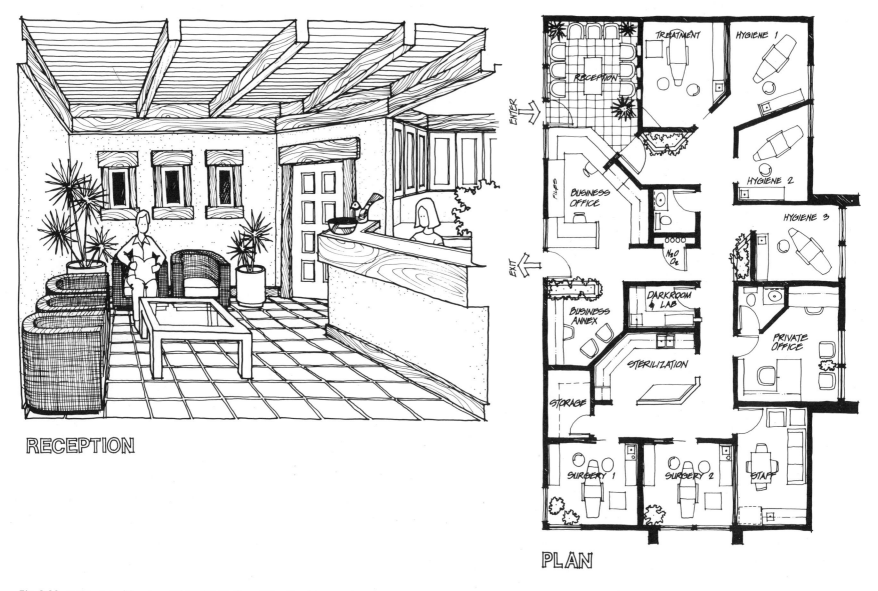

RECEPTION

PLAN

Fig. 8-36. Suite plan. (Courtesy Michael T. Hadley, AIA: Quadrasource.)

224

head and jaw. Orthodontists would often have this type of X-ray unit. There is even a combination panoramic/cephalometric unit. Any X-ray facilities located outside of the operatories, as well as the darkroom, should be located close to the hygientist's area, since he or she is normally the person who takes and develops the X-rays.

If each operatory is equipped for intraoral X-rays, the X-ray head is located on the wall either to the side of the patient or, in an ambidextrous operatory, behind the patient. The relationship of the X-ray mount to the position of the chair is critical since the arm will swing in several positions and will extend 4 or 5 feet. The wall that supports the X-ray mount must have additional reinforcement to support the weight, starting at 36 inches off the floor and terminating at a height of 72 inches. The wall must support up to 1500 pounds off of the center load, depending on the type of machine. Some types of remote X-ray control units (mounted on the wall near the operatories) can control four or five X-ray heads (Fig. 8–41).

Each operatory should be equipped with an X-ray film illuminator, also called a view box. It may be recessed in the wall over the fixed cabinet or it may be a portable tabletop model that sits on the counter. In custom dental cabinets, a view box may be built into the cabinet. These view boxes are small—approximately 6 × 12 inches.

Certain walls of rooms in which X-rays are taken must be lined with lead to shield the operator and passersby from radiation scatter. The Bureau of Radiological Health or a local inspection agency (state) must approve the plans and lead-shielding specifications. Sometimes a radiation physicist must prepare a study based on the position of the office in the medical office

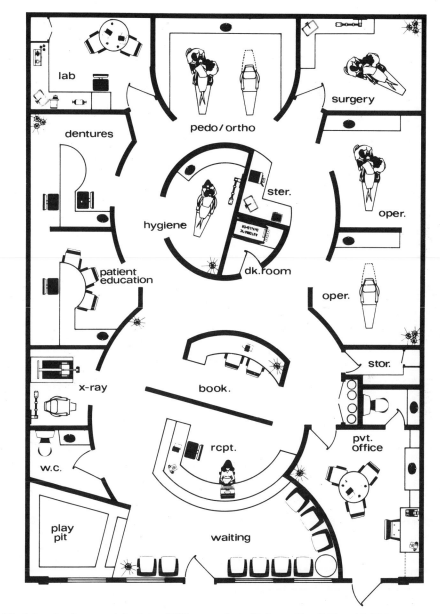

Fig. 8-37. Suite plan for general dentistry, 2200 square feet. (Refer to Figs. 8-33 and 8-49 for wallgraphic treatment of this suite.)

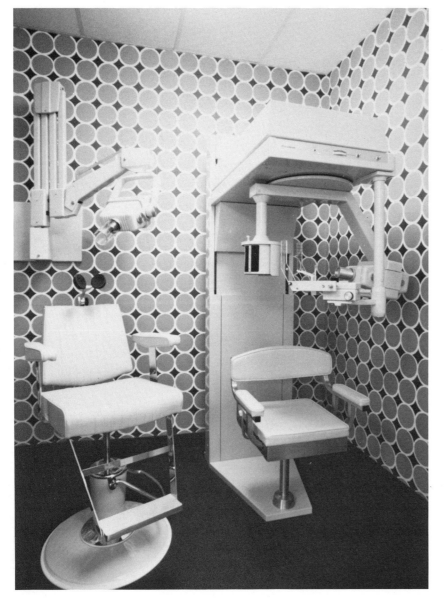

Fig. 8-38. X-ray alcove.

building, the number of films made daily, and the type of equipment used. The radiation physicist's recommendations must then be strictly followed.

Darkroom

A dental darkroom can be as small as 4 × 6 feet. The films may be developed manually or by an automatic processor. However, most dentists who have automatic processors also have manual backup tanks. Maintenance is critical with an automatic processor and it should be located where it is easy to service. The unit usually sits on a 30-inch-high counter (Fig. 8–43). Some are completely enclosed in the darkroom, while others have a chute that fits through a sleeve in the wall and through which finished film is delivered through the wall into a basket or shelf in the corridor sorting area. Some types of processors have daylight hoods for developing film outside of a typical darkroom.

The requirements of an automatic processor include hot and cold water with or without a temperature control valve (some use cold water only and have their own heating units), a waste drain, a 110-volt electrical outlet, and if space permits, a deep janitor's sink with sprayer for cleaning the rollers.

It should be mentioned that some dentists do not have any X-ray equipment. They send all of their patients who need X-rays to a professional dental X-ray lab.

The requirements for manual developing are hot and cold water with a temperature control valve, a waste drain in the floor near the tanks, and a sink. If an automatic processor is not used, the room should be set up with a "wet" and a "dry" side. The room should have two 4 to 5-foot

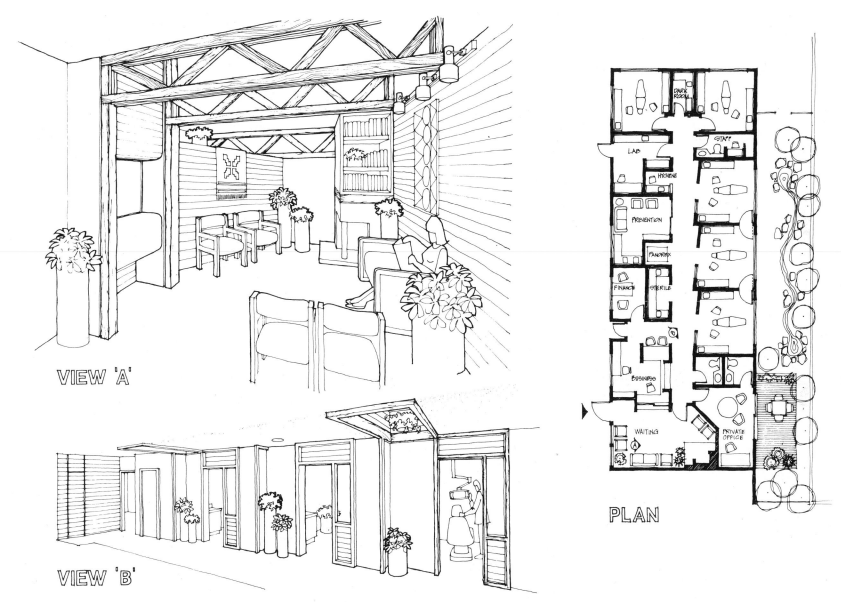

VIEW 'A'

VIEW 'B'

PLAN

Labels within plan: DARK ROOM, STAFF, LAB, HYGIENE, PREVENTION, PANOREX, FINANCE, STERILE, BUSINESS, WAITING, PRIVATE OFFICE

Fig. 8-39. Suite plan. (Courtesy Michael T. Hadley, AIA: Quadrasource.)

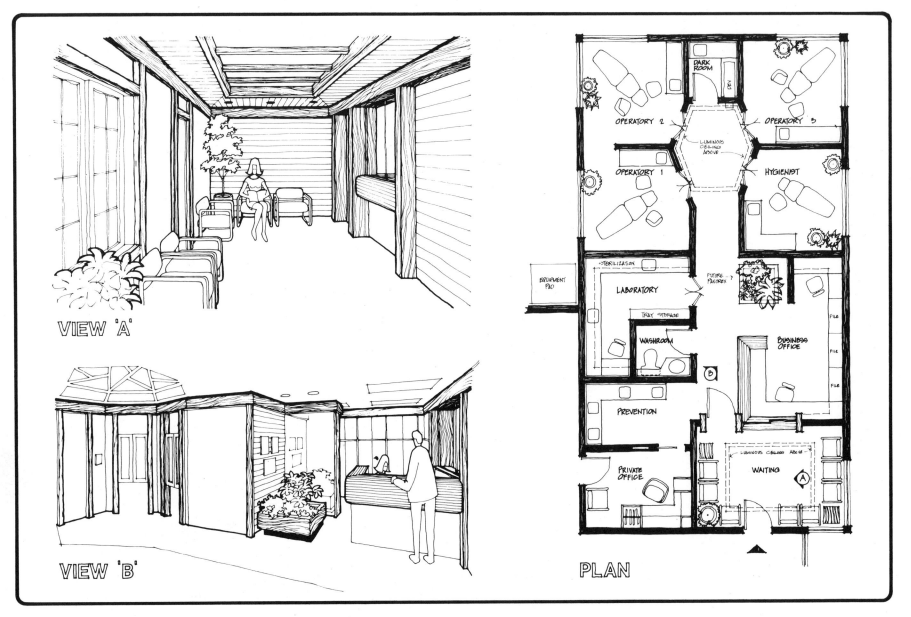

VIEW 'A'

VIEW 'B'

PLAN

DARK ROOM

OPERATORY 2

OPERATORY 3

LUMINOUS CEILING ABOVE

OPERATORY 1

HYGIENIST

EQUIPMENT PAD

STERILIZATION

LABORATORY

FUTURE PANOREX

TRAY STORAGE

WASHROOM

BUSINESS OFFICE

FILE

FILE

FILE

PREVENTION

B

PRIVATE OFFICE

LUMINOUS CEILING ABOVE

WAITING

A

Fig. 8-40. Suite plan. (Courtesy Michale T. Hadley, AIA: Quardasource.)

counters either parallel to each other or at right angles. The wet side contains the sink and developing tank, while the dry side is used for loading and unloading film. Films may be hung in a rack over the counter to air dry or they may be placed in an electric film dryer. The film dryer may be a countertop model or one that slides under the counter, and it requires an electrical outlet. A darkroom needs a timer which may be electric or spring-loaded (wound manually). One outlet should be provided over the counter on both the wet and dry sides. Normally countertops in a darkroom are 36 to 42 inches high, depending on personal preference. Thirty inches will be a maximum height if an automatic processor is contemplated. A 6-inch to 10-inch-deep shelf mounted 12 to 14 inches above the countertop is convenient for bottles of chemicals. There is no need for "closed" storage in a darkroom. All shelves should be open shelves.

A darkroom must have an exhaust fan, and some codes require that the door have a lightproof louver ventilation panel. The darkroom door usually opens in so that if someone tries to enter while developing is in process, the technician can put a foot against the door to prevent it from opening. Some darkrooms have a red warning light over the door that is activated when developing is in process. In a small office, the staff usually know when someone is in the darkroom and there may not be a sufficient volume of X-rays to warrant a more complicated signal system. A darkroom door need be only 24 inches wide and it must have a lightproof seal.

The darkroom must have two sources of light. A 100-watt incandescent light, either recessed or surface mounted to the ceiling, will suffice for normal work, but a safelight must be provided for working with exposed film. The safelight can be

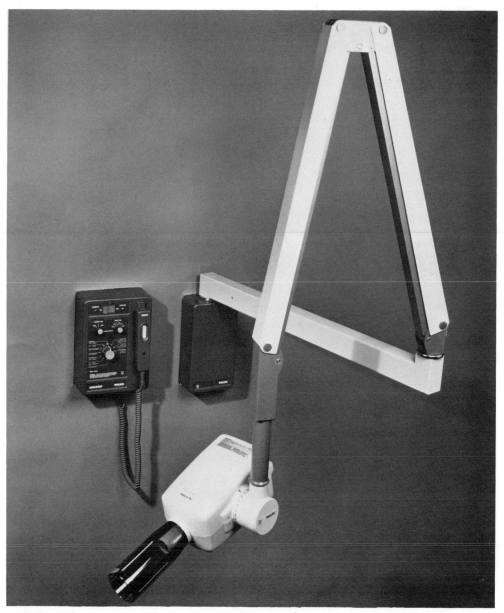

Fig. 8-41. Dental X-ray head. (Courtesy Philips Dental Systems.)

229

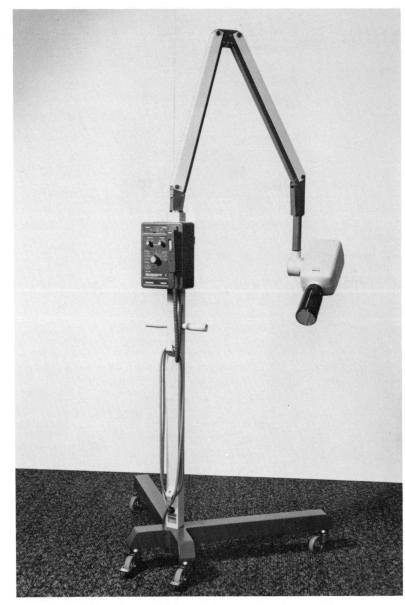

Fig. 8-42. Mobile X-ray. (Courtesy Philips Dental Systems.)

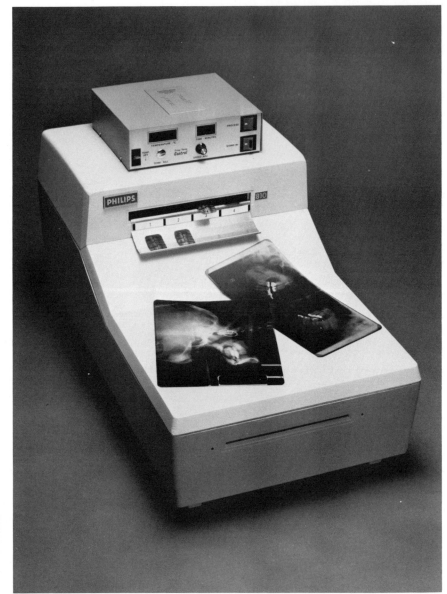

Fig. 8-43. Automatic film processor. (Courtesy Philips Dental Systems.)

plugged into an outlet at 60 to 72 inches off the floor, and it can work by a pull chain or be wired into a wall switch. If the latter, the switch should be located away from the incandescent light switch so that the technician does not confuse them and hit the wrong one while film is exposed. The safelight can also be attached to a pilot warning light outside the darkroom, so that whenever film is exposed and the safelight is activated, the warning light is also activated. Any recessed light fixtures as well as the exhaust fan must have light-sealed housings.

A small viewing and sorting area should be provided outside the darkroom. This may consist of nothing more than a shelf with a view box illuminator to enable the technician or aide to check the films for resolution and clarity before handing them to the dentist.

A note of caution: Local codes normally require a vacuum breaker on piping to all darkroom tanks to prevent the chemical waste from backing up into the water supply. Also, acid-resistant pipe is recommended since the chemical waste is very corrosive.

Unlike the storage of film for medical X-rays, dental X-ray film is stored in lead-lined dispensing units which are either wall mounted in the operatory or stored in a drawer.

Lighting

Good lighting is mandatory in a dental operatory. Some dentists prefer natural light from a northern exposure, but that is not critical since the advent of color-corrected fluorescent lamps. The important considerations are that the illumination be free of shadows and that a brightness ratio of 10:1 be maintained with the operating light. The

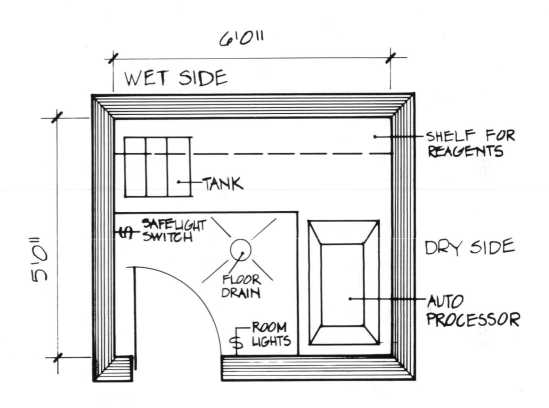

DARKROOM

Fig. 8-44. Plan view of darkroom.

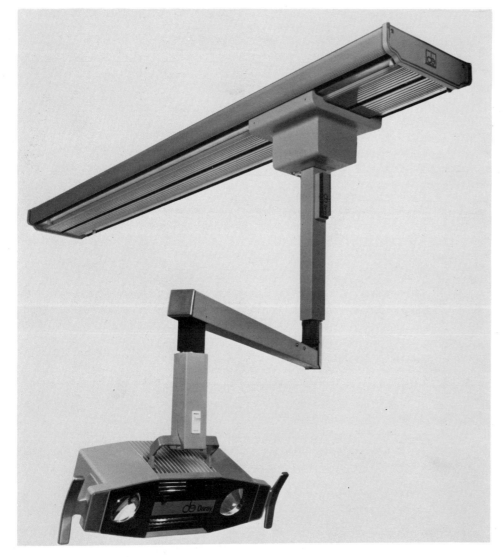

Fig. 8-45. Dental light. (Courtesy Den-Tal-Ez Mfg. Co., Bay Minette, Alabama.)

operating light (Fig. 8–45) may slide in a track mounted in the ceiling, or it may be post mounted to the ceiling or the floor, or it may be mounted to the dental chair or the dental unit. Once again, one encounters the many variables in dental equipment and in practice preference. The quartz halogen operating light delivers a concentrated 1200 to 2500 footcandles of illumination at the oral cavity. Thus the work counters and visual background of the room must receive 200 to 250 maintained footcandles to achieve a 10:1 brightness ratio with the 2500-foot-candle operating light. Two or three four-lamp surface-mounted fluorescent luminaires arranged in a U shape around the chair (Fig. 8–46) will meet this requirement. Of course, the reflectance of the floor, walls, and ceiling have an impact on the footcandle level, as does the ceiling height, the size and shape of the room, and the location of upper cabinets, if any.

Fluorescent lighting around the perimeter of the room is aesthetically pleasing and keeps the glare out of the patient's eyes (Fig. 8–47). However, the number of lamps must still yield the 10:1 brightness ratio. This type of lighting lends itself to a self-contained individual room that is not broken by many openings and doors.

Operatories should not have busy wallcoverings with intense colors because the rooms are small and the reflection of the colors will make it difficult to match shades of teeth for crowns. Soft colors and patterns with little contrast will reduce eye fatigue.

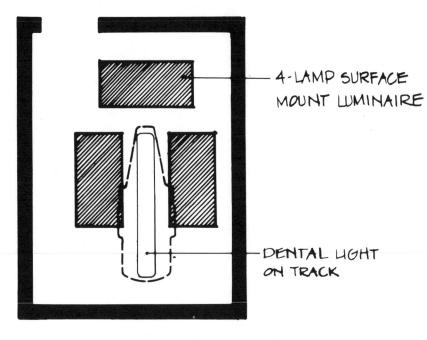

4-LAMP SURFACE
MOUNT LUMINAIRE

DENTAL LIGHT
ON TRACK

OPERATORY REFLECTED
CEILING PLAN

Fig. 8-46. Reflected ceiling plan for dental operatory.

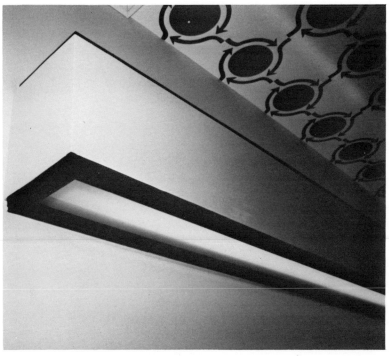

Fig. 8-47. Perimeter lighting, dental operatory.

233

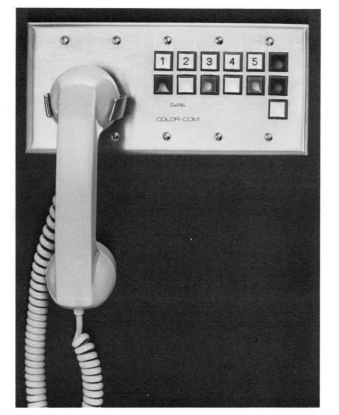

Fig. 8-48. Signal light communication system. (Courtesy Dentek Co.)

Communication Systems

Many small offices do not have a special communication system other than the telephone. In the interests of efficiency, however, such a system can save steps and reduce foot traffic. There are various types of communication systems available. The dealers who sell these products also install them and can tailor a system to the needs of the individual office.

Telephone Intercom. The most basic system is the intercom button on the telephone. This means that each operatory would have to have a telephone just to have the intercom facility. While it enables the receptionist to contact the dentist and speak privately while he or she is working in an operatory, it really does not fulfill the major requirements for communication within a dental office.

Loudspeaker. This has the advantage that the dentist does not physically have to touch a telephone in order to receive a message, but it is unsatisfactory because it is noisy and the patient can hear the message. Also it still does not tell the dentist in which room his or her next patient is waiting.

Colored Signal Lights. A small panel of signal lights is mounted over operatory doors, in the lab and in the sterilizing area, with a control panel in the business office and in the operatories (Fig. 8–48). This system can tell the dentist which room to go to next or whether a phone call or emergency is awaiting his or her attention. Or, if the doctor needs assistance while in the operatory, he or she can activate a light that can be seen by staff outside the room. The limitation of this system is that sometimes the lights go unnoticed.

Buzzers and Chimes. A simple system of communication consists of a soft buzzer that might indicate that the dentist needs assistance (and, if there are not more than three operatories, the room number might be indicated by the number of buzzes) and a chime might signal that the next patient is ready. In a small office, the staff know which operatory the dentist is in and the dentist usually knows in which operatory the next patient can be found, without relying upon an auditory signal. This system is noisy and limited by the number of distinguishable sounds.

Combination System. The most effective communication system for a large office is a combination of all of the above. A chime can be used for the phone. Signal lights, combined with a soft buzzer to call attention to the lights, can be used to get the staff's attention or to indicate which dentist is in which operatory. Twelve signal lights may be combined in groups (controlled by a button block for each series), and these light panels should be set up in strategic locations in the office.

Mechanical Equipment Room

A dental suite will usually fall into one of three categories with respect to location of mechanical equipment: hot-water heater; air-conditioning and heating equipment; air compressor, vacuum pump, or turbine; natural gas connection; and telephone terminal panel.

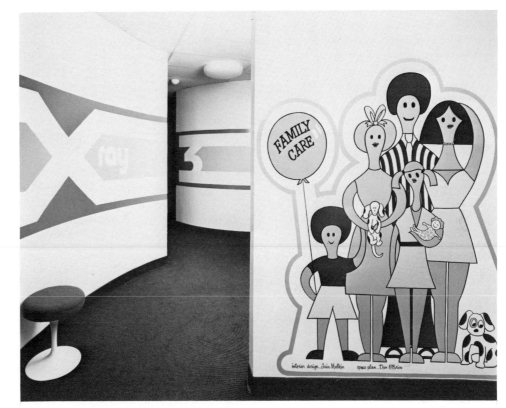

Fig. 8-49. Wallgraphic for general dentistry suite.

235

1. The dental suite is located in a medical office building, and a central mechanical equipment room on each floor will serve the tenants. Thus all of the above equipment will be housed in a remote location and piped to the dental suite, saving the tenant the noise of having a pump and compressor in the office proper, financially saving the tenant from having to pay monthly rent on square footage for a utility room contained within the suite, and further saving the tenant the cost of having to run a gas line into the building or purchase and install an air compressor and vacuum. Many medical buildings offer these utilities to medical and dental tenants and the tenant need only pay monthly service fee for it, or the cost of running the pipes to his or her office.

2. The dental suite is located in a professional office building but not specifically a *medical* office building. In this case, the tenant usually has to bear the expense of piping gas into the building and allotting a sizable room within the suite for the installation of a vacuum pump, air compressor, and possibly a hot-water heater and a telephone terminal panel.

3. The dental suite is located in its own building and, obviously, must bear the expense of running all utilities and services that the practice requires. However, the noisy equipment can be located in a utility room outside the building or off of the public corridor (if there is one).

ORTHODONTICS

Orthodontics is the branch of dentisty that deals with straightening teeth and correcting malocclusions. The majority of patients are children aged 12 to 18, although a sizable number of adults now avail themselves of these services. The orthodontic process is slow, often necessitating weekly visits for months and sometimes years.

Traffic Flow

On the initial visit, the child would be examined and then the orthodontist would discuss the course of treatment with the parents in the private office. Some orthodontists have a fairly elaborate office for making case presentations and some even go so far as to have a sliding panel that conceals a projection screen and a remote control panel near the desk for operating the room lights, the projector, and the sliding panel for the screen. The room should also contain a view box illuminator, and some private offices contain a tabletop for a video cassette instruction unit, to enable parents or patients to view a tape on a particular procedure. If a room for patient education is included in the suite, this is the place where such equipment would be located. The private office or consultation room should be comfortably furnished and have a pleasant ambience. If the dentist does use this room for case presentations, the room lights should be controlled from the dentist's desk.

On subsequent visits, the patient, after being called from the waiting room, would proceed to a vanity cabinet to brush his or her teeth and then would be seated in the operatory bay. After the first few visits, during which the major work is done, the weekly follow-up visits are short. Tightening or otherwise adjusting the devices or appliances in the mouth may take only a few minutes. Thus this is a high-volume practice in which the circulation must be efficiently planned and the waiting room must accommodate a large number of patients. Three or four seats should be provided for each dental chair if space permits.

Operatory Bay

Orthodontists do most of their work in a large communal operatory called a "bay" in which three to eight chairs are arranged with no separation between them. If space permits, the chairs may be arranged like spokes of a wheel with a sterilization station at the hub (Fig. 8–50). But usually the chairs are arranged in a row parallel to each other (Fig. 8–51). Allowing 7 feet for the first chair and 5 feet 6 inches for each successive chair is a rule of thumb for estimating the length of the bay. The location of fixed and mobile cabinets is critical since the orthodontist and assistant must be able to move quickly from one patient to the next with instruments always within reach. The dental units, cabinetry, patient chairs, and dentist's and assistant's stools in Fig. 8–52, Plate 13 are functional and have an uncluttered appearance. Even though the room has a great deal of cabinetry, the neutral color and clean lines make it read as background and keep it from dominating the room.

In addition to the operatory bay, the orthodontist usually has a standard individual operatory (often referred to as a "quiet room") in which he or she may take X-rays, do the initial diagnostic examination, work on a noisy or obstreperous child, or treat an adult patient. This operatory may have special equipment that is lacking in the orthodontic units in the bay (Fig. 8–53).

Table 8-1. Analysis of Program.
General Dentistry

No. of Dentists:	1			2		
Waiting Room[a]		$12 \times 14 =$	168		$16 \times 18 =$	288
Business Office		$12 \times 14 =$	168		$12 \times 16 =$	192
Operatories	2 @	$8 \times 11\frac{1}{2} =$	184	5 @	$8 \times 11\frac{1}{2} =$	460
Lab		$8 \times 10 =$	80		$8 \times 12 =$	96
Sterilizing Alcove		$4 \times 4 =$	16		$4 \times 6 =$	24
Darkroom		$4 \times 6 =$	24		$4 \times 6 =$	24
Staff Lounge		—			$10 \times 12 =$	120
Toilets	2 @	$5 \times 6 =$	60	2 @	$5 \times 6 =$	60
Hygiene Operatory		$8 \times 11\frac{1}{2} =$	92		$8 \times 11\frac{1}{2} =$	92
Panoramic X-ray		$5 \times 8 =$	40		$5 \times 8 =$	40
Audiovisual/Patient Education		$6 \times 12 =$	72		$6 \times 12 =$	72
Private Office		$10 \times 10 =$	100	2 @	$10 \times 10 =$	200
Storage		$5 \times 6 =$	30		$6 \times 8 =$	48
Mechanical Equipment Room		$6 \times 8 =$	48		$6 \times 8 =$	48
Subtotal			1082 ft^2			1762 ft^2
15% Circulation			162			265
Total			1244 ft^2			2029 ft^2

[a] A rule of thumb for estimating the number of seats in the waiting room is to allow 16 to 18 ft^2 per person.

Laboratory

The laboratory should be large with a plaster storage bin and a place to store the considerable number of models accumulated in this practice. Sometimes as many as 4000 models, stored in cardboard boxes 3 × 3 × 3 inches, must be accommodated in the lab, or elsewhere in the suite, on shallow shelves. The reader is referred to *General Dentistry* for further discussion of a dental laboratory.

Other Rooms

An orthodontist's suite would also have a panoramic and cephalometric X-ray machines, a darkroom, two toilet rooms, a fairly large business office, an audiovisual room (Fig. 8–54), and perhaps a private office for a bookkeeper or office manager. Some orthodontists will have only a cephalometric X-ray machine, and since many of these units are designed for a standing patient, they can be accommodated in somewhat less space than can a panoramic X-ray machine with chair. The important thing to remember is that a cephalometric unit requires a 60-inch focal distance for taking head plates plus room for the patient to stand. Thus a space 8 feet long by 3 feet wide is suitable. But many orthodontists use a professional X-ray lab.

Waiting Room

The waiting room may be treated with great imagination since the patient population, adolescents and teenagers, have somewhat homogeneous tastes and appreciate a departure from the norm. The author has designed a waiting room with carpet-covered plywood platforms in-

stead of individual chairs (Fig. 8–55, Plate 13) in order to increase seating capacity of this undersized room and, at the same time, to appeal to the occupants' craving for the unusual. The walls are Levi blue denim and carry photo blowups of children in various stages of orthodontia—*before* (with crooked teeth), *during* (with the rubber bands and appliances) and *after* (with straight teeth and beautiful smiles). The room, although unconventional, was a huge success and contributed to the orthodontist's popularity and the rapid growth of his practice. To further add architectural interest to the room, an artificial skylight fixture was centered over the platforms.

Table 8-2. Analysis of Program.
Orthodontics

No. of Dentists:	1	2
Waiting Room	14 × 20 = 280	16 × 22 = 352
Business Office	12 × 16 = 192	12 × 16 = 192
Bookkeeper/Business Manager	10 × 12 = 120	10 × 12 = 120
Operatory Bay (4 chairs)	12 × 24 = 288	(9 chairs) 12 × 51 = 612
Quiet Room/X-ray	8 × 11½ = 92	8 × 11½ = 92
Audiovisual/Patient Education	6 × 12 = 72	6 × 12 = 72
Lab	8 × 12 = 96	8 × 12 = 96
Sterilizing Alcove	4 × 4 = 16	4 × 4 = 16
Darkroom	4 × 6 = 24	4 × 6 = 24
Staff Lounge	8 × 12 = 96	10 × 12 = 120
Toilet Rooms	2 @ 5 × 6 = 60	2 @ 5 × 6 = 60
Panoramic X-ray	5 × 8 = 40	5 × 8 = 40
Private Office	12 × 14 = 168	2 @ 12 × 14 = 336
Storage	6 × 8 = 48	6 × 8 = 48
Mechanical Equipment Room	6 × 8 = 48	6 × 8 = 48
Subtotal	1640 ft²	2258 ft²
15% Circulation	246	339
Total	1886 ft²	2597 ft²

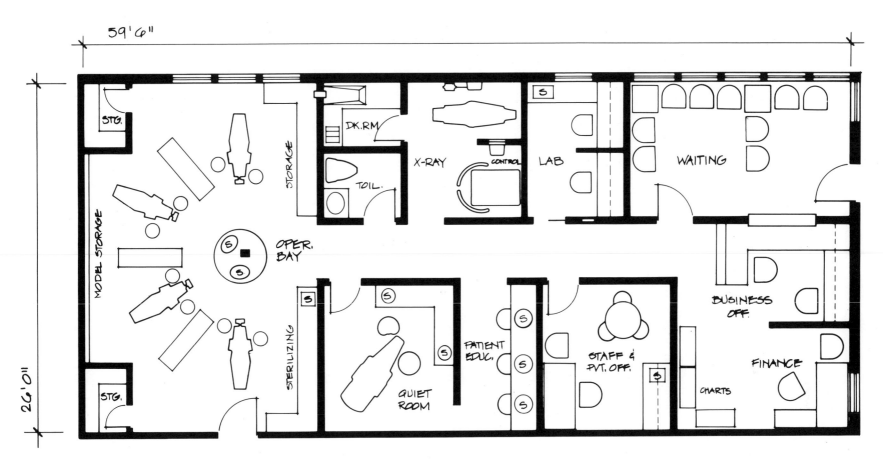

59'6"

26'0"

STG.

MODEL STORAGE

STORAGE

DK.RM

TOIL.

X-RAY

CONTROL

LAB

S

WAITING

OPER. BAY

SERILIZING

S

S

S

PATIENT EDUC.

S

S

S

STAFF & PVT. OFF.

S

BUSINESS OFF.

FINANCE

CHARTS

QUIET ROOM

STG.

ORTHODONTICS
1547 SQ. FT.

Fig. 8-50. Suite plan for orthodontics, 1547 square feet.

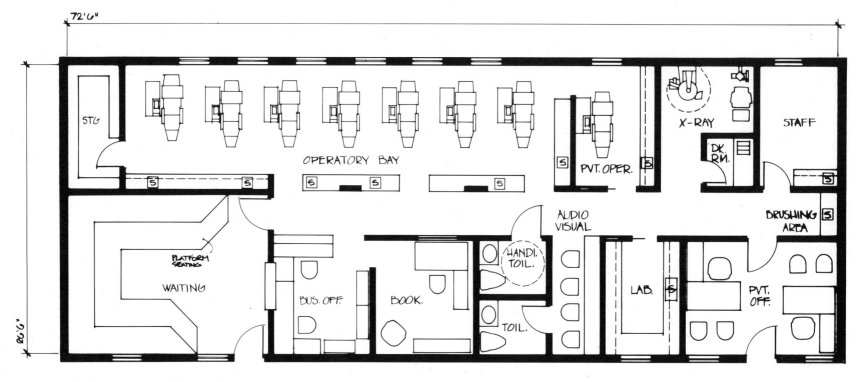

72'6"

20'0"

STG

OPERATORY BAY

PVT. OPER.

X-RAY

STAFF

DK. RM.

BRUSHING AREA

PLATFORM SEATING

WAITING

AUDIO VISUAL

HANDI. TOIL.

BUS. OFF.

BOOK.

TOIL.

LAB.

PVT. OFF.

ORTHODONTICS

1921 SQ. FT.

Fig. 8-51. Suite plan for orthodontics, 1921 square feet.

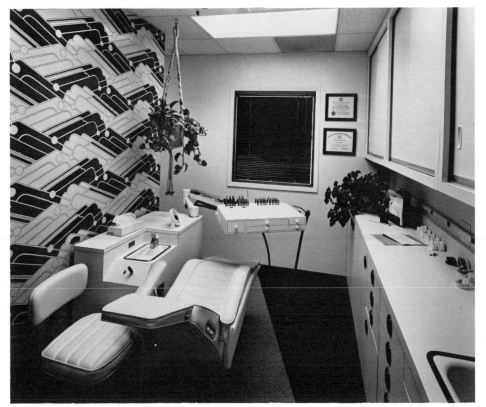

Fig. 8-53. Quiet room.

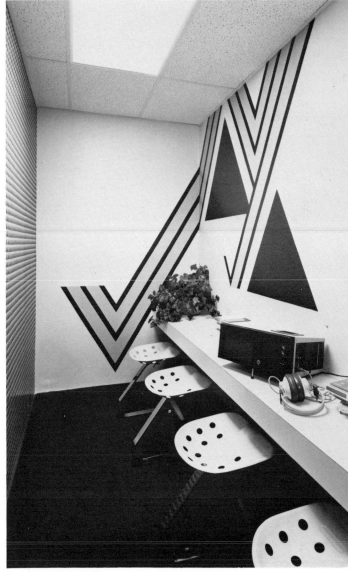

Fig. 8-54. Audiovisual room.

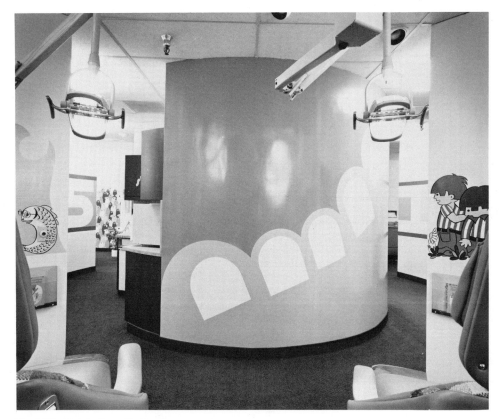

Fig. 8-56. Mural of crooked teeth.

PEDODONTICS

Pedodontics is the branch of dentistry that specializes in children. It is based upon a philosophy of prevention. If the child's teeth are maintained properly from the age of two, it is assumed that there will be no decay and few problems as the child ages. Thus children from the ages of two to twelve visit the pedodontist. Since the children are so young, much of the instruction and care for the child's teeth is entrusted to the parent. The parent (usually the mother) must learn how to floss and brush the toddler's teeth until the child is old enough to do it for himself or herself. Thus a patient education room is required with a built-in bench so that the mother can be seated with the child's head in her lap and the child's body stretched out on the bench. The dental assistant sits near the mother and guides her during the procedure. A plywood bench or banquette, padded and upholstered with carpet (Fig. 8–58, Plate 13), works well and is easy to clean. The room should also have a built-in cabinet with sink, a large mirror, and good illumination (Fig. 8–57, Plate 13).

Traffic Flow

A child and parent, on the initial visit, would be escorted to the operatory and the child's teeth would be X-rayed and examined. Then the parent would usually visit with the pedodontist in his or her private office to discuss the course of treatment and the cost. On subsequent visits, the child would be checked for dental caries or any abnormalities.

Since the visits are typically short, this tends to be a high-volume practice. Thus the circulation patterns should be direct and well planned, and things that little children should not touch should be behind closed doors. The waiting room should be large since each child is accompanied by one or both parents and often one or more siblings. Thus a three-chair operatory bay may account for as many as 14 persons in the waiting room. This is also a function of the socioeconomic composition of the practice. Families with low incomes cannot afford babysitters and tend to bring all the children when one of the children has to visit the doctor. Families with higher incomes have either housekeepers or babysitters with whom to leave the other children.

Waiting Room

This room can truly challenge the designer's imagination. It can be as fanciful as a fairy tale. Children get bored very quickly in a conventional waiting room. Therefore they should be treated to something that captures their imagination, lets them climb around and expend their enormous energies. This has an added payoff: the children will associate a pleasant experience with a visit to the dentist, thus forging what may be a lifelong positive relationship with good dental care. The waiting room in Fig. 8-59 (Plate 14) had no windows or natural light (in fact, the entire office had no natural light; it was remodeled from a former pizza parlor); thus the author decided to enhance this womblike feeling by applying textured fabrics to the walls and ceiling. Felt appliqued banners suspended from the ceiling, built-in carpeted seating platforms, a playpit (Fig. 8-60, Plate 14) for children, and special lighting contribute to the fantasyland ambience. The floor has a design composed of several colors of carpet that are seamed together, with low-voltage lights embedded in the seams outling the shapes. The rear of the room (Fig. 8-61, Plate 14) has a stuffed wall sculpture, which shape, under the accent lighting, is a dominant feature of the room.

A built-in toy bin just under the cashier/check-out counter is welcomed by the children. While the parent is writing a check or booking a future appointment, the child is kept amused by selecting a toy. If space permits, a toilet room should be provided in the waiting room area, in addition to the one in the working area of the suite.

Operatory Bay

The pedo chair is a bit smaller than a standard dental chair (Fig. 8-62). It is standard in this specialty, as in orthodontics, to have the chairs arranged in a communal "bay." Peer group pressure seems to keep the crying to a minimum. The room should have cabinetry similar to that of the orthodontist, and the room should be gaily decorated with circus posters and other artwork that appeals to children on the walls where the children can see it (Fig. 8-63).

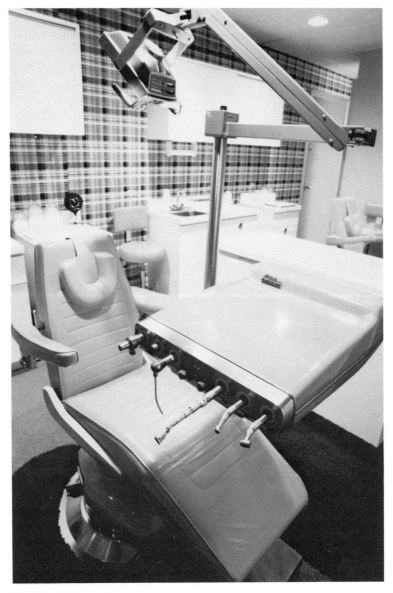

Fig. 8-62. Pedodontic operatory.

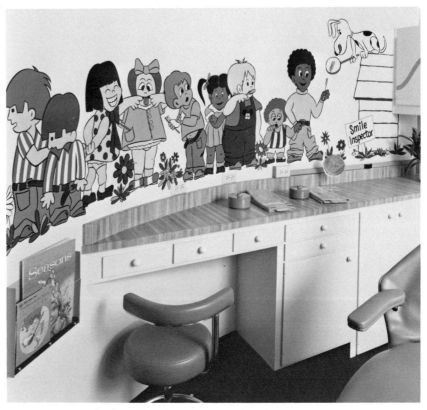

Fig. 8-63. Pedodontic wallgraphic.

244

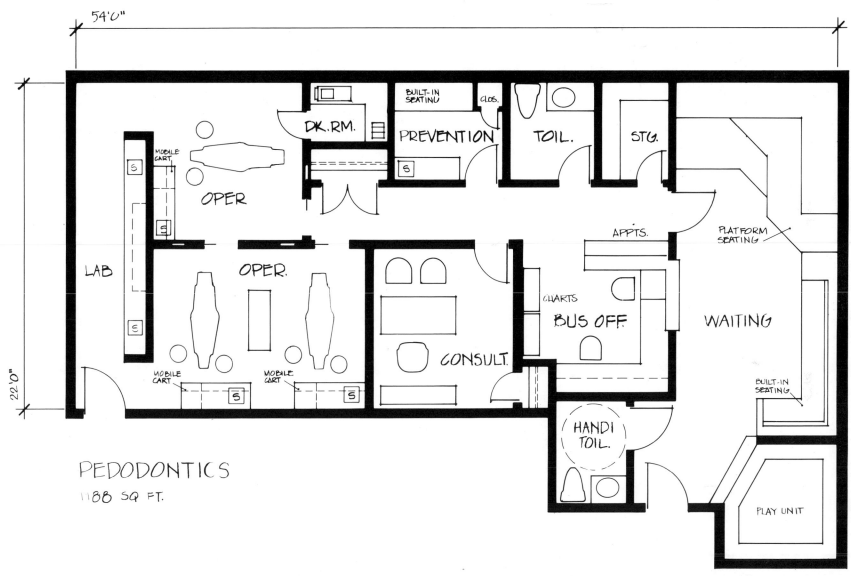

54'0"

22'0"

MOBILE CART
S

OPER

LAB
S

S

OPER.

MOBILE CART
S

MOBILE CART
S

DK. RM.

BUILT-IN SEATING

CLOS.

PREVENTION
S

TOIL.

STG.

APPTS.

PLATFORM SEATING

CHARTS

BUS OFF.

WAITING

CONSULT.

HANDI TOIL.

BUILT-IN SEATING

PLAY UNIT

PEDODONTICS
1188 SQ FT.

Fig. 8-64. Suite plan for pedodontics, 1188 square feet.

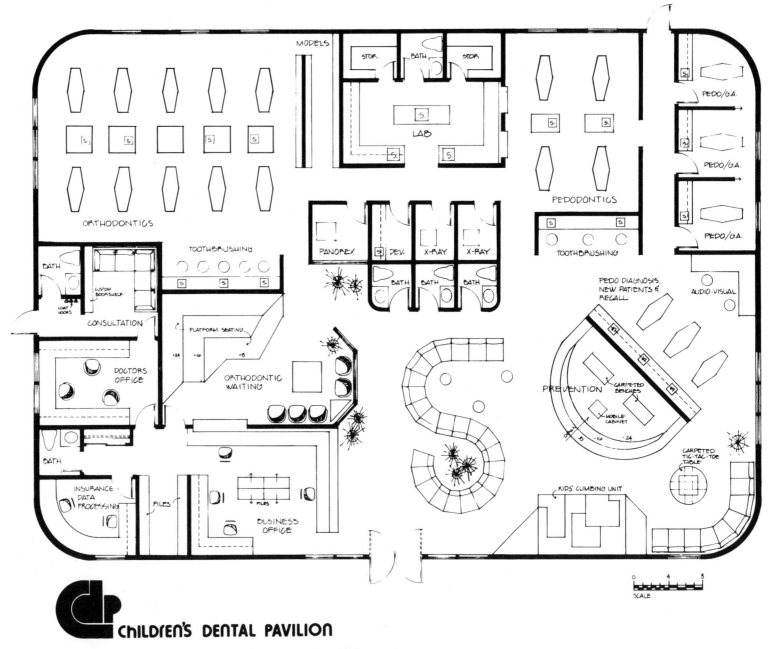

MODELS

STOR. BATH STOR

LAB

ORTHODONTICS

PEDODONTICS

PEDO/G.A.

PEDO/G.A.

PEDO/G.A.

TOOTHBRUSHING

BATH

CUSTOM BOOKSHELF

COAT HOOKS

CONSULTATION

PANOREX DEV. X-RAY X-RAY

BATH BATH BATH

TOOTHBRUSHING

AUDIO-VISUAL

PEDO DIAGNOSIS, NEW PATIENTS & RECALL

PLATFORM SEATING

DOCTORS OFFICE

+24 +16 +8

ORTHODONTIC WAITING

PREVENTION

CARPETED BENCHES

MOBILE CABINET

+8 -16 -24

CARPETED TIC-TAC-TOE TABLE

BATH

INSURANCE - DATA PROCESSING

FILES

FILES

BUSINESS OFFICE

KIDS' CLIMBING UNIT

0 4 8

SCALE.

Children's Dental Pavilion

Fig. 8-65. Suite plan for group practice, pedodontic/orthodontic HMO, 5000 square feet.

Other Rooms

The suite will require a business office and dental records area, a darkroom, perhaps a panoramic X-ray unit, a storage room, a lab/sterilization area with a minimum of 12 lineal feet of countertop, and at least three chairs either in an open operatory bay or in individual operatories (Fig. 8-64).

**Table 8-3. Analysis of Program.
Pedodontics**

No. of Dentists:		1
Waiting Room	14 × 20 =	280
Business Office	12 × 16 =	192
Operatory Bay (3 chairs)	12 × 18 =	216
Quiet Room/X-ray	9 × 11 =	99
Sterilizing/Lab	8 × 12 =	96
Darkroom	4 × 6 =	24
Staff Lounge	8 × 12 =	96
Toilet Rooms	2 @ 5 × 6 =	60
Prevention/Patient Education	10 × 12 =	120
Panoramic X-ray	5 × 8 =	40
Private Office	10 × 12 =	120
Storage	6 × 8 =	48
Mechanical Equipment Room	6 × 8 =	48
Subtotal		1439 ft²
15% Circulation		216
Total		1655 ft²

ORAL SURGERY

An oral surgeon's work is composed primarily of two functions: diagnosis and surgery. On a patient's initial visit an examination and diagnosis will be made. Then the patient will be scheduled for surgery. For a solo practitioner, two small operatories will suffice for examination and diagnosis, and these same operatories will be used for postoperative procedures and checkups. One or both of these operatories will be equipped for intraoral X-ray in addition to the panoramic X-ray area. A small darkroom should be located near these operatories as should the consultation room or private office. If all of these rooms are located at the front of the suite, near the waiting room, only surgical patients need enter the rear of the suite.

Surgical Operating Rooms

Two surgical operating rooms with a prep/cleanup room between them will be required for a solo practitioner. Although these rooms should be large (11 × 12 feet), some oral surgeons use a room as small as 8 × 11 feet. The room should have a sink with foot-pedal controls, and vacuum, oxygen, nitrous oxide, nitrogen, electricity, and compressed air must be available in the room. Oral surgeons use nitrogen for their surgical drills because it is a totally pure propellant which can deliver up to 100 pounds constant pressure. Most will still need an air compressor for their more conventional drills. The analgesic gases may be portable or may be piped into the room through degreased, sealed copper tubing (using only silver solder) to a flow meter in each surgery. *Building and fire codes are very strict regarding where and how medical gases are stored.* The reader is referred to *General Dentistry* for a detailed discussion of this topic.

Some oral surgeons work from a mobile cabinet in the surgery room, with no fixed cabinetry. Other prefer at least 8 lineal feet of fixed cabinetry and countertop, in which case the room should be large—approximately 12 × 12 feet. The cabinetry need not be located near the operating chair since a portable electric engine or air drill is commonly used, but the utilities must be properly located in the room in relation to the chair. In addition, the room should have several general electrical outlets and a nurse call buzzer. (See Fig. 8–66.)

Some oral surgeons use a special chair, but others use a standard operatory chair with an armboard attachment for administering Sodium Pentothal. Tray setups of sterile instruments can be passed from the prep area to the operatories without someone entering the room (refer to *Tray Set-Ups, General Dentistry*).

Recovery

Another factor in determining the size of the surgery is the surgeon's preferred method of transferring the patient to the recovery room. Some surgeons transfer the patient from the operating chair to a gurney cart (a 2 × 6-foot wheeled stretcher) and then wheel him or her to a nearby recovery room where the patient may remain on the cart or may be transferred to a recovery bed. Some surgeons transfer the patient via a wheelchair. Others effect the transfer by putting an arm around the sedated patient and helping him or her to walk the short distance to the recovery room. Thus one can see that if gurney carts are used, surgeries, corridors, and recovery rooms would have to be large enough to accommodate this type of maneuvering. In addition, there must be a place to store the gurney carts or wheelchairs when not in use.

A solo practitioner with two operating rooms will usually have three or four recovery cubicles. Each should have a built-in or freestanding bed, or just be an empty room if the patient remains on the gurney. In many cases, a built-in platform with a thick vinyl-upholstered pad is used for the recovery bed. In addition, there should be a place for a friend or relative to sit, a hook or locker for clothes or personal items, a vanity mirror and shelf, a tissue box, a wastebasket, and a blanket and pillow. The opening to the room may be closed off by a cubicle curtain. The recovery rooms should be near a toilet and also near a rear, private exit so that the patient does not have to pass through the waiting room after surgery. The recovery area must be located so that the staff can observe the patients while going about their cleanup and prep duties.

Sterilization/Lab

This may be a separate room or an alcove convenient to the front operatories in addition to a prep/cleanup room near the surgeries, or the latter may serve the entire suite.

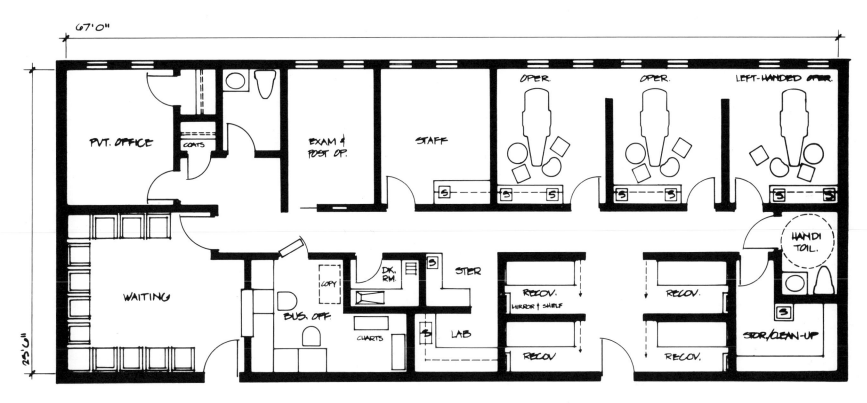

ORAL SURGERY
1708 SQ. FT.

Fig. 8-66. Suite plan for oral surgery, 1708 square feet.

Other Rooms

A small staff lounge is desirable due to the demanding nature of the work. The private office can be small since patients usually do not enter it. The suite should contain at least two toilet rooms, a storage room, a darkroom, and a small to medium-size business office. The volume of patients is low, so neither the business office nor the waiting room need be large. As with any surgical specialty, the waiting room should be conservatively furnished in subtle colors, avoiding flamboyance and frivolity. The surgeon's image should be that of a serious person who is skilled and successful at his or her profession.

* The author wishes to thank Harv Baron of City Dental Co. for his generous assistance in reviewing and editing the material in this chapter.

Table 8-4. Analysis of Program. Oral Surgery

No. of Dentists:		1
Waiting Room		$12 \times 14 =$ 168
Business Office		$12 \times 14 =$ 168
Examination Operatories		2 @ $8 \times 11\frac{1}{2} =$ 184
Surgical Operatories		2 @ $12 \times 12 =$ 288
Prep/Cleanup[a]		$8 \times 10 =$ 80
Recovery Rooms	4 @	$5 \times 8 =$ 160
Panoramic X-ray		$5 \times 8 =$ 40
Sterilization/Lab[a]		$6 \times 8 =$ 48
Darkroom		$4 \times 6 =$ 24
Staff Lounge		$8 \times 12 =$ 96
Toilet Rooms	2 @	$5 \times 6 =$ 60
Private Office		$10 \times 10 =$ 100
Storage		$6 \times 8 =$ 48
Mechanical Equipment Room		$6 \times 8 =$ 48
Subtotal		1512 ft²
15% Circulation		227
Total		1739 ft²

[a] These areas may be combined.

Chapter 9
Color and Its Impact on the Medical Environment

HISTORICAL BACKGROUND

In early civilizations, man made color holy. He saw intimations of life's mysteries in the spectrum, and assigned it power—so that each color became emblematic of divine forces in a world that so integrated art, ritual, and myths with everyday life that each was suffused with the other. Color was a language in itself; hieroglyphic paintings of vibrant blues, reds, greens, and purples could be interpreted as clearly as words are today. Recent comparative cultural studies have shown similar symbolic uses of color among peoples who could not possibly have had contact with one another. Birren has reported that the points of the compass in China, for example, were represented by black for north, white for west, red for south, and green for east, and that the people of ancient Ireland and also the Indians of North America used the identical designations.

Now the old myths have been dismissed as superstition, color has been stripped of its early and specific symbolism, we can no longer precisely "read" a color painting. But just as it is the task of psychologists and mythologists to plumb the depths of the human consciousness from which came those primal myths, from which our dreams still come, so that we may arrive at a greater knowledge of our common inner life, it is also important to learn how color has always held humankind in its sway—so much so that we hallucinate color if deprived of it too long—and most important, to gauge scientifically its specific influences upon our behavior. The color gold no longer carries the power of the Egyptian sun-god, but research indicates that its perception does have an effect upon the entire human organism, not only the optic nerve. And the implications of this—the differentiated influences of colors, real and measurable—are manifold in regard to environmental design, and just beginning to be recognized.

The history of color theory and research is long and variegated, with most of the early work done by philosophers and artists. Aristotle was the first to pose a systematic theory of color, one that is no longer considered relevant. In the early part of the eighteenth century the German poet Goethe expressed his views on color harmony and the symbolic values of color in his book, *Farbenlehre*.

The most obvious weakness of Goethe's work was that of most color studies before the twentieth century; he dealt with hues, failing to consider saturation and brightness. Nevertheless, he did make an observation which—scores of studies and tests later—has been accepted as valid: that red, yellow, and orange—longer wavelength colors at the warm end of the spectrum—are exciting and "advancing" colors, they seem to come towards one and draw one out; while blue, green, and purple—shorter wavelength colors at the cool end of the spectrum—are "retreating" colors and induce a more quieting, inward-drawing response.

Artists have had their own theories of color and its effect, and they have often been penetrating and insightful, but always based on one person's trial and error, or impression, rather than vigorous scientific investigation. Nineteenth-century artist Odilon Redon made dazzling explorations into color. Other artists famous for their research in color theory include Paul Klee, Wasily Kandinsky, and Josef Albers. Dozens of others—among the more well known are Munsell, Ostwald, Chevreul, Bezold, and Wundt—toward the close of the nineteenth century and the beginning of the twentieth, postulated color theories and laws of harmony along less subjective lines than the often empirical studies of the artists. In the first quarter of the twentieth century investigators even began testing color preferences for many different groups of people.

COLOR PREFERENCE TESTS

The obstacles confronting all of these color preference enthusiasts, however, were considerable: Color samples were not yet standardized,

nor were there backgrounds, nor was the light of their viewing conditions similarly controlled. Furthermore, there is the difficulty inherent in any test of color and "affect," or feeling—since an individual does not respond to a hue as pure color, but as something that evokes myriad and unique associations with objects, with experiences, and these are psychological processes that resist measurement. It is hardly surprising, then, that in 1925 one well-known researcher reviewed the mass of contradictory preference findings in his own and others' studies and declared that all hope of finding consistent reactions to color would have to be abandoned.

It was not. In the 55 years since that pessimistic dictum, a great variety of studies on color responses have been conducted. The number of color preference studies—on normal persons, feeble-minded persons, psychotics, males, females, the old, the young, in all parts of the world—is probably equal to the total of all other studies on "color and affect" combined. While the findings are often contradictory, certain agreement has been reached among numerous investigators. The difficulty in testing for color preference lies in not being able to control the many variables. Too many articles have been published on the results of market research, and these findings represent current fads rather than scientific investigation. Many of the "conclusions" extracted from these spurious studies are either obvious or dubious.

Color preferences develop as a reaction to culture, education, experience, and genetics. People see the world in different ways and process the environment according to their own needs and drives. Thus it has been postulated that there is a relationship between a person's color responses and his or her emotional state.

But is is difficult to test reactions to color because so much depends on the subject's verbal assessment of what he or she sees and colors are so symbolic, carrying highly personal connotations. If, as a child, a person had always been punished in a blue room, that person may dislike blue as an adult. Therefore any studies of color preference on "normal" subjects must be based on large samples so that individual biases due to highly personal experiences do not bias the results of the study, which may have been designed to test *cultural* color preferences, *age* color preferences, or some variable other than pathologically based color preferences or aversions. There is also the physiological problem that people often do not see a color alike. One person may see a dark green as having more yellow, one may see it as having more blue.

Because the color preferences of adults are so much a result of learning, many researchers have preferred to work with children to minimize the effects of learning and experience. Various studies have corroborated that young children prefer the warm, exiciting colors of red and yellow, but when they get older they prefer cool colors—blues and greens—as they become less impulsive and more reflective and intellectual.

The researcher Ellis, however, noted in primitive societies a continuing preference for the brilliant hues of red and yellow from childhood into adulthood—and hypothesized that "the apparent trend away from yellow as a revered color among early Greeks and Romans was largely due to the taboo placed upon it by the Christian church, as the symbol of sin and gaiety." Another researcher in the preference field, T. R. Garth, conducted tests among children of six different groups—white, Negro, American Indian, Filipino, Japanese, and Mexican—and found that the preference differences were minimal among them; he concluded that the differences that do appear in adulthood are due to nurtural factors.

Finally, Eysenck, in a critical review of numerous other color preference studies conducted all over the world, and also of his own experiments, concluded that there is a high degree of agreement among investigators, and that a general order of preference is as follows: blue, red, green, violet, orange, and yellow. He furthermore concluded that there are no sex differences, apart from a slight preference among women for yellow over orange, and among men for orange over yellow.

How can such uniformity of color preference be explained? Researchers Guilford and Smith have attributed it to innate biological factors, while others have emphasized the role of culture, learning, and experience. The truth probably lies in a balance between the two, a combination of innate and cultural factors. In other words, it is not yet known exactly what determines color preferences, only that a marked similarity does exist among all peoples.

COLOR-FORM PREFERENCE

In child-development evaluation, various color-form preference categorization tests are among the most often used measures of the abstraction phenomenon—that ability to single out specific elements from a pattern on the basis of similar factors. The classic color-form preference measure has been used mainly with young children, and has demonstrated that most children reach the peak of color dominance around four and a half, that the median age of transition from color to form dominance is five, and that form dominance is usually established by the age of nine.

The Rorschach inkblot method has also been used, with its results consistently showing that pure color responses dominate among young children, color-form dominates in the older child, and from late childhood through adolescence and adulthood, form-color responses dominate. Explanations for the color-form dominance phenomenon include maturation, increased personality differentiation from the affective to the intellectual, increased meaningfulness of the environment in terms of utility, less concern for primitive characteristics, increased verbal skills, and introduction to reading and writing.

Furthermore, since 90% of the adult population *is* form-dominant, color-dominant persons have been considered deviates. One of the most commonly held theories is that since color is a primitive response, the adult color-dominant personality is impulsive, immature, egocentric, and less intelligent than his or her form-dominant and therefore mature, socially adjusted peers. A child who retains his or her color dominance after classmates have switched over, therefore, is considered regressive and is subjected to academic and cultural programs to change his or her orientation.

What is interesting, however, is that some recent studies of creativity have indicated that the color-oriented child is more likely to emerge as an artistic, creative adult, far more innovative than his or her form-dominant peers, who will tend to deal well with analytical work in the traditional mold. One of the ingredients of that creative ability is to be free of that mold, to see with fresh eyes and envision new relationships, untried combinations. If further studies support this theory, then it will be clear that a disservice has

been done to those who have not fit the conventional mold, and who should be encouraged in their different way rather than pressed into a constricting and uniform shape.

One of the most interesting tests concerned with the connection between specific colors and emotion in children was performed by Alschuler and Hattwick at the University of Chicago. Noting that preschool children express themselves generally at the abstract, nonrepresentational level and reveal more of their affective lives than older children, they studied the expressive outlets of two-, three-, and four-year-old children in easel painting, crayons, clay, blocks, and dramatic play over an extended period of time. They concluded that color gave the clearest insights into the child's emotional life. Color preferences and color patterns gave clues to the child's emotional orientation. *Red,* found to be the most emotionally toned color, carried associations of both affection and love as well as aggression and hate. *Blue* was associated with drives toward control.

COLOR AND MENTAL DISORDERS

A variety of color tests—among them the Rorschach and the color pyramid test, devised by Swiss psychologist Max Pfister in 1950—are used as diagnostic tools in determining normality/abnormality. Because so many tests involving color preference, response, and placement have been made on the mentally and emotionally ill, with such a plethora of conflicting results, it is clear that the data must be interpreted cautiously and in conjunction with those from other tests. The most abused area here is probably preference, as some have not hesitated to link preference for

254

specific colors to specific disorders, in irresponsible and unproven attribution. Eric P. Mosse, as quoted in Birren,* reveals:

> We generally found in hysterical patients, especially in psychoneuroses with anxiety states, a predilection for green as symbolizing the mentioned escape mechanism.... Red is the color of choice of the hypomanic patient giving the tumult of his emotions their 'burning' and 'bloody' expression. And we don't wonder that melancholia and depression reveal themselves through a complete 'blackout.' Finally, we see yellow as the color of schizophrenia. ... This yellow is the proper and intrinsic color of the morbid mind. Whenever we observe its accumulative appearance, we may be sure we are dealing with a deep-lying psychotic disturbance.

Faber Birren, a noted color historian, disagrees. "Yellow may be looked upon as an intellectual color associated both with great intelligence and mental deficiency." He claims that schizophrenics prefer blue. The contradictions are legion. A study done by Warner, in which 300 patients were tested including diagnosed anxiety neurotics, catatonic schizophrenics, manics, and depressives, found in most cases no significant correlation of preference with psychiatric disorders.

How does the Rorschach contribute to clinical diagnosis? Rorschach's hypothesis was that color responses are measures of the affective, or emotional, state and he noted that neurotics are subject to "color shock," (rejection) as manifested in a delayed reaction time when presented with a color blot. He also stated that

Light, Color and Environment, by Faber Birren (New York, Van Nostrand Reinhold, 1969).

red evoked the shock response in neurotics more often than did other colors. Schizophrenics also suffer color shock when presented with the chromatic or color cards (following the black and white cards) of the Rorschach. Birren postulates that color may represent an unwanted intrusion on their inner life.

In the realm of color research, however, nothing goes uncontested, and the Rorschach is no exception. Two major criticisms of it are the lack of work with normal subjects as a criterion against which pathological groups could be compared, and also the basic postulate that the way in which a person responds to color in inkblots reflects his or her typical mode of dealing with, or integrating, affect. In fact, researchers Cerbus and Nichols, in trying to replicate Rorschach's findings, found no correlation between color responsiveness and impulsivity, and no significant difference in use of color by neurotics, schizophrenics, and normals. Nevertheless, the weight of evidence still favors the Rorschach color-affect theory.

Color and Depression

There exists almost unanimous agreement on the depressive's total lack of interest in color. However, some studies indicate that depressed persons prefer dark colors of low saturation and others claim they prefer bright, deeply saturated colors. Probably both conclusions are accurate since color can be either a stimulant or compensation for lack of excitement and dreariness as well as a reflection of one's inner state. Seen in another light, the depressive's attraction for bright colors may be an expression of homeostasis—the organism's subconscious striving for balance or equilibrium.

Compton Fabric Preference Test

Another test done with the mentally ill that deserves mention is the Compton fabric preference test. Sharpe reports that Compton tested the fabric and design preferences of a group of hospitalized psychotic women, in terms of the relationship between concepts of body, image boundary, penetration of boundary, and clothing preference. It was anticipated that persons with mental and emotional problems would be likely to suffer some aberrated form of body image, and it was found that persons with weak body boundaries tended to reinforce them with fabrics of strong figure-ground contrasts and brighter, more highly saturated colors—thus allowing them to feel less vulnerable to penetration, in a sense armored by the "strength" of the color and pattern.

BIOLOGICAL EFFECTS OF COLOR

At the dawn of civilization color was a biological necessity for locating food and observing predators. It is nature's survival kit for plants and animals—it attracts, camouflages, and protects them. Today color permeates our entire existence. Every aspect of our life involves color: Traffic is directed by color, instrument panels are regulated by color, electrical wires are color coded, advertising is printed in color, medicines and capsules are in color, office file folders have colored tabs, clothing has color, uniforms have color, the list is infinite. Biological or physiological reactions to color are the most susceptible to testing and the most valuable from a pragmatic point of view, particularly in relation to design. Kurt Goldstein, a highly regarded researcher, attributes the ambiguity of so much research on color to the fact that the tests were not performed from a "biological point of view," for color, he has stated, affects the behavior of the entire organism.

Goldstein is criticized primarily for having worked with a small sample of brain-damaged persons, but he presumes—and later studies appear to support his position—that these sensations occur in "normals" also, but are brought to the fore in extremely sensitive persons, such as artists, or in psychotics and neurotics. One of his most famous examples of color and effect is that of a woman who had cerebellar disease and resultant disturbance of equilibrium; when she wore a red dress, her symptoms increased to the point of her falling down.

Other effects of *red* that Goldstein noted in other patients were myopic refraction, abnormal deviation of the arms when held out from the body, errors in cutaneous localization, and again, increased loss of equilibrium. In all of these cases, *green* had the opposite effect, that of reducing the already present abnormal conditions. Goldstein states, "The stronger deviation of the arms in red stimulation corresponds to the experience of being disrupted, thrown out, abnormally attracted to the outerworld." Green stimulation resulted in withdrawal from the outerworld and meditation.

Goldstein also noted a large variety of differential motor reactions displayed by his patients under the effects of red and green. Movements executed with the same intention were performed much more exactly in green than in red light; handwriting, for example, was nearer to normal with green ink than with red. And estimates of length, as well as weight and time, were better under green light than red.

Other investigators have noted that blood pressure and respiration increased during exposure to red light, but decreased in blue illumination. Red light has been said to reduce the pain of rheumatism and arthritis. It dilates the blood vessels and produces heat in the tissues. Birren postulates that the red color of mercurochrome may be effective in the healing of wounds due to its absorption of blue light. Blue lights aids headaches and lowers blood pressure, and its tranquilizing effect may even aid insomniacs. Blue light is currently used with high success in the treatment of jaundice—bilirubinemia—in newborns. Yellow has been said to stimulate the appetite and to raise low blood pressure associated with anemia.

Finally, supporting the work of Goldstein and others, tests done with the GSR (galvanic skin response, commonly called the lie-detector test) produced significant relationships between GSR response and the colors that have been rated high in excitatory value, mainly reds and yellows.

COLOR AND PERSONALITY

Another major area of color research has focused upon the interaction between color and personality. Many of these "tests" take the form of informal questionnaires in popular magazines—both irresponsible and exploitative. More serious tests include the Rorschach inkblot, and the color-form tests discussed previously. Although color has been associated with personal characteristics since antiquity, it was not until the publication of the Rorschach, in Switzerland in 1921, that a systematic exploration of the relationship between color responses and personality, or emotional pattern, was begun.

In Germany in the mid-1930s, Jaensch developed a personality type theory correlating "systems of emotion" with "systems of color vision." Jaensch began by observing that in daylight vi-

sion there is increased sensitivity for red and yellow, and in twilight vision there is increased sensitivity for green and blue; then he went on to classify individuals according to their predominance of warm or cold vision systems.

Persons of the "warm color type" supposedly meet the external world with warm feelings; those of the "cold color type" are closed off from their surroundings and inwardly integrated. Before puberty, Jaensch asserted, most individuals are of the "outward integration" type, but in maturity the distinction between Nordic and Mediterranean types appears: Nordic being of the cold system, Mediterranean of the warm. As spurious as Jaensch's theories seem, they have not been universally repudiated by those concerned with color research. Faber Birren, noted author of dozens of books and articles on color, corroborates Jaensch's findings but substitutes "blond complexion type" for Nordic and "brunet" for Mediterranean, perhaps to make the "theory" seem more universal. Whatever the label, such notions seem far too generalized to be taken seriously.

Others have recognized the potential for opportunism and exploitation in color, since it strikes the public imagination and its maze of contradictory research offers "scientific findings" to support practically any theory or commercial gimmick. In 1969, a book appeared by Max Luscher called the *Luscher Color Test,* which subsequently reached the ranks of the best-seller list, and which relates the various personality characteristics to a person's ranking of several series of colors. The reader is led to believe that through these projective devices he or she can determine his or her personality structure, his or her strengths of weaknesses, within just a few minutes.

257

Some believe that this kind of instrument, used in conjunction with many others, can be useful; others question any validity. What is inarguable, however, is that the *Luscher Color Test,* issued as a popular text, is grossly misleading, although Luscher's test seems to be highly regarded by many professionals in the field. His latest book, *The 4-Color Person,* tantalizes readers of the September 1979 *House & Garden* with an "intriguing color quiz" [*sic*], which promises to reveal the key to the reader's "four dominant feelings of self—self-confidence, self-respect, self-satisfaction, and self-development." Various categories (furniture, modern art, music, architecture, etc.) of preference are listed. Upon scoring the quiz the reader becomes aware that the four preference choices of each category have been related to red, yellow, blue, or green, depending upon the assumed "affect" qualities of each color. Thus a preference for a "mobile by Calder" registers a point for yellow (self-development, imagination, independence), a preference for "Chopin" a point for blue (romance, trust, love, and peace), a taste for "cymbidium orchids" rates a point for green (self-respect, responsibility, persistence), and a preference for "riding a bike" over "joining a car pool" rates a red (passion, vitality, self-confidence).

Such personality quizzes are too simplistic and do not take into account those who have broad interests and catholic tastes. A gardener, for example, might prefer cymbidium orchids over daisies, because he or she has a greenhouse and has had good luck with that plant. Sometimes the questions on these tests are ridiculous: Would you rather read a book to a sick friend, eat in an Italian restaurant, or go dancing? Do you prefer filet mignon, duck flambé, imported cheeses, or homemade soup? Do you prefer florals, geometrics, or batik fabrics? A sophisticated person may like all of the choices equally depending upon the proper context. Such examples of popularized color theory are analogous to newspaper astrology. Home-decorating magazines frequently carry articles that offer such illuminating clues to one's inner life as, "If you like red, you are a strong personality with a craving for action, and are compatible not only with other reds but 'sun yellow' and 'wild iris.' "

Researchers have even hypothesized that people express their personalities through the clothes they wear. Sharpe reports, "An overview of the research suggests that the more *secure* individual tends to favor colors that range from neutral to cool (green, blue, beige and gray), of medium value tending toward dull, whereas the more *insecure* individual tends to select warm, bright colors (red, yellow) that range from the extremes of light and dark."

Such generalizations are narrow since they overlook many obvious reasons people dress as they do (education, upbringing, climate, budget, artistic expression, professional impact) and do not take into account the many people to whom clothing is completely unimportant, or those who economically cannot afford to express themselves sartorially, or that large group of people who wear anything that is "fashionable" at the moment regardless of whether it suits them. Perhaps those to whom clothing is unimportant are secure since their ego gratification is not dependent upon others' visual assessment of them. Those who cannot afford to buy the clothes they might like to buy may fall anywhere along the secure-insecure scale. Those who must continually buy and wear what is fashionable at the moment perhaps are the most insecure since this expresses a strong desire to be accepted and to conform. Thus it seems that clothing is not a valid indicator of personality: There are too many variables.

COLOR AND HARMONY

In the last two decades many of the old color taboos have been lifted, and the archaic laws have become obsolete—especially that of *complementary* colors (mainly, those diametrically opposite one another on the spectrally ordered color wheel)—as the *only* basis for color harmony. For according to traditional colorists, complementary colors equaled harmony equaled balance; to which the modern school of colorists added that noncomplementary colors equaled asymmetry equaled tension.

But adherence to such rigid formulas began to give way in the sixties, when the color revolution, paralleling others, exploded in bursts of psychedelic light, furthering a lasting acceptance of a vastly wider range of color combinations, as well as more vivid, brilliant color. The psychedelic movement helped to create among designers a more eclectic approach, one that accepts the dictates of neither school but rather relies on creating the color environment most appropriate to the specific situation, taking into account the size of the space, its architectural form, the proposed use of the space, the age of the occupants, the natural light, and the tasks to be performed there.

Color harmony is not just a function of the relationship of hues but depends largely upon the quantity of color, the intensity, balance, and weight. Certain color combinations create ten-

sion or movement. The goal of color is not always harmony; sometimes it is used to excite, stimulate, manipulate, create tension, or expand or contract a space.

THE COLOR WHEEL

The old color wheel (Fig. 9–1, Plate 15), based on arbitrary paint-mixing color qualities has been displaced by a new color wheel (Fig. 9–2, Plate 15) in which colors are based on the true color perception qualities of vision. The new color wheel has additional advantages in that it is accurate in explaining subtractive, additive, and partitive color mixing. Thus in the new color wheel, the complement of yellow is blue, not violet. The complement of green is magenta, not red. Although it has been widely accepted (based on the old color wheel) that red is the complement of green and vice versa, this is visually incorrect. The afterimage of green is magenta and the afterimage of red is cyan (blue).

The three color mixing systems are defined as follows.

Subtractive: Transparent colors placed on top of each other or in front of each other form a third color. Yellow and blue mixed make green. The mixed color is always darker than any of the component colors.

Additive: The cumulative effect of colored lights mixed together. The mixed color is always lighter than the lightest component color. Yellow and blue light equal white.

Partitive: The averaging of several colors as in pointillism style paintings. Adjacent spots in three-color printing and color T.V. are "mixed" by the eye and read as solid colors. The total effect of a fabric woven of different-color threads is a color different from any of the component threads individually. The mixed color has the average brightness of all the colors mixed.

It is not within the scope of this chapter to discuss in detail the highly technical aspects of color theory or the rationale that supports the development of the new color wheel. The reader is referred to an extraordinarily fine and highly readable book on the subject, *The Theory and Practice of Color,* by Frans Gerritsen (New York, Van Nostrand Reinhold, 1974).

LAWS OF PERCEPTION*

Sensitivity to Light and Color

The human eye can distinguish up to nine million colors with normal vision and mutual combinations of the three eye primaries, blue, green, and red (short, medium, and long wavelengths, respectively) and the three eye secondaries, yellow, magenta, and cyan. Color is light energy after it hits the eye. *Rods and cones,* the light *receptors,* are located in the retina. There are many more rods than cones. The rods are clustered on the periphery of the retina and the cones in the center, generally speaking. Since the cones are concentrated in the center of the retina, color sensitivity *decreases* toward the periphery of the retina until it reaches the edge where only light and dark can be discriminated. *Translating this into a more practical application, the greatest values (brightnesses) and the warm, active colors (yellows, reds, and oranges) should be placed in the center of attention. Lower brightnesses and*

* A good deal of the material presented under *Laws of Perception* has been adapted from *The Theory and Practice of Color,* by Frans Gerritsen (New York, Van Nostrand Reinhold, 1974).

cool, unsaturated colors (dark green, dark blue, dark brown) should appear on the periphery of the visual field. This knowledge is particularly important for the design of graphic signage, posters, large paintings, exhibitions, displays, and interior design. One may lead people from one room to another by the skillful arrangement of successive values and colors.

Simultaneous Contrast

Simultaneous contrast is the change in appearance of a color due to the influence of a surrounding contrasting color: Larger color masses influence smaller ones. If two spots of a neutral gray are surrounded by a larger area of white and of black, respectively, the gray surrounded by white will *appear* to have less brightness than the gray surrounded by black. This happens because the local adaptation of the eye is less sensitive to high brightness in a bright surrounding, thus more sensitive to low brightness or value. Against the bright white background, then, the gray will be evaluated as having less brightness than it actually has. However, the eye, against a black background, will be less sensitive to low brightness and will evaluate the gray spot as being very bright. This is true not just of white and black but of most colors in which a strong contrast exists (Fig. 9–3).

Successive Contrast and Afterimage

When the eye is adapted to the value and color of an environment, this will influence the brightness and color of what is seen directly thereafter. For example, if the eye is adapted to a blue background of a stage set and a performer wearing a yellow costume suddenly appears, the costume will appear much brighter yellow than if the eye had not first been adapted to yellow's complementary color, blue. If one concentrates on a green surface and then looks away at a white one, an afterimage of magenta will appear. One is in effect seeing the white surface *minus* the green to which the eye has already adapted. Looking at a certain color produces an *afterimage* of its complement (Fig. 9–4, Plate 16). A practical application of this principle is the surgical operating room where the walls and the garments are always blue-green because the eye is concentrated on a red spot (blood), and when the surgeons look up from their work, they see afterimages of blue-green. If the walls and their garments were white, they would see green spots before their eyes every time they looked away from their work. Thus the blue-green walls and gowns act as a background to neutralize these afterimages.

Another example of afterimage can be experienced if one walks through a corridor that has yellow walls, a warm-toned floor, and incandescent (warm) light—essentially a yellow-hued environment. When leaving the corridor, perhaps entering a lobby, one will see afterimages of blue, the complement of yellow. *This is very important for interior design.* An understanding of this concept can prevent a designer from creating undesirable color relationships.

Metameric Color Pairs

Metameric color pairs are those that are alike only under certain conditions. For example, if two color chips of turquoise blue paint fabricated by two different paint manufacturers seem identical under incandescent light, they may appear vastly different from each other under a different source

of light due to the absorption curves of the color surfaces. The vast number of chemical formulas and varying compositions of pigment and binder will produce colors that, although they may appear to match another color in a certain light, actually have different short and long wavelength areas. Thus the colors would look quite different under a different source of light due to the differences in absorption.

A practical application of this principle occurs daily in the offices of architects and interior designers. Frequently the carefully selected paint colors specified by an architect or designer will be met by the contractor's request for a substitution of manufacturer. While seemingly harmless, provided the substituted manufacturer has a high-quality comparable product, the possibility of "mixing to match" the designer's original palette of colors is almost impossible.

It is highly unlikely that the two manufacturers would use the same chemical formula and exactly the same type of pigment. The colors will probably be "mixed to match" under cool white fluorescent light in the paint store. While they may appear to match perfectly there, they will not match in the incandescent light or warm white fluorescent of the job site. *The pigment molecules of one formulation will be sensitive to and absorb different wavelengths than the other formulation.* Colors that have identical chemical formulations will look identical in all sources of light even if the samples were mixed at different times. It is critical that colors always be evaluated under the lighting conditions where they will be used.

Reflectance

The colors of a room are influenced by the reflection of the natural light entering the room as well as by artificial sources of light. An example of the first condition is a room with a large expanse of window facing a garden. The green grass will absorb most of the long wavelengths of the daylight (the reds and oranges) and permit the short wavelengths (greens and blues) to be reflected through the window onto the walls of the room. If the walls are white, they will have a green tint. The green tint can be neutralized by painting the reflection wall a *complementary* color in the magenta or red family.

An example of the second condition (artificial light) is a corridor with red carpet, white walls, and white ceiling, with recessed incandescent light fixtures. The carpet absorbs most of the wavelengths of the artificial light except for the long waves of the red-orange spectrum. Thus the floor reflects an intense red light on the ceiling, making it appear red. A way to avoid this condition is by lighting the ceiling from below.

Purkinje Effect

The Purkinje effect was named after its discoverer, a Czechoslovakian physician, who observed that at twilight, color impressions are shifted to favor the short wavelength area of the spectrum. Thus reds, oranges, and yellows become colorless and darker, greens and blues become clearer.

Color Constancy

This phenomenon refers to the relationship between the eye and the brain to translate visual information in a constant manner. For example, if one looks at a piece of white paper while standing in front of a red wall under daylight, the paper will still appear white, but a colored photograph would show the paper to be pink. In other words, intellectually the brain knows the paper is white and so translates it as white in spite of perceptual information to the contrary.

Advancing and Receding Colors

Goethe's observation, mentioned earlier, that warm colors seem to advance while cool colors recede, can be explained by optic laws. Red—being only slightly refracted by the lens of the eye—focuses at a point behind the retina, and the lens, in order to see it clearly, grows more convex, thus pulling the color forward. Blue, on the other hand, is more sharply refracted and causes the lens to flatten out, thus decreasing its size by pushing its image back.

Figure-Ground Reversal

This phenomenon is a principle of Gestalt psychology and refers to the optical illusion apparent particularly in geometric patterns in which the figure seems to be in front of the background. Obviously, both figure and ground are printed on the same surface. Warm colors (red, orange, yellow) tend to be seen as figure since they advance, and cool colors (green, blue, purple) as ground since they recede. But whether a color is seen as figure or ground also depends on the value (light advances, dark recedes) and the saturation (high advances, low recedes).

COLOR SYMBOLISM

Emotional evaluations of color are a function of time, place, culture, nationality, age, fashion, and even gender. Colors conjure up highly personal images and meanings, making it difficult to predict and understand preferences. Furthermore, emotional evaluations of colors are made in relation to an object. While "apricot" may be a fashionable color this year for residential interiors, it is unlikely to be considered tasteful in an automobile or a toaster. People usually like colors associated with pleasurable experiences. Those who like modern art usually like the brilliant colors found in such paintings. Those who prefer the old masters usually favor a more subdued palette.

The symbolic nature of color is expressed in color names, which are often made up of the basic color plus an adjective: *black magic, snow white, spice beige, chocolate brown, shocking pink, red hot, true blue (loyal)*. Paint manufacturers often express sheer whimsy in naming colors such as "Persimmon" for an olive green or "Touch of Love" which tells one nothing about the color.

Colors, through the ages, have come to be associated with certain emotions or personality traits. Some of the more common follow.

Blue: Tranquility, cool, solitude, intelligence, soothingness, truth, divinity, quiet, melancholy, calm, sincerity, generosity, serenity, hope, conformity, control, suppression of feelings, constancy, accomplishment, devotion, introspection.

Yellow: Joy, gaiety, harvest, brilliance, morbidity, cowardice, disease, fruition, regality, hope, jaundice.

Orange: Warmth, glow, sociality, friendliness, good cheer, good nature, gregariousness.

Red: Heart, blood, tragedy, cruelty, war, heat, hatred, power, bravery, love of life, courage, fire, fury, purgatory, passion, beauty, truth, shame,

destruction, anger, danger, stop, love, excitement.

Green: Peace, youth, hope, victory, jealousy, life, nature, immortality, safety, conventionality, good adjustment, balance.

Orange-Brown: Deceit, distrust, inconstancy, treachery.

Red-Brown: Strength, solidity, vigor, sadness, maturity, simplicity, sturdiness, reliability, rationality.

White: Truth, innocence, purity, virginity, chastity, modesty, humility, light, love, temperance, friendship.

Black: Evil, gloom, death, terror, horror, darkness, crime, melancholy, secrecy, mystery, wickedness, witchcraft, mourning, solemnity, potency, social status.

Gray: Penance, humility, sadness, age, sobriety, death, fear, dreariness, bleakness, sterility, maturity, emotionlessness, isolation.

PRACTICAL APPLICATIONS OF COLOR PSYCHOLOGY

Where does all this investigation—preference and personality, color shock and loss of equilibrium—bring us in terms of design? Clearly, much of the research that has been reviewed here is at yet inconclusive. Many conclusions propagated about the effect of color and its link to emotional patterns have not been scientifically proven; so the real investigation of the effect of color upon human behavior has only just begun. Early state of the science notwithstanding, however, certain practical applications in design do suggest themselves.

1. *Reds and yellows,* for example, should be used in settings where creative activity is desired,

greens and blues in areas that require more quiet and extended concentration—and the appropriate combinations of these colors in classrooms, hospitals, and offices.

2. Cool colors should be used in the surroundings of the hysterical, hypertensive, and anxious, red in the depressive's environment. Highly saturated colors should be avoided with autistic schizophrenics, as should red with those afflicted—like Goldstein's classic case—with organic brain disease.

3. Rousing, bright colors should be used with the aged rather than pastels, which are barely visible to those with failing eyesight.

4. Strongly contrasting figure-ground patterns and extremely bright colors should be avoided in the rooms of psychotic patients since these—when not worn by the patients but impinging upon them from their environment—might be thought to have an overwhelming, even intimidating and threatening effect.

5. The knowledge of color preference and usage can be employed in cultural liaison and trade with foreign countries. Knowing which colors are taboo and which carry religious or symbolic associations in each country is mandatory for expanded marketing and trade relations.

6. Under *warm* colors, time is overestimated, weights seem heavier, objects seem larger, rooms appear smaller. Under *cool* colors, time is underestimated, weights seem lighter, objects seem smaller, rooms appear larger. Thus cool colors should be used where monotonous tasks are performed to make the time seem to pass more quickly, and red, for example, should be used in an employees' restroom to reduce the amount of time spent there.

7. Under *warm* colors with high illumination, there is increased alertness and outward orientation—good where muscular effort or action are required such as a physical therapy gym. Under *cool* colors and low illumination, there is less distraction and more opportunity to concentrate on difficult tasks, an inward orientation is fostered. Noise induces increased sensitivity for cool colors, probably because the tranquility of these colors compensates for the increased aural stimulation. One becomes less sensitive to warm colors under noise since they offer additional stimulation rather than less.

COLOR AND ITS EFFECT ON OUR PERCEPTION OF SPACE

The various laws of perception discussed previously can be translated into the following guidelines for interior design and architecture.

1. To prepare people for the color of a room they are about to enter, the entry should be painted a *complementary* color.

2. Color modifies architectural form—it can expand, shorten, widen, lengthen, and give the illusion of lowering or raising a ceiling. Color can

change the appearance of the environment to lift the individual out of reality.

3. Bright colors seem lighter in weight. Ordered from "heavy" to "light" they are: red, blue, purple, orange, green, yellow.

4. Bright objects are overestimated in size. Yellow appears the largest with white, red, green, blue, and black in descending order.

5. A light object appears larger against a dark background. A dark object will appear smaller against a light background.

6. The wall opposite a window should generally be kept light or it will absorb much of the daylight.

7. A window wall and frame should be light so as not to contrast too much with the sky—high contrast can result in headaches and eye strain.

8. If a red wall is placed next to a yellow wall, the yellow wall will appear greener than it actually is due to the afterimage of red: cyan. The blue afterimage of the yellow will cause the red to appear more purple.

9. Warm colors advance, cool colors recede.

10. Light colors and small patterns visually enlarge a space. Dark colors and large patterns make it appear smaller.

11. The absence of variety in the visual environment causes sensory deprivation. Those who are confined to nursing homes, hospitals, and institutions desperately need changes in lighting, accent walls, and artwork in order for their nervous systems to function properly. Monotonous white walls devoid of interesting graphics of artwork deprive the brain of the constantly changing stimulation it requires to remain healthy.

12. In low levels of light (under 30 footcandles), object and surface colors will appear normal when the light source is slightly tinted with pink, orange, or yellow. As higher light levels are reached, a *normal* appearance for object colors will be found with cooler light; it is best to stay warm at low levels and go cooler at high levels* (Kruithof's principle).

Since lighting and color influence each other greatly, the reader is referred to Chapter 10 for additional information.

SUMMARY

The old strictures are loosening, and more attention is focusing on the environment's vital influence and the powers inherent in design. In the past, different disciplines were rigidly separate; social scientists concentrated on the influence of the social environment, psychologists were absorbed with rat behavior and isolated stimuli in the sterile confines of their laboratories, and designers and architects strove, in the main, for aesthetically pleasing functionality. What is now emerging, however, is a more interdisciplinary, holistic approach, for we have begun to perceive people in their total environment, to realize that behavior is influenced by space, structure, color, lighting, activity, and other participants, as well as by our own inner being—in sum, that everything has its effect in an environmental process that works as a kind of circular feedback. With this understanding, design becomes in a sense akin to social action: We can either stimulate learning or dull the requisite desire and concentration; enhance recuperation or impede it; encourage vital social interaction or hinder it; improve mental and emotional well-being or further listless torpor. While an awareness of these influences through emerging reseach in the field is important for *any* design, be it private home or public facility, it is *crucial* in the planning of societal structures—schools, hospitals, mental and penal institutions, factories, offices buildings—that contain large masses of people over sustained periods of time, thus giving shape to the moments and the course of their lives.

* *Light, Color and Environment,* by Faber Birren (New York, Van Nostrand Reinhold, 1969) p. 25.

Chapter 10
Interior Finishes and Furniture

The interior design of a medical or dental office is critical to the patients' assessment of the physician or dentist and the level of anxiety the patient experiences. These topics have been covered in depth in Chapter 1; thus the present discussion will be limited to specifications of interior finish materials and furniture items that are particularly well suited to medical and dental offices.

All too often interiors are designed to residential standards with materials that are not intended to withstand the use of a high-volume office. A door that, in a residence, may be opened and closed 3000 times in a year, may be opened and closed 100,000 times a year in a medical office. Similarly, shag or cut pile carpet designed for residential use does not hold up well. It is difficult to clean and may show wear sooner than a commercial carpet.

If budget permits, all walls should receive a commercial vinyl wallcovering (see Chapter 13 for classification characteristics). Gypsum board walls make a good substrate for application of vinyl wallcoverings provided they have not been textured. A light texture is desirable, however, if one intends to paint the walls, since the texture helps to conceal the drywall taping and nail heads. A heavy stucco or sand finish texture is to be avoided since it collects dirt, and it is difficult to clean. Special wall treatments for decorative purposes such as wood paneling, grasscloth, or woven fabrics are fine in limited areas such as consultation rooms.

A suspended acoustic tile ceiling is more suitable than a sprayed acoustic ceiling because it gives access to the electrical and mechanical equipment above it and it is easier to clean. Where sanitation is of extreme importance, a plastic-coated acoustic tile should be used.

Flooring may be carpet, vinyl asbestos tile, sheet vinyl, or a combination of all three. Vinyl asbestos tile is the least expensive flooring and is very durable, but it does need to be waxed. Sheet vinyl is recommended for wet areas such as bathrooms if the budget does not allow for ceramic tile. Sheet vinyl is also recommended in minor surgeries or anywhere sanitation is a concern because it has fewer seams than VA tile and a self-coved base.

It is increasingly common to find entire medical offices carpeted. Carpet, if selected properly, is easy to maintain and adds warmth to the appearance of the office. It provides a much-needed acoustic function as well. And it prevents serious accidents caused by people slipping. Volumes have been written on carpet fibers, the density of construction, pile height, and the other numerous factors that must be considered in the selection of a carpet. Suffice it to say that the toughest fiber is nylon and the most serviceable of the nylons is the third generation, Dupont's Antron III, Dow Badische's Zeflon and Allied Chemical's Anso-X, with soil-hiding properties actually designed into the chemical structure of the yarn. A brand-new Anso IV has just been introduced which adds the feature of permanent stain repellency to the third generation product. The third and fourth generation nylons are permanently antistatic, a very important feature for medical and dental facilities.

Acrylic fibers resemble wool and are delustered (nylons have a sheen that is sometimes objectionable), but they tend to pill or fuzz from abrasion and do not hold up as well as nylon. There are, however, combination yarn systems which feature the delustered wool-like look of acrylic and the durability of nylon. Dow Badische's Zefran blend CR-4 yarn is an example. Actually, commercial carpets have never been better. Technology has made available nylon carpets that are delustered and resemble richly textured wool Berber carpets. Practically any color or texture one would want to see in commercial carpet is presently available. Carpets with a synthetic backing (instead of jute) are desirable particularly where there is a possibility of water leakage. The synthetic backing will not rot or leach out its color as does jute. When jute gets wet the dye in it sometimes leaches out to the surface of the carpet, and it is very difficult, if

ever possible, to remove it. Dental operatories are often prone to plumbing accidents, so it would be especially important to have a carpet with a synthetic backing here.

A level loop pile is the most serviceable for high-traffic areas, although a combination loop and cut pile will work well in most medical facilities. There are even a number of high-traffic commercial-use cut piles on the market. The rule about shag carpet not being desirable in a medical office can be disregarded in a pediatric waiting room. There, a thick cut pile or short shag is preferable because mothers may be embarrassed to report accidents and it may be days before urine or drops of milk or grape juice are discovered—dried and caked. A high pile tends to hide these discolorations well and, it all else fails, the carpet can be snipped to remove the stain.

Carpet is best installed in a medical or dental office glued directly to the slab with no pad. This provides a firm footing, making it less likely that people will trip. Direct glue-down is the recommended installation method in hospitals and many other commercial facilities. In offices, it often eliminates the need for acrylic chair mats since it is firm enough to allow chairs and carts to roll freely. Where a pad is desired, as in a consultation room, a dense rubber slab pad is preferable to a foam waffle pad, which tends to "bottom out." Omalon is a high-quality pad with long life that works well where a pad is desired in a commercial facility.

Furniture

Offices that are located in cities with inclement weather must provide an area near the entrance to the waiting room for removing boots, rubbers,

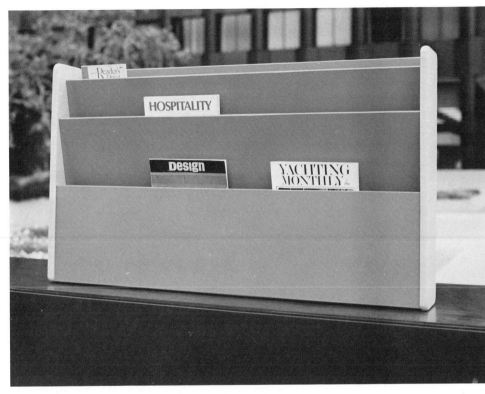

Fig. 10-1. Magazine rack. (Courtesy Peter Pepper Products Co.)

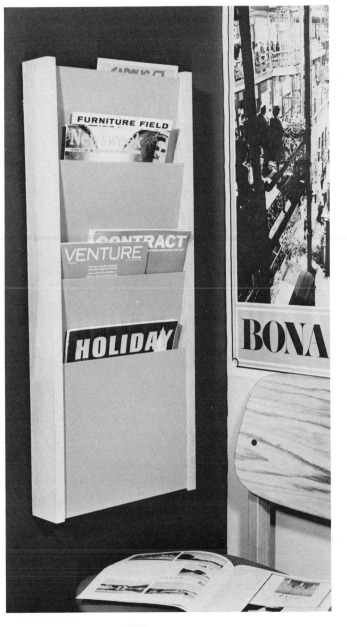

Fig. 10-2. Magazine rack. (Courtesy Peter Pepper Products Co.)

269

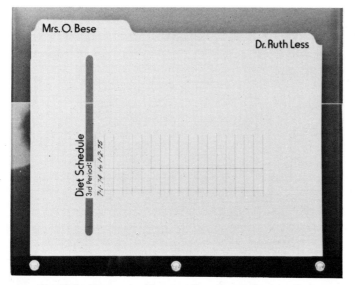

Fig. 10-3. Chart rack. (Courtesy Peter Pepper Products Co.)

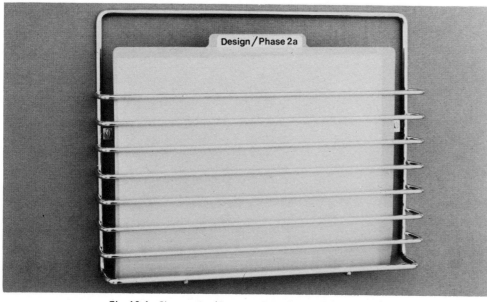

Fig. 10-4. Chart rack. (Courtesy Peter Pepper Products Co.)

and winter apparel. An umbrella caddy and coat hooks (some low enough for children) are also necessary. For the comfort of those waiting, it is desirable that the coat area be visible from the waiting room. Offices in California and other states with a temperate climate usually do not have entry vestibules or coat closets.

To eliminate the clutter of magazines being strewn about the room, the waiting room ought to have a magazine rack. A wall-hung unit is most functional. Those in Figs. 10-1 and 10-2 are decorative and well suited to a medical or dental office.

The doors of medical exam rooms require a chart rack. Those in Figs. 10-3 and 10-4 function well and are available in a number of accent colors.

There is great latitude in the selection of waiting room seating. The main criteria are that a suitable number of individual chairs with arms be provided and that the chairs not be too low or hard to get out of. The chairs in Figs. 10-5 through 10-8 are examples of chairs that are well suited to medical and dental waiting rooms.

It is important for the parents' and the staffs' sanity to keep children occupied—patients and siblings alike. A small table or work counter will provide space for coloring or playing games. Proper stroage for toys will encourage the children to replace toys after use. Creative Playthings of Princeton, New Jersey, designs and manufactures marvelously inventive toys for children.

Educational exhibits or artwork can be put to good use in a medical waiting room. The subject matter could provide useful information about the facility or its physicians or history, or explain birth defects, sports injuries, or other medical conditions.

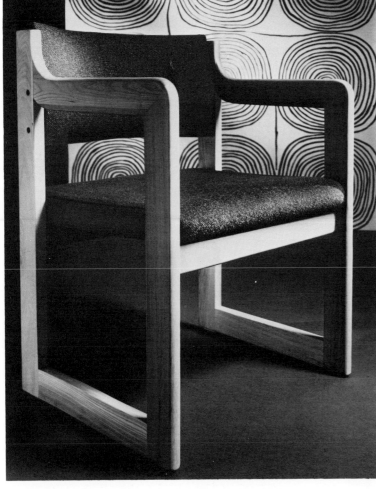

Fig. 10-5. Waiting room chair. (Courtesy Thonet Industries.)

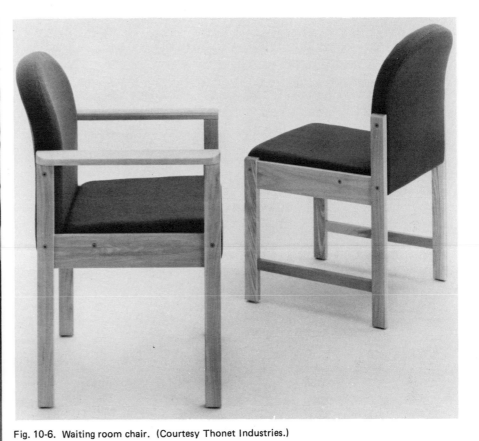

Fig. 10-6. Waiting room chair. (Courtesy Thonet Industries.)

271

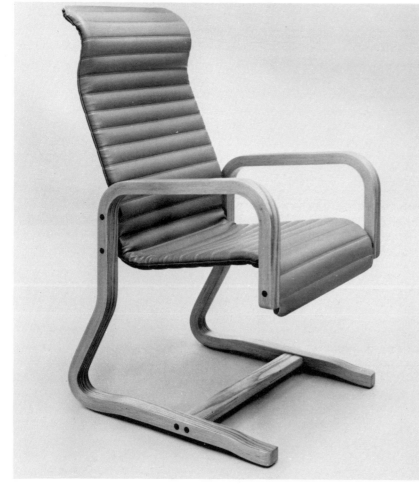

Fig. 10-7. High-backed chair for geriatric patients or those with orthopedic problems. (Courtesy Thonet Industries.)

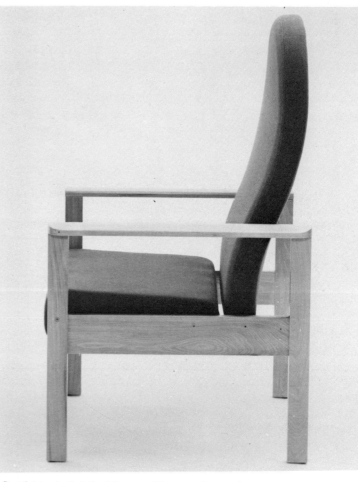

Fig. 10-8. High-backed chair. (Courtesy Thonet Industries.)

Chapter 11
Lighting

BIOLOGICAL EFFECTS OF LIGHT

Traditionally lighting engineers and those in the design professions have been concerned with lighting in terms of either vision or aesthetics. What has been overlooked until recently is the biological significance of light. Incandescent and fluorescent lamps are presently fabricated according to the assumption that persons will be exposed to sunlight as a normal part of each day and not be confined to a habitation of artificial illumination. These lamps emit a narrow spectrum of light that does not include ultraviolet. Fluorescent light is a light without heat whereby ultraviolet radiation is converted into radiation of a longer wavelength (since the human eye is not sensitive to UV radiation, these wavelengths are lengthened by phosphors to which the eye is sensitive). Different phosphors create different tints of fluorescent light. Thus fluorescent lamps, in simplistic terms, are nothing more than glass tubes the inner surface of which has been coated with phosphor powders which, when excited by ultraviolet energy created within the arc stream, give off visible light. As an aside, all fluorescent lamp tints cost the same to manufacture, although thanks to marketing demand, cool white always costs less than the more appealing colors.

If persons are to be confined for long periods away from sunlight, a balanced light that emits a fairly full spectrum of wavelengths is desirable. The illumination of our environment acts as both an inducer and a timer of glandular and metabolic functions, affecting, among other things, milk produced, the quality and quantity of eggs laid, and stimulation or inhibition of sexual activity. Light dilates blood vessels, thereby increasing circulation. Sudden exposure to bright light stimulates the adrenal gland. Our biological time clocks—our circadian rhythms—are manipulated by light. Studies have shown that subjects who are forced to live in darkness for prolonged periods suffer sensory deprivation. The loss of environmental cues that tell the body what to do throws the body systems out of kilter.

As populations increase, and pollution likewise, those in urban centers will increasingly be forced to live in indoor environments. Persons confined to nursing homes or institutions who are not able to get outdoors are similarly dependent on their indoor environment to supply a well-balanced light that includes some ultraviolet. Those who design such environments will have to be aware of not just the biological effects of light, but also the psychological mood-inducing effects as well as the visual quality of the light.

Perhaps the optimal solution to lighting in offices, homes, restaurants, hospitals, and hotels, would be a system of changing light levels and tints. Since natural light changes throughout the day (warm and rosy at dawn and dusk and bright with a bluish cast at midday), should we not try to imitate these day-night cycles in our built environments?

TECHNICAL DATA

The sensation that we call color and light is our psychological interpretation of certain portions of the electromagnetic spectrum. How well we see colors depends on how closely the ingredients of our artificial light source match the ingredients of sunlight. Artificial sources of light have varying degrees of each color—some have more warm wavelengths and some more cool. An incandescent bulb, for example, is high in orange and red and low in blue and violet; thus it imparts a warm glow, but it is far from the color of daylight. The most efficient lamp is probably the sodium vapor lamp, but its color rendition is so distorted that it cannot be used in interior environments.

Fluorescent lamps are far more energy efficient than incandescent. Typically, fluorescents produce about 72 lumens (the amount of light generated at the light source) per watt, compared with 17.5 lumens per watt produced by a 100-watt general service incandescent lamp. The fluorescent has an average life of 15,000 hours versus 750 hours for the average incandescent. Furthermore, it takes 60 gallons of oil to burn one 100-watt bulb continuously for one year. With the energy shortages which have become a fact of life, it seems irresponsible to use more than a smattering of incandescent just for special effects when fluorescent will not do.

Fluorescent lamps have been improved in recent years, and over 20 different colors are presently available. But one must select carefully and only after consulting the manufacturer's lamp specification catalog because bulbs of the same wattage do not necessarily have equal lumen counts. And often there are other quantitative differences on a particular lamp from one manufacturer to another. Fluorescent lamps are selected on the basis of lumen output, color temperature, and color rendition. The *color temperature* is expressed in degrees Kelvin. The higher the color temperature, the bluer the appearance and the closer to daylight; the lower the color temperature, the redder the appearance. The *color rendering index* (CRI) describes the ability of a lamp to render objects as they would be seen in outdoor sunlight, which has a CRI of 100. Thus a lamp with a CRI of 80 renders the object 80% as accurately as outdoor sunlight. Below is a list of the most commonly used fluorescent lamps plus a few unique ones.

Cool white lamps are approximately 4100°K and CRI 68%. They intensify white, gray, blue, and green and do not blend well with incandescent.

Warm white lamps are approximately 3000°K and CRI 56%. They slightly distort all colors and have a pink glow but mix well with incandescent.

Warm white deluxe lamps are 3000°K and CRI 71%. They greatly intensify warm colors, are not as pink as standard warm white, and blend well with incandescent.

Daylight lamps are 6500°K and usually have a CRI of 75%, but Duro-Test Corp. makes one with a CRI of 92%. This lamp produces a cold blue-white light, unflattering to warm colors and incandescent light but useful in a room where a large quantity of natural light is present.

Standard white lamps are 3500°K and CRI 64%. These lamps fall between cool white and warm white, so they are a good middle-of-the-road choice where budget does not permit a more quality lamp. The one with the highest CRI number is best. These lamps blend adequately with incandescent light.

Vita-lite lamp is 5500°K and has a CRI of 91%. This is a high-quality lamp made only by Duro-Test Corp. It is a bright white lamp that simulates the full color and ultraviolet spectrum of sunlight.

Ultralume 3000 lamp is 3000°K with a CRI of 85%. Made by Westinghouse, this lamp is flattering to warm colors and has a better color rendition than warm white deluxe.

Optima 32 lamp is 3200°K and has a CRI of 82%. Manufactured by Duro-Test Corp., this is a general purpose lamp with the warmth of incandescent but better color rendition.

Optima 50 lamp is 5000°K and CRI 91%. Made by Duro-Test Corp. and recommended where visual acuity is required and where color matching is performed.

For comparison, an incandescent lamp is 2800°K and daylight (although it does vary with the time of day and the time of the year and whether the sky is sunny or cloudy) is arbitrarily established at 6500°K. The reader is encouraged to write to the Duro-Test Corp. in North Bergen, New Jersey, and to Westinghouse in Bloomfield, New Jersey. Both manufacturers have excellent technical literature on their lamps. The General Electric Co. in Nela Park, Ohio, also publishes a number of interesting booklets.

ENERGY CONSERVATION

Worse than not enough light is too much. More is not better. The designer, if not qualified to do the lighting calculations, may wish to retain a lighting consultant or an electrical engineer. A high level of general illumination tends to wash out textures and colors. Much more interesting, not to mention energy efficient, is an interplay of high and low levels of illumination. In offices, we now light the task, not the entire room. Lighting, skillfully handled, can set up a rhythm of patterns, light, and shadow, which can transform an otherwise commonplace interior into something quite spectacular.

Another practical way to prune watts is to install fixtures with dimmer controls (fluorescents must be ordered specifically with dimming ballasts). An attempt to save electricity by removing two of the four lamps in a four-lamp fixture without changing the ballast saves nothing. One should specify only acrylic lenses, never polystyrene, which is less expensive but yellows with age.

The maintenance of light fixtures is extremely important to their performance. Technical equations permit one to calculate the light loss factor, which takes into account temperature and voltage variations, dirt on the lens, lamp depreciation, maintenance procedures, and atmospheric conditions. The ceiling height and the reflectance of walls and floor also affect the footcandle level

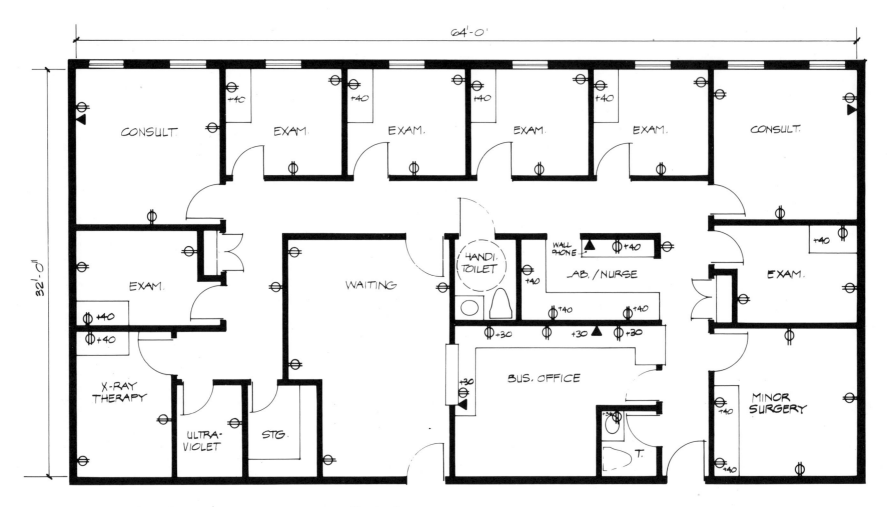

ELECTRICAL & TELEPHONE PLAN
DERMATOLOGY SUITE

Fig. 11-1. Electrical plan (for dermatology suite in Fig. 4-43.)

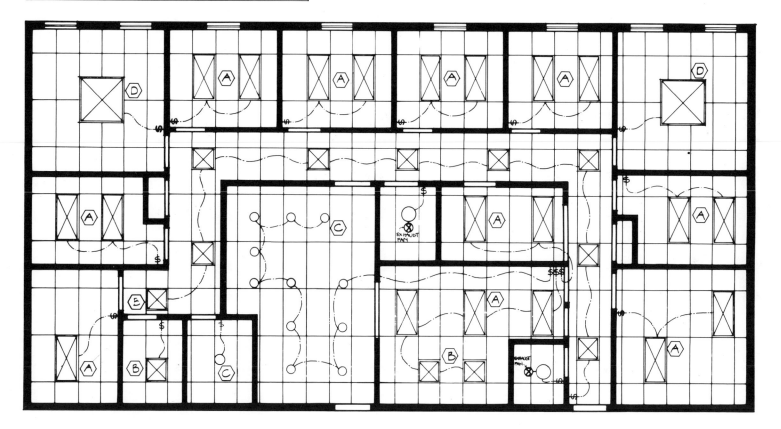

REFLECTED CEILING PLAN
DERMATOLOGY SUITE

Fig. 11-2. Reflected ceiling plan (for dermatology suite in Fig. 4-43.)

A 2×4 FLUORESCENT LAY-IN FIXTURE · 4 LAMP
B 2×2 FLUORESCENT LAY-IN FIXTURE
C INCANDESCENT RECESSED CAN
D 4×4 SURFACE MOUNTED FLUORESCENT

277

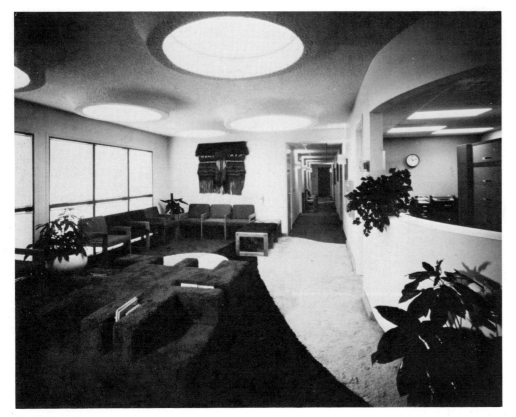

Fig. 11-3. Waiting room lighting.

(the measurement of light that reaches a given surface). Thus when one speaks of a requirement of 100 *maintained* footcandles at a given task, one must start with a number of lamps somewhat in excess of that measurement to take into account the light loss factor and the interior finishes of the room.

ELECTRICAL AND LIGHTING REQUIREMENTS FOR MEDICAL OFFICES

The electrical and lighting requirements for medical and dental offices differ greatly with the specialty and are discussed somewhat under each chapter. Chapter 8 discusses thoroughly the requirements of dental operatories, so that information will not be repeated here. Figure 11–1 shows the recommended electrical outlets for the dermatology suite first introduced in Fig. 4–43.

Exam rooms need a maintained light level of 100 footcandles. This can be achieved by two four-lamp (2 × 4-foot) luminaires, either recessed (lay-in) or surface mounted. Physicians who require a high-intensity light for examinations will have a portable lamp or other light source for that purpose.

Nurse stations also require a maintained illumination of 100 footcandles. A lower light level is appropriate for waiting rooms (30 to 50 footcandles), and the concentration of illumination should be where people are reading. The lighting may be indirect downlights or fluorescent luminaires, or perhaps an artificial skylight. Figure 11–3 shows an interesting use of fluorescent. These custom-built fixtures have square housings (so that they take standard fluorescent lamps) and 30, 36, and 48-inch-diameter disks of

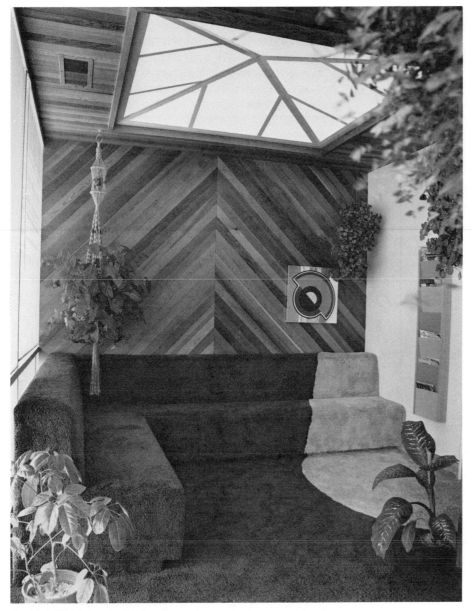

Fig. 11-4. Waiting room lighting.

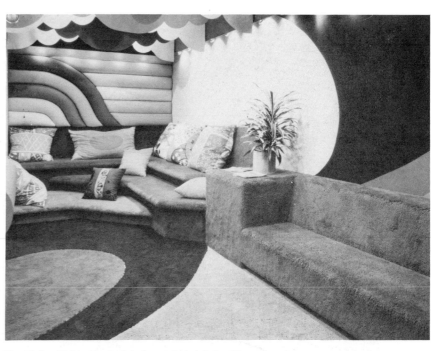

Fig. 11-4a. Waiting room lighting, pedodontist's office.

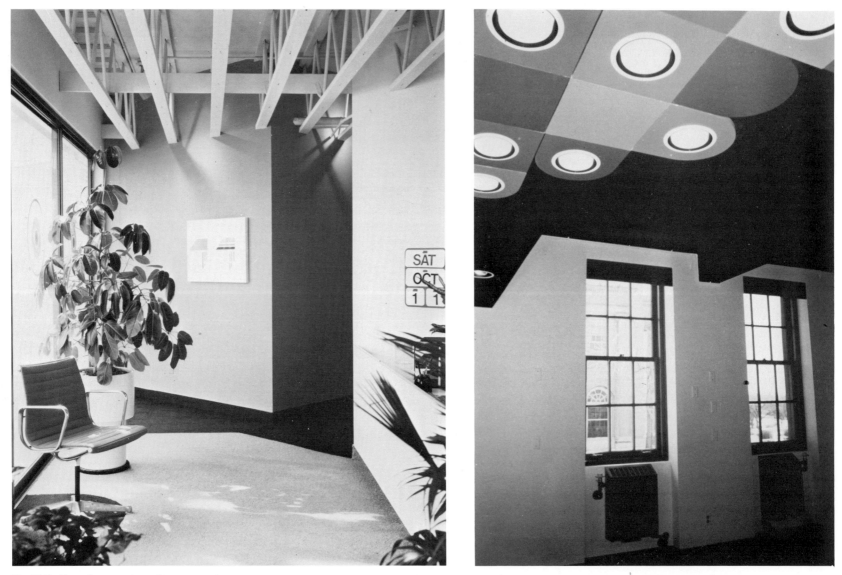

Fig. 11-5. Entry foyer, orthopedic surgery suite.

Fig. 11-6. Lighting detail at entry to CAT scanner wing.

translucent cast sheet acrylic. The ceiling is furred down around them to give a sculptured dimension to the ceiling. Figure 11-4 shows how a recessed artificial skylight fixture opens up a tiny room, gives illumination, and at the same time adds architectural interest. Figure 11-4a shows how incandescent lamps, properly placed, can create patterns of light as interesting as any artwork. Similarly, Fig. 11-5 shows an entry foyer of an orthopedic surgery suite, utilizing incandescent lights tucked away in the exposed truss joists to create a sculptural interplay of light on the walls. Another interesting lighting treatment for an entry foyer is that of Fig. 11-6. This is the entry to the CAT scanner wing at Milwaukee County Hospital. Standard downlights but with a closed opal glass lens (to keep glare out of the eyes of patients being wheeled in on stretcher carts) are worked into custom wood modules which are fastened to the ceiling. A nurse station, which is actually the core of this orthopedic surgery suite (Fig. 11-7), has a wood ceiling to add warmth and recessed downlights which, instead of giving uniform illumination, create pools of light and interesting drama. (The writer wishes to note that this suite was designed years before the energy conservation legislation was enacted.)

Corridors need only about 20 footcandles of illumination, and the light certainly need not be confined to the ceiling. In fact, lighting mounted on the walls of a corridor often give better color rendition to interior finishes than would those same lights mounted on the ceiling. Also, there is more glare when lights are mounted on the ceiling. Figure 11-8 shows a prefabricated fluorescent fixture (slimline with a remote ballast)

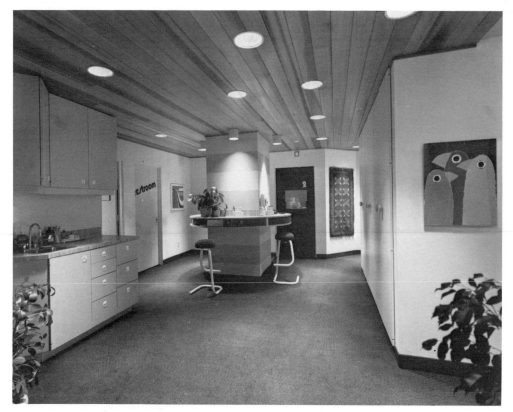

Fig. 11-7. Nurse station, orthopedic surgery.

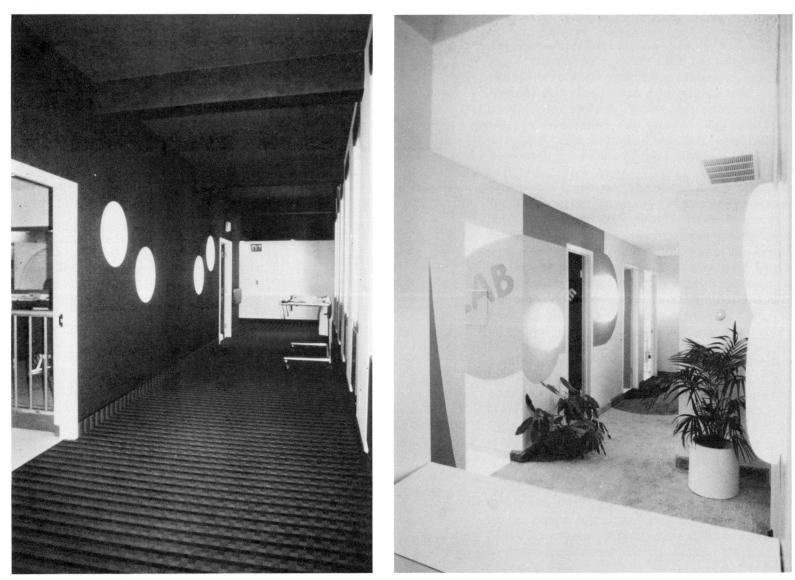

Fig. 11-8. Hospital corridor lighting.

Fig. 11-9. Corridor lighting, dermatology suite.

mounted in the wall of this hospital corridor. Not only is it interesting, it assumes a dimension of artwork. Functionally, it was initially designed because the ceiling was a rated fire enclosure and could not be penetrated. Due to the code requirement that hospital corridors be a net 8 feet wide, with no intrusions allowed, a lighting soffit or any surface-mounted fixture was out of the question. It seems that sometimes the most stringent restrictions lead to the most creative solutions. Figure 11-9 and 11-10 show a similar design treatment, except that the fixtures are surface-mounted fluorescent which take a circline lamp. Since these are cool to the touch, there is no problem locating them at heights where people might touch them. They can even be successfully worked into a graphic design as was done in these two installations, one a corridor of a dermatologist's office and the other a playpit for children in a dentist's office. Figure 11-11 shows a lighting treatment for exposed truss joists where there is no place to hide electrical wiring or bury the housing for a recessed fixture. A light track fastened to the chord of the joist lends itself well to the informality and vitality of the exposed truss architectural treatment.

The consultation room requires approximately 50 footcandles of light with the concentration of it over the desk. Figure 11-12 shows two oak-framed surface-mounted fluorescents of commercial manufacture butted together to form a larger and more imposing fixture unit. Additional lighting in a consultation room may be used to accent diplomas or artwork if the room is large enough to handle additional lighting.

The minor surgery room requires from 100 to 150 maintained footcandles, depending upon the detail of the procedures performed. Most minor

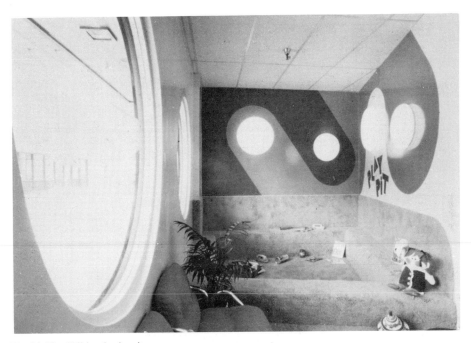

Fig. 11-10. Children's playpit.

surgery rooms will have a ceiling-mounted high-intensity surgical light, in which case two four-lamp fluorescents often will suffice, providing the lumen ouput of the specific lamp is high enough.

The lighting requirements of specialized rooms such as refracting rooms or radiology rooms is discussed under these specialties, as are any special considerations concerning the type or level of illumination for the individual suite as a whole.

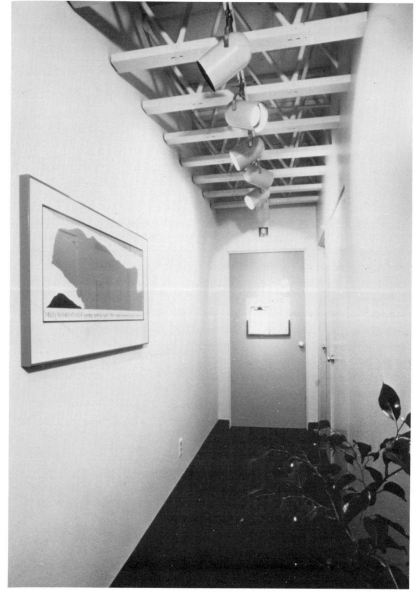

Fig. 11-11. Corridor lighting.

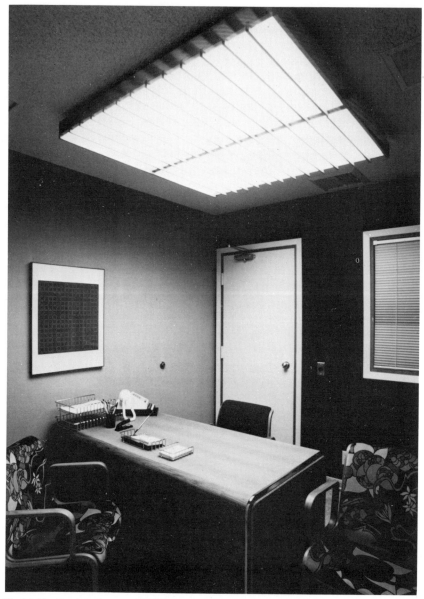

Fig. 11-12. Consultation room lighting.

Chapter 12
Construction Methods and Building Systems

HEATING, VENTILATING AND AIR CONDITIONING (HVAC)

The mechanical requirements of medical and dental offices are quite specialized in that the physical comfort of staff and patients is very important and there are a great many variables in terms of room function, often within a small area. An examination room, for example, is typically 8 × 12 feet in size, and the patient (who spends more time in the room than the doctor) is usually undressed. The waiting room, by contrast, is designed to accommodate many people and often they have sweaters or coats on their laps which add to their body warmth. Not only does this room have a higher density (one person per 16 to 20 square feet compared with one person per 96 square feet in an exam room) but the occupants themselves generate heat. A nurse station or business office, where fully clothed persons are busily moving about, has yet a different requirement. The dental operatory, typically 100 square feet, usually has three occupants in addition to a high level of illumination. These rooms each have different comfort requirements in

terms of temperature and varying load characteristics. The lighting load for a waiting room will be approximately 2 watts per square foot, for an examination room 3.3 watts per square foot, for a dental operatory 10 watts per square foot, for a nurse station or business office 2.5 watts, and for corridors 1 to 1.5 watts per square foot.

The factors that must be considered in designing a functional HVAC system are:

1. The lighting load.
2. The room occupancy.
3. The equipment load.
4. The comfort level based on room function.

The type of HVAC system (equipment and method of distribution) may vary, but often it is a ducted air system which supplies heated, cooled, and fresh air. The system should be designed with maximum concern for sound control. Thus each room may have its own supply and air return; undercutting doors and the use of transfer grilles for return air are to be avoided. There are a number of ways that the sound carried through the ducts of a ventilation system can be reduced.

285

A certain amount of sound will naturally be absorbed in the duct wall lining and some will pass through the duct walls into the plenum. Additional insulation, duct linings, or package attenuation units can produce even a greater degree of sound control. However, a certain amount of "white noise" produced by the mechanical system is desirable for masking conversation from room to room.

CONTROL OF ODORS

To prevent the spread of odors from the radiographic and fluoroscopic rooms, darkroom, toilets, cast room, laboratory, or other areas, the ventilation system should be designed so that a negative air pressure relative to the adjoining corridors will be maintained in these rooms. This can be accomplished by exhausting more air from these rooms than is supplied to them, and by reversing this procedure in the corridors. Air from fluoroscopic radiography rooms should not be recirculated when these rooms are in use unless adequate odor removal equipment is incorporated in the ventilation system.

PLUMBING

The plumbing in a medical or dental facility is not essentially different from that in other types of commercial buildings, but by their very nature, medical office buildings have a *high density* of plumbing fixtures, and provisions must be made to locate them anywhere except along the perimeter of the building. Plaster traps should be supplied in sinks of cast rooms, clinical laboratories, barium prep areas, dental operatories, surgeries, and laboratories, and sometimes in minor surgery rooms. Darkrooms and clinical laboratories should have acid-resistant waste piping.

MEDICAL GASES

Certain suites—dentists, oral surgeons, plastic surgeons—require medical gases. Building and fire codes are very strict with regard to where and how medical gases are stored. The gases may be in mobile tanks that are wheeled from room to room as needed, or the gases (nitrous oxide and oxygen) may be stored in tanks in a nearby room designed for that purpose and piped through degreased, sealed copper tubing (using only silver solder) to a flow meter in each room where gases are needed. If the gases are located outside of the suite, a pressure gauge must be located within the suite to monitor the supply. The reader is referred to Chapter 8 under *General Dentistry* for a complete discussion of this topic.

Certain suites require compressed air and central suction. Usually each tenant will have his or her own vacuum pump and air compressor located in a small mechanical equipment room within the suite. But some medical buildings provide these utilities and pipe them to the suites. Vacuum piping is PVC Schedule 40. Suites requiring these utilities include dentists, oral surgeons, clinical laboratories, and dental laboratories.

SOUND CONTROL

Sound control is of utmost importance in a medical office especially with regard to examination rooms and consultation rooms. Unfortunately, all too many medical buildings are constructed with profit rather than function as the prime motivation, and the partitions terminate at the finished ceiling and have no sound attenuating properties. There are, however, several ways to reduce sound transmission without spending a great deal of money:

1. All partitions should terminate 6 to 8 inches above the suspended ceiling. Thus each room has its own ceiling, rather than dropping the suspended acoustic ceiling over the entire suite with only the demising walls continuing above it.

2. Sound can be absorbed near its source through the use of carpet, wallcoverings, draperies, and acoustic ceiling tile.

3. Solid-core doors should be used.

4. Fiberglass batting should be added inside partitions between studs.

5. To control passage of sound through walls, floors, and ceilings, acoustical holes should be avoided, such as those created by use of pocket doors or when electrical outlets on opposite sides of a partition are positioned too close to each other, when doors are poorly fitted, when plumbing pipes or heating ducts are improperly fitted, or when partitions do not make proper contact with the ceiling.

6. A certain amount of "white noise" from the ventilation system will mask soft conversation from room to room.

7. A piped-in music system will also mask normal conversation. An AM-FM tuner or cassette deck located in the business office with speakers in the waiting room and corridors is preferable to the well-known brand of prerecorded "background" music.

8. Recessed light fixtures should be avoided.

9. Certain rooms, such as psychiatrists' consultation rooms and audio rooms for hearing tests, need a high level of sound control. These partitions should be constructed of 5/8-inch gypsum board with a sheet of 1/2-inch sound board on both sides of the partition, staggering the seams.

MEDICAL OFFICE COMMUNICATION SYSTEMS

The reader is referred to Chapter 8 for a discussion of communication systems for the dental office.

Many offices over 1500 square feet have some sort of interoffice communication system other than the telephone intercom. There are three conditions for which some sort of signal is required:

1. To tell the doctor which room has the next patient.
2. To call the doctor to the telephone.
3. To call a nurse or aide when the doctor is in the examining room.

A small panel of signal lights mounted above the exam room doors can indicate to the doctor when a patient has been prepared for examination. When the patient is ready, the nurse turns on the light code for a particular doctor. When the doctor enters the room, he or she turns off the light. This system requires additional modification for large busy practices, since several patients may be prepared and waiting for an individual doctor who will have to have some way of knowing the sequence.

The receptionist who handles the phone must know in which room each doctor can be found. A toggle switch for each doctor must be located in each exam, treatment, or consultation room the doctor(s) uses. When the doctor enters the room he or she trips the switch, which lights a panel located at the reception desk.

Some offices do not use signal lights. A variety of "homemade" systems may be devised, one of which follows. Assume for our example, a group of three orthopedists: each physician is assigned a color and a set of Plexiglas chips 4 × 5 inches in size. Each chip has a large number 1 to 3 (since each has the use of three exam rooms). The chips are stored in a wall-mounted rack at the centrally located nurse station. When a nurse readies a patient, she puts that doctor's color chip in a slot on the door; thus each doctor knows, by the color of the chip, if the patient in that room is his (or hers), and by the number, the order in which to examine the patients.

In order to call a nurse or aide when the doctor is in the exam room, a signal light can be used, but it has the disadvantage of not being noticed. Thus a preferred system is an annunciator panel, although it is limited by the number of sounds a person can reasonably discriminate. Each doctor would have a distinctive buzz or chime. When the nurse hears the signal, she consults a panel to determine what room the doctor is in and she proceeds to that room.

There are a variety of other interoffice communication systems available. The dealers who sell these products also install them. They can design a system to suit the needs of the individual office and can furnish the designer with the electrical specifications. A leader in this field is Executone Systems with offices throughout the country.

CHECKLIST

The following is a construction checklist to jog the designer's memory. It is not intended as a complete inventory of requirements.

Code Review
- Occupancy load
- Number of required exits, location of exits
- Illuminated exit signs
- Radiation shielding
- Fire separations
- Handicapped bathrooms and other requirements

Partitions
- Sound control
- Continuation past suspended ceiling
- Fiberglass batt
- Verify construction of partitions with contractor when planning offices in a building not designed by the space planner. (One may find that the contractor, in order to come in with a low bid, based his bid on 2 1/2-inch

studs, giving a finished wall that has to be "thickened" wherever plumbing occurs.)
- Verify or specify texture of finished wall
- Spec semigloss enamel for walls for durability and cleanability
- Spec special ceiling heights, if required
- No texture for walls that will receive wall-covering

Doors
- Hollow vs solid core
- Pocket doors
- Gate or Dutch doors
- Door closers
- Hardware, keying of locks
- Door finish: painted or stained, plastic laminate
- Door stops
- Verify or spec door frame
- Spec width and height of doors
- Spec carpet height (plus pad, if any) for cutting doors

Plumbing
- Plaster traps
- Wrist or foot pedal control faucets
- Acid-resistant waste pipes
- Spec sizes of sinks, china, or stainless steel
- Vacuum breakers (darkrooms)
- Separate shutoffs for each fixture

- Floor drains in cystoscopy, darkrooms, hot-water heater room
- Temperature regulators in darkrooms

Communication Systems
- Telephones
- Intercom
- Signal lights
- Annunciator panel
- Music system: provide speakers
- Locate telephone terminal panel (requires electrical outlet)

Mechanical Systems
- Locate air compressor and vacuum
- Locate medical gases, natural gas
- Locate hot-water heater (if electric, requires outlet) and floor drain
- Exhaust fans (bathrooms, darkrooms, labs, cast rooms)

Casework
- Spec style of construction, type drawer glides, hardware
- Detail typing wells in business office
- Trash slots in exam cabinets, as required
- Spec type and finish of hinges
- Spec wood blocking in walls (or ceiling) to support X-ray view boxes, cassette pass boxes, dental operatory lights and X-ray heads, special light fixtures, upper cabinets,

and certain pieces of medical equipment

Lighting
- Do switching diagram
- Spec dimmers as required (fluorescent fixtures require dimming ballasts)
- Spec color fluorescent light tubes
- Spec lamp wattages
- Spec lenses of fixtures
- Spec color of grid (spline) in suspended acoustic ceiling
- Spec size and texture acoustic tile

Electric
- Note special outlets, 200 lines, floor receptacles
- Spec height of outlets.
- Outlets over countertops should run horizontally
- Locate circuit breaker panel
- Locate intercom and phone, note wall phones

Miscellaneous
- Locate scale spaces, as required, noting any that are to be recessed in the slab

Chapter 13
Researching Codes and Reference Materials

Codes are designed to ensure life safety. As health care services have become increasingly more complex and sophisticated, the design and construction of these facilities has become more specialized. Paralleling the increasing sophistication in health care is the development of numerous codes and standards designed to limit risk and make buildings relatively safe. The problem is that codes occasionally contradict one another and the language is frequently subject to interpretation. Often, the level of protection is a value judgment. The minimum standards per code may be inadequate for a facility serving the elderly, for example. Or, the corollary may be true: The minimum standards may occasionally be excessive for a particular project. The cost of implementing them may make the project unfeasible. Thus codes must be evaluated in terms of: (1) *What is an acceptable level of risk in terms of life safety?* (2) *Is the cost of that level of protection warranted or within the budget for that facility?* (3) *Are the codes or standards applicable to that facility redundant?*

Further complicating these issues is the fact that codes are written by one body and enforced by another. The local agent, who is responsible for interpretation and compliance, does not always understand the intent of the codes, and agents within the same office may disagree on interpretations. Nevertheless, codes are an important part of medical work and designers need to be familiar with them. If anything, the next ten years will bring more codes and regulations, not fewer.

Codes cover these general areas:

FIRE PROTECTION

1. Flammability of Materials: especially carpet, wallcoverings, draperies, upholstery fillings and fabrics, carpet and wallcovering adhesives.

2. Exiting Requirements: number of exits, travel distances between doors of exiting, corridor separations, sizes of doors and stairwells, construction of doors and walls, illumination of fire exits.

3. Storage: how and where medical gases are to be used and stored; storage of combustible solid supplies.

4. Fire-Fighting Equipment: locations of wet and dry standpipes, chemical fire extinguishers, and in high-rise buildings, smoke evacuation shafts and central control station for fire department use.

5. Electrical Systems: standards for wiring, equipment, emergency power systems.

6. Fire Detection Devices: locations of sprinklers, smoke detectors, and alarms.

HANDICAPPED

(Both federal and state codes provide for the handicapped.)
1. Location of ramps, curb cuts, parking stalls; placement of exits and design configurations.
2. Dimensions of elevators and restrooms, door widths, and placement of restroom fixtures and accessories.

SANITATION

1. Cleanability of wallcovering, flooring, and other interior finishes.
2. Asepsis (ability to support bacteria) of interior finish materials.

MINIMUM CONSTRUCTION REQUIREMENTS

1. Minimum sizes of rooms and minimum sizes of various departments (within a hospital, for example), location and number of windows, minimum ceiling heights, relationship of various rooms to each other.
2. Planning and programing decisions with regard to function.
3. Accommodation of equipment: spaces for gurneys, drinking fountains, public telephones. Minimum requirements for laundries, kitchens, laboratories, operating rooms, etc.

ENERGY CONSERVATION/ ENVIRONMENTAL IMPACT

State and local codes govern energy conservation and the ecological impact of a proposed building on its environment.

The above code classifications may fall under the jurisdiction of city, county, state, or federal codes in addition to these nationally recognized standards:

Life Safety Code. Published by the National Fire Protection Assn.

National Electrical Code. Published by the National Fire Protection Assn.

The Rehabilitation Act of 1973. Concerns the handicapped.

Building Officials and Code Administrators (BOCA)

Joint Commission on Accreditation of Hospitals

"Minimum Requirements—Construction and Equipment/Hospitals and Medical Facilities," published by the U.S. Dept. of Health, Education and Welfare.

National Bureau of Standards (U.S. Dept. of Commerce)

American Society for Testing and Materials (ASTM)

Underwriters' Laboratories

Recognized state building codes include:

Uniform Building Code (used by many western states)
Southern Standard Building Code
National Building Code

Some states have their own building code, others use a regional code that serves several neighboring states.

CERTIFICATE OF NEED

Prior to building any new health care facility or remodeling or adding to an existing one, a local health systems agency must endorse the project with a Certificate of Need. In California, any project costing more than $150,000 must go through the Certificate of Need process. The CON is designed to prevent duplication of highly specialized facilities and equipment and to keep a lid on rising health care costs. States receiving federal funds under the National Health Planning and Resources Development Act of 1974 were required to introduce CON programs by 1980.

CODES RELATING TO MEDICAL OFFICE BUILDINGS

The code requirements for medical and dental offices are minimal compared with hospitals. The local building code will determine the type of construction for a particular medical building and site, the zoning requirements, and the fire zone.

Although state building codes vary, the following items are generally pertinent to planning *individual* medical and dental offices within a medical office building.

- Minimum width of corridors
- Number of exits
- Handicapped bathrooms
- Separation of exits
- Maximum length of dead-end corridors
- Minimum ceiling height
- Construction of partitions
- Fire separations
- Radiation shielding
- Fire detection devices or sprinklers

Some of these items apply only to suites in excess of a specified square footage. Suites over 3000 square feet, for example, in the Uniform Building Code, 1976 Edition (current as of 1980 in the City of San Diego) must have at least two exits "separated by a distance equal to not less than one-half the length of the maximum overall diagonal dimension of the area to be served measured in a straight line between exits," and no more than a 20-foot dead-end corridor. With an occupancy load of 30 or more, the suite would have to have corridor walls that are one-hour fire-resistive construction, and the ceilings must be no less than what is required for a one-hour fire-resistive floor or roof system. The codes applying to medical occupancy (medical office buildings) deal mainly with fire prevention and exiting in case of fire. The principles, in terms of space planning and construction, are easy to understand:

1. Isolation of Risk

If a facility is divided into sections by corridor

separations, fire-resistive stairwell enclosures, and sealed vertical openings, the fire may be contained and prevented from spreading.

2. Required Exits

The number of exits is based on the proposed occupancy load or the number of persons using the space. Approved exits must lead directly out or to other means of egress, and doors must open in the direction of egress. Exits may not be through a room unless that room is a lobby or reception room. Thus people will not be trapped in a building, and all exits will be clearly marked and accessible in case of fire.

3. Separation of Exits

If exits are separated by a specified distance proportional to the size of the space, persons located at each end of the suite will have an accessible exit.

4. Stairs and Doors

Stairwells with fire-resistive enclosures and self-closing fire doors are intended to be smokefree evacuation towers in case of fire. The stairs must be of sufficient width to enable stretchers to be evacuated if necessary.

5. Fire Warning or Extinguishment Devices

Sprinkler systems are required in many facilities, particularly in laboratories, boiler rooms, large storage areas, or hazardous areas that are often unoccupied. Smoke or heat detectors and alarms are good warning devices where sprinklers are not feasible.

FLAMMABILITY TESTING

Building codes, regulations, and local ordinances are designed to restrict the use of flammable materials on walls, floors, and ceilings of buildings. The flammability characteristics of various interior finish materials influence the behavior of a fire. Although it is impossible to make a building and its furnishings absolutely "fireproof," it is desirable to limit the risk to a reasonable standard by ensuring that the major interior finishes will not support flame or generate smoke. The Life Safety Code (NFPA 101) specifies the *flame spread, smoke density,* and *fuel contributed* standards for floors and walls of hospitals.

Carpet

The flame retardance of a carpet is a significant factor in its selection for a health care facility. Carpet fibers have different melting points: (acrylics 420°F to 490°F, nylons 415°F to 480°F, modacrylics 275°F to 300°F; polypropylene fuses at 285°F to 330°F; wool, which does not melt, scorches at approximately 400°F.) Four factors affect the flammability of a carpet:

1. Type of face yarn
2. Type of construction and texture
3. Pile density
4. Underlayment or pad

There are three tests of carpet flammability:

The Pill Test (Dept. of Commerce #DOCFF-1-70). A methenamine pill (a timed burning tablet)

294

placed on the carpet is used to determine if a carpet will burn when ignited by a small incendiary source. Since April 1971 all carpet sold in the United States must pass the pill test.

The Steiner Tunnel Test (E-84). This has been the standard test of carpet and wallcovering flame spread although its validity for testing the flammability of carpet in a realistic situation has been widely disputed. This test is required by H.E.W. for all carpets installed in hospitals receiving Hill-Burton Act funds. The carpet sample is mounted on the ceiling of a tunnel and exposed to a front flame. The results are published as a flame spread rating. Normally a flame spread rating of 75 or less is required for hospital corridor carpet.

Flooring Radiant Panel Test. This is the newest and most accurate test for carpet flammability. Local fire marshals in some cities are still unfamiliar with this test and insist upon a tunnel test rating. However, many new commercial carpets now have only radiant panel test ratings; thus it seems probable that in a couple of years this test will completely replace the Steiner tunnel test. The radiant panel test evolved from extensive corridor fire test programs. The test measures the *critical radiant flux* (the minimum radiant energy necessary for a fire to continue to burn and spread) in watts per square centimeter (watts/cm^2). The lower the number, the greater the capacity for flame propagation.

0.45 watts/cm^2 is the minimum critical radiant flux recommended within corridors and exitways of hospitals and nursing homes.

0.22 watts/cm^2 is the minimum critical radiant flux recommended within corridors and exitways

of other occupancies except one-family and two-family dwellings.*

These values provide a level of safety for a carpeted hospital corridor equal to or in excess of that now required in the NFPA 101 Life Safety Code. Smoke density is as important as flame spread since many people are killed by the smoke generated from a fire.

Wallcoverings

Interior finish materials (including wallcoverings) are grouped into three classes, according to their flame spread and smoke development characteristics. The code will qualify rooms by occupancy and specify which class of finish is applicable.

Class A Interior Finish. Flame Spread 0-25, Smoke Developed 0-450.
Class B Interior Finish. Flame Spread 26-75, Smoke Developed 0-450.
Class C Interior Finish. Flame Spread 76-200, Smoke Developed 0-450.

Where Class C is specified, Classes A and B are permitted; where Class B is specified, Class A is permitted.

Wallcoverings are also classified according to weight and texture. Smooth surfaces—less apt to support bacterial growth or collect dirt—are required for surgeries, isolation rooms, nurseries, and other high-risk areas. Heavily textured wallcoverings may be used in lobbies, waiting rooms, or administrative offices.

* *Flammability Testing for Carpet,* by I. A. Benjamin and S. Davis (Washington, D.C., The National Bureau of Standards, U.S. Dept. of Commerce, April 1978).

It is the designer's responsibility to verify the codes pertinent to a particular project. Swatches of all interior finish materials must be attached to a copy of the laboratory test data (supporting the flame spread classification claimed) and submitted to the state fire marshal for approval.

Wallcovering Specifications. Fabric-backed vinyl wallcoverings are classified into three general categories:

Type I. In accordance with Federal Specification CCC–W–408a, Type I must weigh a minimum of 7 ounces per square yard and may weigh up to 13 ounces per square yard. It usually has a lightweight scrim backing. Type I materials are acceptable for light commercial use such as offices and corridors with moderate traffic.

Type II. In accordance with Federal Specification CCC–W–408a, Type II must weigh a minimum of 13 ounces per square yard and may weigh up to 22 ounces per square yard. It usually has an Osnaburg or Drill tear-resistant fabric backing. Type II materials are suitable for general commercial use in public corridors of hospitals, lobbies, waiting rooms, dining rooms, cafeterias, and other areas of high traffic and above-average abuse.

Type III. In accordance with Federal Specification CCC–W–408a, Type III must weigh in excess of 22 ounces per square yard. It usually has a Broken Twill fabric backing for maximum strength and tear resistance. Type III materials are suitable for areas receiving exceptionally hard wear and abrasion such as elevators, stores and shops, hospital corridors, stairwells, etc.

Wallcoverings in high-traffic areas can be ordered with a Tedlar coating to give walls even greater protection. Tedlar is a registered tradename for a tough preformed film of polyvinyl fluoride which is laminated to the face of the vinyl wallcovering to make it resist stains such as lipstick, ball point pens, silver nitrate, and other indelible substances. Even harsh solvents and cleaning solutions will not mar the Tedlar coating, making it ideal for use in psychiatric hospitals, pediatric wards, and other institutional facilities where walls are subject to graffiti and high abuse.

Chapter 14
Humanizing the Hospital Environment

Florence Nightingale's dictum that the first requisite of a hospital be that it do the patients no harm may not have been intended to apply to the visual environment but should be extended to that context today. The rationale behind hospital design until recently has been based upon a puritanical attitude toward comfort. One has but to enter any of our large urban hospitals to experience the awesome scale and impermeability of the architecture. Like government buildings, our hospitals are designed to look strong and be resistant to human imprint. This bureaucratic "no frills" theory represents a popular prejudice against pleasantries in public facilities.

There are those who believe that providing a pleasant environment may even reward or reinforce illness. These neo-behaviorists suggest that people may not avoid illness unless they associate it with some form of punishment. Fortunately, the past ten years have produced many studies contradicting the behaviorist viewpoint. An age of enlightenment is upon us, and at last hospital administrators and designers of such facilities are trying to humanize them. Cheerful colors and intimate spaces occasionally break

the institutional tedium. Creative lighting can interject a rhythm in a seemingly endless corridor. Naked walls now carry textured wallcoverings and attractive works of art. All of these amenities help to break down the barrier between the patient and the institution.

In the author's opinion, after many years of working in hospitals and extensive interviews with patients and staff, cheerful colors, carpeted corridors, and other cosmetic treatments greatly benefit morale and speed patient recovery. But cosmetics are, by definition, applied and can only go so far. The best solution is to start with humane architecture. Certain architects have challenged the physical structure of the hospital and have devised imaginative spaces flooded with natural light, views of lush gardens or atriums filled with trees and sky, and patient rooms that are angled to given the patients better views of the outdoors as well as improved communication with the nursing staff. The space planning in these award-winning hospitals is not only functional but visually stimulating, with interesting spaces and intimate lounges where ambulatory patients and visitors may chat inform-

297

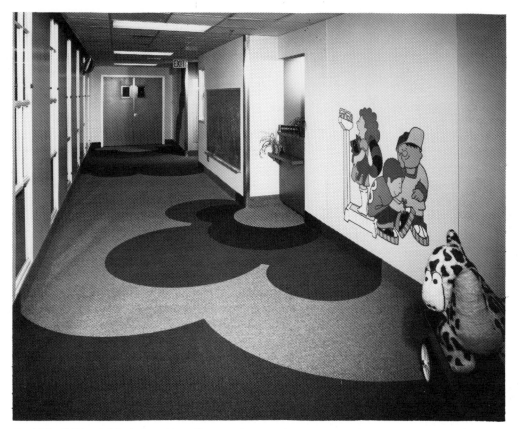

Fig. 14-1. Children's hospital corridor. (Cartoon characters by Don DeMars.)

ally. Color and form are an inherent part of the design, not just a cosmetic application.

Thus we see that the architect and interior designer have a grave obligation to research the psychological and emotional complexities of health care before developing their design program. Failure to fully understand the behavioral component implicit in medical treatment and rehabilitation may lead a designer to unknowingly create a dehumanizing environment.

Conversely, a sensitive designer may create an environment so soothing and so tailored to occupant needs as to actually expand the dimensions of a patient's hospital experience. The patient may leave the facility in some way spiritually enriched or better educated in responding to a future health crisis. Patients have less apprehension of a return visit. One may speculate that more persons will seek medical care earlier instead of waiting until a disease has progressed to advanced stages.

Patients entering a hospital are under stress. They fear the unfamiliar and are squeamish about medical procedures. They experience a loss at being separated from family, friends, and their usual routine. This break with routine is especially difficult to accommodate when the body's normal defenses are already under attack due to illness. A feeling of helplessness accompanies an enforced confinement. Worries about the cost of their medical care and the outcome of the diagnosis or surgery intensify patient stress. Added to this is the embarrassing loss of personal privacy which hospital patients must endure. One's personal intimacies must be shared with strangers.

The designer must be aware of these factors. They apply in greater or lesser degree in different areas depending upon whether one is dealing with the emergency room, nursing areas, outpatient services (radiology, physical therapy, renal dialysis, lab), maternity, burn unit, pediatrics, or intensive care unit. Obviously, patients with incurable diseases (and their families) face stresses the average patient does not experience. Common sense would dictate the specific frustrations and needs of patients or visitors to each area.

Hospitals are an architecture of corridors with small rooms sprouting off of them. Relieving the montony of such a landscape requires empathy and imagination. Institutional corridors, devoid of warmth, may be transformed into cheerful avenues to coax recuperating patients from their rooms. Such corridors in nursing areas become informal meeting places where ambulatory patients may greet each other and socialize. The more ambulatory the patient, the speedier the recovery and the less chance of postoperative complications. In addition, ambulatory patients require less staff care, which in turn cuts spiraling hospital costs.

A sterile patient room that resembles a prison cell will do little to encourage recovery. One may analogize a patient room in a hospital to that in a hotel. A hotel room is institutional in that it not only has a proscribed furniture arrangement, heavy-duty, low-maintenance materials, and a fixed color scheme, but it also has a certain warmth about it and a resemblance to home. A hospital room need not *look* like home to *feel* like home. The analogy is more apt that one might first imagine. Both a hotel and a hospital provide maid service and meals. Even hospital linens and meal trays could utilize some color. Hospital china could be designed with a border or accent

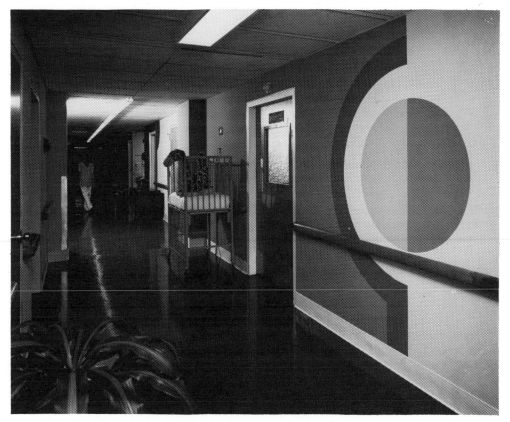

Fig. 14-2. Children's hospital corridor: Geometric wall designs are done with vinyl wallcovering.

299

color on a white plate. Molded plastic trays in cheery colors would do much to revive faltering appetites. We might think of patients as guests rather than inmates.

The lobby is a visual introduction to the hospital and a circulation focal point. It, as well as other waiting areas, should not be overly dramatic or complicated. Visual instructions to users must be clear—not confusing or ambiguous. Furniture should be inviting but simple. There ought to be a suitable number of individual chairs so that strangers need not endure forced intimacy. Seating should be clustered to permit several related people to sit together. Furnishings must be easy to maintain. Fabric upholstery is preferable to vinyl in most waiting areas (except perhaps pediatrics) for its warmth and domestic touch. Fabrics should be tightly woven nylons specifically engineered for institutional use. Colors should be dark enough or tweedy so that they do not quickly appear soiled.

Furthermore, it is a good idea for the designer to prepare a book for the hospital housekeeping staff with small swatches of all materials used and the manufacturer's recommended instructions for cleaning and maintenance. Of course, all fabrics and materials used in a hospital must meet the flammability code and they must be submitted to the fire marshal with a copy of the manufacturer's test data to support the flame spread classification they claim. The Public Health Department at the city and the state level have certain guidelines for sanitation of materials used in hospitals. The designer must research and be familiar with the many codes pertaining to materials used in hospitals.

To further enhance waiting areas, incandescent lighting may be used whenever practical.

The author prefers ceiling-mounted fixtures, but a combination of ceiling and table lamps may be used, depending upon the design scheme of the room. Recent energy conservation codes in many states make it difficult to use anything but fluorescent lighting. However, a designer working with a qualified architect at the inception of the project can usually negotiate some sort of a trade-off on the amount of glass (heating/cooling load) and the energy required for a certain amount of incandescent lighting. All the more reason for an interior designer and an architect to begin working together on a project early.

In all areas it is important to provide psychological escape routes via windows, graphics, and artwork. They interest, amuse, and distract. In addition, people have a need to be physically stimulated when walking through an interior, and this may be real (stairs, articulations in partitions; or in pediatrics, ladders or structures for climbing) or implied (a view through a window or via a photo mural or wallgraphic).

Lack of color (white) is frightening as it does not simulate a familiar environment. Paint in attractive accent colors costs slightly more than white (or traditional hospital pale green) and is the least expensive way to introduce some vitality to a lackluster interior. One frequently encounters some resistance from conservative staff members when a proposal for some cheerful accent walls is presented to a hospital board of directors. They conjecture that one might tire of accent colors or a specific wallgraphic. As if one did not tire of the endless miles of pale green corridors and gray tile floors! Even a wallgraphic that people disliked would be better than nothing as it would at least draw a reaction from passersby and stimulate their senses and intellect.

Dining rooms, cafeterias, lobbies, and other public areas can take stronger color and bolder accents than nursing areas, although it is the author's preference to color-adapt people with a neutral buffer zone before and after an area of strong color.

Carpeting, in all areas that permit it, does wonders to buoy morale, and its acoustical properties hush the rattle of carts and voices. In addition, it eliminates the sloppy water bucket and mop in a patient's room every morning. Carpeting should be a continuous-filament soil-hiding nylon such as Antron III, tightly woven, level loop, low pile height, with a direct glue-down installation. The last prevents shifting and stretching under wheelchairs, carts, and gurneys. Antron III nylon is permanently antistatic, which is mandatory in a hospital carpet.

Much controversy accompanies the use of carpet in patient rooms. Many hospitals have tried it and enthusiastically support its use. Others complain it is difficult to clean, supports bacteria, and is not worth the trouble. When a patient vomits, it is much easier to wipe it from a hard-surface floor than from carpet. And it is the nurse who usually performs this task because in most hospitals it would take housekeeping too long to respond.

The author's experience has been that many of the hospitals that objected to carpet on the basis of past performance had not purchased the proper carpet. In most cases they had bought inexpensive goods that were not intended for high-traffic hospital use. Today one can purchase aesthetically beautiful carpeting that will meet the most stringent maintenance and durability standards. Several mills have introduced third-generation nylon carpets with woven construc-

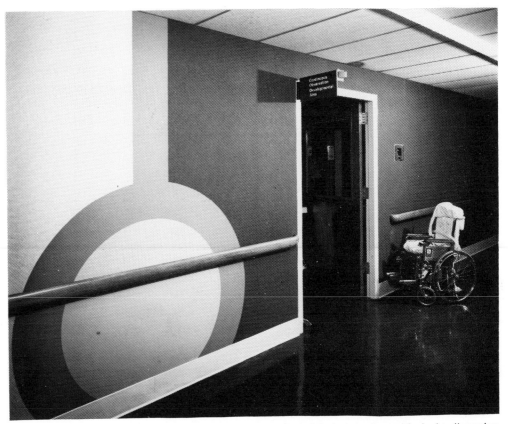

Fig. 14-3. Children's hospital corridor: Geometric wall designs are done with vinyl wallcovering.

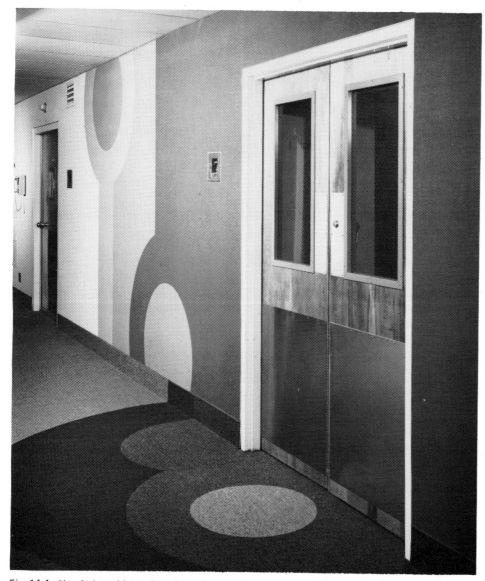

Fig. 14-4. Hospital corridor wallgraphic: Geometric wall designs are done with vinyl wallcovering.

tion, synthetic backings (do not mildew or bleed when wet as does jute), and mottled coloring which closely resemble an acrylic or wool carpet.

A designer may create exciting corridors or lobbies by using several colors of carpet (solid colors) seamed together in an original design of stripes or other geometric shapes. Instead of the standard 4-inch or 6-inch rubber top-set base in corridors, one may fabricate a base of carpet by cutting the appropriate length strips and finishing the raw edge in a binding machine with ribbon tape that matches the carpet color. Carpet base is easier to maintain than rubber base because it does not scuff. Visually, it provides for continuity between floor and wall.

The type of window treatment in patient rooms depends on the decorative scheme, the size and location of the window, as well as the building's maintenance priorities. The most functional window covering appears to be either a vertical or horizontal slat window blind. The horizontal type are available in a 1-inch slat, are fabricated of metal, and are enameled in many attractive colors. A clear plastic wand rotates the slats. The advantage of this type of blind over drapes is that one may block the sun without entirely cutting off the view or natural light.

The vertical style slat or louver is typically 4 inches wide and is fastened at the bottom and the top of the window frame. It may be fabricated of metal or heavy fabric such as canvas. The principle is more or less the same as for the horizontal blinds; however, the wide louvers collect dust a bit more than do the narrower metal slats. Some hospitals actually have a double-glazed window with vertical louver blinds installed between the two panels of glass. It does keep the blinds dustfree although it lends an institutional ap pearance. Draperies are still preferable in some cases where the window treatment may be the only viable way of injecting a cheerful pattern into the room or where the window itself is large enough and with some wall area on either side of it so that the stacking drapery fabric does not obscure the view when the drapes are open. Drapery fabric does collect dust and needs to be cleaned more frequently than does either type of blind.

Isolation rooms, used for those with contagious diseases, are best handled with metal slat blinds or a washable pull-down window shade, both of which can be disinfected with an antiseptic solution more easily than a drapery fabric can be cleaned. In pediatric or geriatric rooms a drapery is aesthetically preferable as a splashy print is more comforting and reminiscent of home.

An additional window blind is available for specific areas such as a surgical room or observation area—a place where the strictest hygienic requirements must be observed—which is made of PVC (polyvinyl chloride). The individual slats are approximately 1/4-inch wide and, unlike the blinds discussed previously, it rolls up when one pulls a cord. The PVC material is inherently flame retardant and can be subjected to an antiseptic scrubbing when required.

All patient rooms have cubicle drapes, and that is an item that is available in an almost unlimited selection of attractive stripes and plaids or solids in deep tones as well as pastels. Cubicle drape fabric is manufactured by several mills, and all fabric of this classification must be inherently flame retardant as well as be able to withstand numerous washings at temperatures that would ruin most fabrics. Additionally, the stripes or

design are woven into these fabrics rather than printed on the face of it, so one has the advantage of having two "right" sides—they look the same from both sides.

Wallcoverings can add vitality to patient rooms, waiting areas, and corridors. It is smart to put all accent colors in commercial wallvinyl and keep the painted surfaces a neutral ivory color. This plan enables the hospital maintenance crew to use only one paint color for touch-ups and repairs. All wallvinyl should be Tedlar coated if the project can afford the small additional cost. This coating, now available on many commercial vinyls, is resistant to ball-point pen, lipstick, crayon, and many other indelible substances.

Type II or Type III weight classification wallvinyls with a fabric back should be used in corridors and other areas where there exists the probability of heavy carts bumping into the walls. A major maintenance (as well as visual) problem in hospital corridors is the damage done to the walls due to heavy carts, gurneys, and hospital beds bumping into them. Most hospitals have wooden or vinyl bumper guards along the walls. The heavier the vinyl wallcovering, the less likely it is to puncture when hit.

Patient rooms can benefit greatly from an accent wall be it a patterned wallvinyl or paint. The pattern ought to be a stripe or a subtle design that is easy on the eyes. The designer must continually remember that people are confined to a hospital room and may not be able to leave at will. Therefore any designs or patterns or colors must be universal enough to be pleasing to any age, male or female, person. Realizing that the person occupying a particular room may suffer from any number of medical disorders, the colors or patterns must not interfere with the patient's recovery.

Care must be taken to avoid a figure-ground reversal. This type of optical illusion is caused by the lens of the eye trying to focus contrasting colors of differing wavelengths side by side in one pattern. Hence the lens vacillates back and forth causing the pattern one is viewing to vibrate. This type of visual rhythm can be experienced if one looks at stripes of primary red and blue. The eye cannot focus on both colors at once and quickly focuses on one then the other until the stripes pick up a visual rhythm. This could be extremely distressing and perhaps even cause seizures in persons with certain neurological disorders.

If a selected wallcovering pattern seems too stimulating to stare at all day, it could be put on the headboard wall in a patient room rather than at the foot of the bed where a patient might have to focus on it for long periods. The same principle holds for a painted accent wall. This bit of color does much to brighten the monotone of bed linens, hospital gowns, and medical equipment. Three or four room color schemes may be alternated among patient rooms on a floor. Similarly, corridors and public areas of each floor may be varied in color and treatment to give the staff a change of scenery as they move about the facility. A person departing an elevator might be greeted by a unique piece of artwork or a different color scheme to give a visual identity cue at each floor.

In pediatric areas a designer can use strong color and pattern. Unlike adults, children are delighted and distracted by busy designs and contrasting colors. Whimsical wallpapers and custom-designed furniture that the children can manipulate may be used in corridors and playrooms. Stuffed animals or soft objects upon which children might teethe or drool must be avoided in an effort to control the spread of bacteria. With a little imagination there is no end to the wondrous things a designer might dream up for a pediatric hospital. A child might be pulled down to X-ray or therapy in a specially designed red wagon, rather than a conventional wheelchair, for example. The walls the child passes on the way might be decorated with whimsical characters from fairy tales, and the nurse might give the child something to look forward to on the trip back such as: "On the way back you'll be seeing Pinocchio." Above all, *it is important to locate pediatric wallgraphics at a child's eye level.* All too often, they are placed at the adult's eye level and if even seen by young children, are viewed at a distorted angle.

Sexist color stereotyping should be avoided in nurseries and pediatric areas. Forty years of baby blue for boys and pink for girls is enough. Babies, studies have shown, prefer strong primary colors even at infancy. Researchers have learned that such colors stimulate an infant's awareness to such a degree that the infants recognize shapes and forms months before they had developmentally been able to do so in previous testing.

In psychiatric areas, unusual architectural spaces should be avoided, as such unexpected stimuli compete with patients' fears rather than soothe them. All design in such an area should be uncomplicated and pull no punches. Lighting, even in lobbies and sitting rooms, should be even and without shadows and contrasts. A constant, secure environment is what will encourage recovery here. When the mind is in crisis, it is reassuring to find a warm, secure environment that does not change and has no surprises.

The overall architecture, however, should be planned to coax patients from their rooms into central socializing areas. This, too, aids recovery. As for color, red should be avoided. It is a stimulating color and may incite an unstable person to violence. In addition, this color carries heavy emotional connotations of blood. Yellow would create the same warm ambience as red, but without the negative emotional overtones. Orange, gold, green, and blue are other good colors for use in these areas. Particular attention should be given to any patterns in flooring and wallcoverings. High contrasts in color, texture, or pattern should be avoided. Paranoid persons might imagine all sorts of frightening images suggested by the pattern, texture, or contrasts.

Every area of the hospital benefits from good graphics and artwork. Art should be varied and represent subjects with appeal for all ages and cultural backgrounds. Art enriches the spirit. But this is not the place for subject content that might offend, threaten, or make people feel culturally insecure. This is not a place to make political statements. The artwork should decorate and highlight public corridors, elevator lobbies and any other places where people spend any amount of time waiting. A selection of original graphics, watercolors, framed panels of colorful fabric, or weavings may be used together to provide interesting variation. Inexpensive artwork may be reproduced for patient rooms by the silk-screen method: One or two designs may be varied by color and position of the screens.

A good signage program should be part of every hospital. A competent graphic designer should be retained to study traffic flow and make recommendations for positioning signs throughout the institution. The colors, sizes, and typeface should be coordinated with the overall interior design scheme.

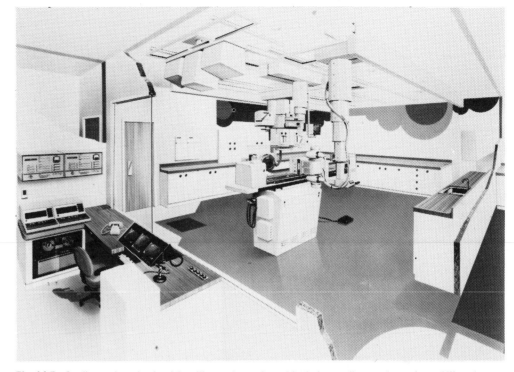

Fig. 14-5. Cardiac catheterization lab utilizes color and graphic design to distract the patient. Milwaukee County Hospital. (Equipment by General Electric Co., Medical Systems Div.)

In summary, a designer has a serious obligation to research the physiological and psychological effects of color and design in any facility where patients are confined—*they are subjected to their environment whether they like it or not.* The color blue, for example, slows respiration and may be soothing to some patients but deadly to others. Yellow, in a recovery area, may cast a reflection on a patient's skin tone and create an appearance of jaundice. Red, researchers have shown, is universally and cross-culturally favored by children.

Above all, a hospital's design ought to reflect the character of the community it serves. A rural hospital should not look like an urban hospital, as that would be unfamiliar to the occupants. All design planning should be based upon a realistic appraisal of the quality of the hospital's housekeeping procedures in order to determine just how practical materials must be. The facility's program must be analyzed—the age of participants, average length of stay, and type of medical services offered. The appearance of a room should signal the room's function and use to visitors. Simple uncomplicated spaces are best.

A modern hospital must utilize the latest technology, yet should not deny the psychological needs of the patient. It should appear friendly—with a design that does all possible to preserve human dignity at a time when flagging spirits most require it.

Appendix

HANDICAPPED TOILET

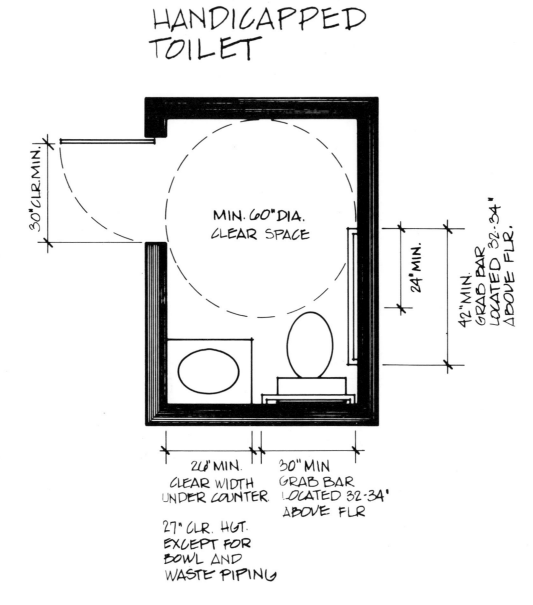

30" CLR. MIN.

MIN. 60" DIA.
CLEAR SPACE

24" MIN.

42" MIN.

GRAB BAR
LOCATED 32-34"
ABOVE FLR.

26" MIN.
CLEAR WIDTH
UNDER COUNTER.

30" MIN
GRAB BAR
LOCATED 32-34'
ABOVE FLR

27" CLR. HGT.
EXCEPT FOR
BOWL AND
WASTE PIPING

Handicapped toilet.

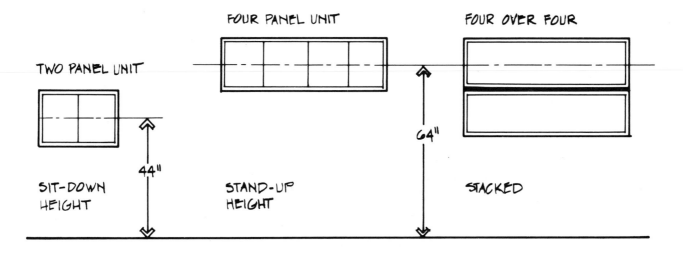

TWO PANEL UNIT

FOUR PANEL UNIT

FOUR OVER FOUR

44"

64"

SIT-DOWN
HEIGHT

STAND-UP
HEIGHT

STACKED

SUGGESTED MOUNTING HEIGHTS
VIEW BOX ILLUMINATORS

View box illuminators.

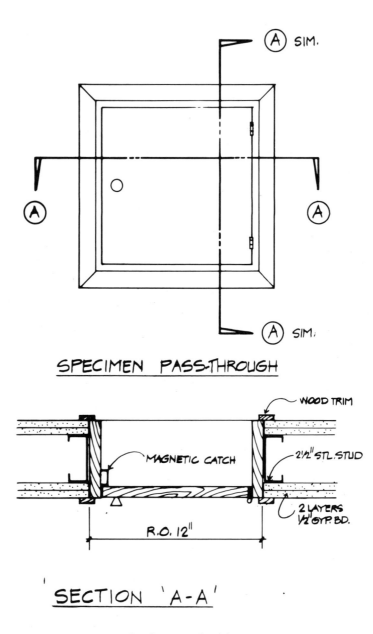

SPECIMEN PASS-THROUGH

SECTION 'A-A'

Specimen pass-through.

310

CLIENT INTERVIEW FORM (MEDICAL)

DATE:_____

JOB TITLE_____

DOCTORS PRESENT AT INTERVIEW:

Dr._____

Address _____

Phone _____

Dr._____

Address _____

Phone _____

Dr._____

Address _____

Phone _____

Dr._____

Address _____

Phone _____

Dr._____

Address _____

Phone _____

Dr._____

Address _____

Phone _____

** CONTACT DOCTOR

SUITE DESIGN REQUIREMENTS

EXISTING OFFICE

Number and size of exam rooms_____,_____x_____

Number and size of cons. rooms_____,_____x_____

Number of seats in waiting room _____

Number of toilets _____

Size of business office _____

Special rooms and equipment:

Number of doctors working at one time _____

Existing staff: Medical _____

                 Business _____

General comments:

311

CLIENT INTERVIEW FORM (MEDICAL)

PROPOSED SUITE REQUIREMENTS

GENERAL:

Doctor _____

Specialty _____

Average Number of Patients/Day _____

Composition of Patients _____

_____

_____

Office Hours: From_____To_____

Days Office is Open: From_____Through_____

Suite Location Requirements Within Building _____

_____

ROOM & SIZE:

Waiting Room_____No. of Seats_____

Exams_____

Consultations _____

Minor Surgery/Treatment _____

Nurse Station _____

    Combined with Lab_____

    Separate_____

Lab _____

Staff _____

Toilets_____

Conf./Library_____

Storage _____

X-Ray _____

    Type of Films_____

    Viewing _____

    Darkroom _____

    Barium Prep _____

EKG_____

Pulmonary Function _____

Procto/Sigmoid _____

Cast Room _____

Physical Therapy_____

Audio Room _____

Allergy Test Rooms _____

Refraction Rooms _____

Field Room _____

Drop Room _____

Miscellaneous Rooms _____

_____

_____

CLIENT INTERVIEW FORM (MEDICAL)

PROPOSED STAFF:

ADMINISTRATION:

Reception _____

Telephone _____

Insurance _____

Bookkeeping_____

Manager_____

_____

_____

MEDICAL:

_____

_____

_____

PROPOSED BUSINESS OFFICE:

MEDICAL RECORDS:

Size _____

No. Per Inch _____

Filing System _____

Existing Lineal Footage—Active _____

Inactive _____

New Record Growth _____

_____

Plan for_____Years Growth

Plan for_____Lineal Feet

FILM FILES:

Size _____

No. Per Inch _____

Filing System _____

Existing Lineal Footage—Active _____

Inactive _____

New Growth _____

_____

Plan for_____Years Growth

Plan for_____Lineal Feet

BOOKKEEPING METHOD: _____

_____

SPECIALIZED EQUIPMENT:

Xerox _____

_____

_____

_____

_____

_____

_____

_____

CLIENT INTERVIEW FORM (DENTAL)

DENTAL INTERVIEW FORM

Date:_____

Dr's Name(s)_____

DBA:_____ Phone: Office_____ Home_____

Type of Business (circle): solo practitioner, corporation, partnership.

Office Address:_____

Dental Equipment Dealer:_____ Phone:_____

Salesperson to contact:_____

Sq. Footage Existing Office:_____ Sq. Footage New Office:_____

Dental Specialty:_____ Dr. is Right-handed_____ or Left-Handed_____.

Type of Present Delivery System:_____

Type of New Delivery System: Over Chair_____, Behind Chair_____, Cabinet_____,

Split Carts_____, Pedestal Unit_____.

OFFICE PERSONNEL:

Dentists_____ Secretary_____ Receptionist_____ Hygienist_____ Full Time Chair

Assistants_____ Part Time Chair Assistants_____ Dentist Associates_____ Lab techs

_____ Others _____.

Total personnel:_____(including dentists).

Number Operatories in Present Office:_____.

Number Operatories in New Office:_____.

Number of patient appointments per day:_____.

Answer the Following Questions for Each New Operatory:

CHAIR:

New_____ Existing_____? Mfg.:_____ Color:_____.

SINKS:

Number_____ Location_____ Wall-hung_____ Built into Cabinet_____.

CABINETS:

Fixed (Built-in)_____ Mobile_____ Modular_____.

DENTAL UNIT OR OTHER DELIVERY SYSTEM:

New_____ Existing_____? Mfg.:_____ Color:_____.

UTILITY REQUIREMENTS:

Waste_____ Water_____ Air_____ Gas_____ Electric_____.

DENTAL INTERVIEW FORM

X-RAY:

New_____ Existing_____? Mfg.:_____ Model:_____ Stationary_____

Mobile_____? Intraoral_____ Panoramic X-ray Alcove_____ Cephalometric_____.

OPERATING LIGHT:

On Dental Unit_____ Ceiling Track_____ Wall Mounted_____ Post Mounted

to Floor_____ Post Mounted to Ceiling_____.

VACUUM:

Cuspidor____ Wall Outlet____ In Fixed Cabinet____ In Mobile Cabinet____ On Dental Unit____.

NITROUS OXIDE AND OXYGEN:

Mobile tanks_____ Piped Through Wall_____.

STERILIZING:

In room_____ Outside of Room_____ Autoclave_____ Ultrasonic_____ Dry Heat_____.

ASSISTANT'S CART:

Electric_____ Gas_____ Air_____ Suction_____.

DENTIST'S CART:

Electric_____ Gas_____ Air_____ Suction_____ Built-in X-ray View Box_____.

LABORATORY:

Number Technicians_____ Number sinks_____ Electric_____ Gas_____ Air_____

Vacuum_____ Plaster Bin_____ Model Trimmer_____ Lathe_____ Hand Pieces_____

Dental Engine_____.

DARKROOM:

Manual tanks_____ Automatic Processor_____ Mfg.:_____ Model:_____ Film

Dryer_____ Sink_____.

OTHER ROOMS:

Staff Lounge:_____ With Sink Cabinet_____ With Toilet Room_____.

Patient Education Room:_____ Or Alcove_____ With Sink_____.

Business Manager:_____ Private Office_____

Doctor's Private Offices ____Separate ____Shared ____With Toilet Room ____With Shower.

EQUIPMENT ROOM:

Inside Suite_____ Outside Suite_____ On Roof_____.

MISCELLANEOUS:

Office Communication System Required:_____.

INDEX

flammability testing, 295–296
sanitation, 292
specifications, 296
use of, 303–304. *See also* discussion under medical
specialties

X-ray room, 44–45, 128, 135. *See also* Radiology

3·2·84

37·45   VNR # 24963